Workplace: Fertility Clinic

Monika Bals-Pratsch · Stefan Dieterle · Frank Nawroth

Workplace: Fertility Clinic

Essential Knowledge for Medical Assistants and Nursing Professionals

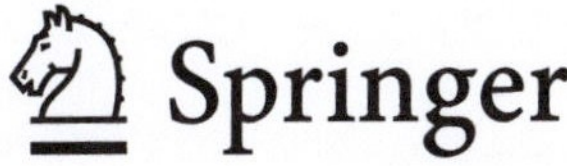

Monika Bals-Pratsch
KinderwunschWissen
Regensburg, Germany

Stefan Dieterle
Überörtliche Berufsausübungsgemeinschaft
Kinderwunsch Dortmund, Siegen, Dorsten,
Wuppertal GbR
Dortmund, Germany

Frank Nawroth
Facharzt-Zentrum für Kinderwunsch,
Pränatale Medizin, Endokrinologie und
Osteologie, amedes MVZ Hamburg
Hamburg, Germany

ISBN 978-3-662-73034-8   ISBN 978-3-662-73035-5   (eBook)
https://doi.org/10.1007/978-3-662-73035-5

Translation from the German language edition: "Arbeitsplatz Kinderwunschzentrum" by Monika Bals-Pratsch et al., © Der/die Herausgeber bzw. der/die Autor(en), exklusiv lizenziert an Springer-Verlag GmbH, DE, ein Teil von Springer Nature 2025. Published by Springer Berlin Heidelberg. All Rights Reserved

This book is a translation of the original German edition "Arbeitsplatz Kinderwunschzentrum" by Monika Bals-Pratsch et al., published by Springer-Verlag GmbH, DE in 2025. The translation was done with the help of an artificial intelligence machine translation tool. A subsequent human revision was done primarily in terms of content, so that the book will read stylistically differently from a conventional translation. Springer Nature works continuously to further the development of tools for the production of books and on the related technologies to support the authors.

This Springer imprint is published by the registered company Springer-Verlag GmbH, DE, part of Springer Nature.
The registered company address is: Heidelberger Platz 3, 14197 Berlin, Germany

If disposing of this product, please recycle the paper.

I dedicate this book to my mentors and role models during my studies, my further training, and my professional career. Professor Frank **Lehmann** (1940–1992) not only founded the German IVF Registry (D·I·R) in 1982, but also inspired my interest in gynecological endocrinology and reproductive medicine while I was still a student. During this time, the first IVF babies in Germany were born, with his involvement. He was also my doctoral advisor and shaped my scientific and clinical focus in gynecological endocrinology and reproductive medicine, as well as in practical obstetrics. Professor Eberhard **Nieschlag** (1941–2025) established, defined, and advanced andrology as a clinical specialty not only in Germany but also internationally, purposefully and consistently from the beginning of his career until the end of his life. From him, I learned internal medicine endocrinology and andrology. I am proud to be part of our Münster "Nieschlag family." His outstanding scientific achievements have been recognized worldwide with awards and honors. For his life's work, he received the Federal Cross of Merit. This honor was recently also bestowed upon my friend Professor Liselotte Mettler (b. 1939), whom I had the pleasure of meeting during my active time in professional politics. She is a very active person and is among the successful pioneers in reproductive medicine. In addition, she played a key role in establishing pelviscopy. Her scientific career was not easy. Despite her advanced age, she continues to travel to scientific congresses worldwide and remains a sought-after clinical advisor not only at the Women's Clinic in Kiel but also internationally. Reproductive medicine in Germany could no longer be conducted at an international level without the patient-friendly interpretation of the Embryo Protection Act (ESchG). This is essentially the achievement of Professor Monika **Frommel** (1946–2025). The criminal law expert from Kiel showed us reproductive medicine specialists about twenty years ago the interpretive leeway within the Embryo Protection Act. Laws are formulated in such a way that their interpretation can adapt to new findings and societal change. Through my numerous personal contacts with her at reproductive medicine and professional policy meetings, and through joint publications, a friendship developed. In the process, I realized that I can only bear my legally mandated medical responsibility for the treatment of germ cells in the IVF laboratory through in-depth embryological knowledge. This was the reason for me to study clinical embryology alongside my professional work.

I would like to thank my family, especially my husband and my children, for their support and understanding during my more than 40 years of active professional work in reproductive medicine. With this book, I also hope that my grandchildren will be able to read about the exciting era in which I was professionally active in a rapidly developing field.

Prof. Dr. med. Monika Bals-Pratsch, M.Sc.

Preface

Medical assistants, nurses, and members of other medical support professions play a crucial role in fertility centers. They support and relieve reproductive physicians and reproductive biologists in the diagnosis and treatment of infertility. The better their qualifications, the smoother and more successful the care provided to couples seeking to conceive.

In 2022, the German Medical Association adopted the "Model Continuing Education Curriculum in Reproductive Medicine for Medical Assistants." This curriculum was previously coordinated with the Professional Association of Reproductive Medicine Centers of Germany (BRZ) and the German Society for Reproductive Medicine (DGRM). The specialization qualification "Reproductive Medicine" is offered as eLearning and webinar, and is supplemented by a one-day practical training session at a fertility center. Upon successful completion, the Westphalia-Lippe Medical Association issues a nationally recognized certificate.

This book was created to provide both course participants and medical assistants, nurses, and support staff in fertility centers, gynecological clinics and practices with a practical compendium for reproductive medicine. The "Model Continuing Education Curriculum in Reproductive Medicine" serves as the "guiding thread." It complements the eLearning and webinar content provided by the lecturers (reproductive medicine specialists, reproductive biologists, andrologists, and social educators). In addition, it imparts in-depth knowledge where it is relevant for understanding reproductive biology.

Since reproductive medicine is a young field, new aspects continually emerge. Methods that have not yet been fully scientifically evaluated are also mentioned, in order to ensure preparedness when caring for couples with fertility desires. In these cases, scientific literature has been deliberately included, as fertility patients search for information on the internet and often specifically inquire about new methods at fertility centers.

We hope that this book will help medical assistants, nurses, and other healthcare support staff to provide even better support to physicians in fertility centers, clinics, and practices. In doing so, this book on contemporary reproductive medicine fills a gap in the book market, situated among the various relevant medical specialties and the challenging legal regulations.

Prof. Dr. med. Stefan Dieterle

Prof. Dr. med. Frank Nawroth

P.S. For reasons of readability, the masculine form is predominantly used. It is expressly intended to refer to all genders equally in the interest of equal treatment. The shortened form of language is used solely for editorial reasons and does not imply any value judgment.

The electronic version of this Book contains supplementary material, which can be accessed via the following link [(c) Bals-Pratsch, et al. (2025). Workplace Fertility Center. Springer, Berlin, Heidelberg. https://doi.org/10.1007/978-3-662-71659-5].

Acknowledgments

This book is based on the model continuing education curriculum for medical assistants "Reproductive Medicine" of the German Medical Association from 2022. It covers the required knowledge in reproductive medicine for the specialization qualification

The initiator of the specialization qualification was Prof. Dr. med. Stefan Dieterle, who played a key role in initiating and designing this advanced training for medical assistants, nurses, and other medical support staff. Special thanks are also due to Ms. Elisabeth Borg, Head of the Continuing Education Department of the Westphalia-Lippe Medical Association (ÄKWL), for her support in developing the curriculum and planning the training at the Academy of the ÄKWL and the KVWL. Contributions were also made by Prof. Dr. med. Barbara Sonntag, German Society for Reproductive Medicine (DGRM), and Priv.-Doz. Dr. med. Ulrich Alfred Knuth, Professional Association of Reproductive Medicine Centers of Germany (BRZ).

The curricular advanced training has been conducted annually since 2023 by the Academy of the Medical Association of Westphalia-Lippe (ÄKWL) and the Association of Statutory Health Insurance Physicians of Westphalia-Lippe (KVWL). The scientific direction is provided by Prof. Dr. med. Stefan Dieterle together with Dr. med. Caroline Niehoff and Prof. Dr. med. Frank Nawroth. Special thanks are due to Mr. Martin Wollschläger-Tigges from the Academy of the ÄKWL and the KVWL, who, with great personal commitment, organizes and leads the implementation of the specialization qualification, ensuring that course participants are excellently supported and accompanied in all respects. Thanks are also extended to all lecturers for preparing the training materials for eLearning and the online webinars: Prof. Dr. med. Monika Bals-Pratsch, M.Sc., Dr. rer. nat. Dunja Baston-Büst, Dr. rer. nat. Dagmar Gutknecht, Prof. Dr. med. Katharina Hancke, Dr. med. Aida Hanjalic-Beck, Dr. med. Nora Holtmann, Dott. Mag. Ershela Kazazi, Prof. Dr. med. Frank Köhn, Prof. Dr. med. Frank Nawroth, Dr. med. Caroline Niehoff, Dr. med. Thilo Schill, Dr. med. Andreas Ott, Prof. Dr. med. Barbara Sonntag, Dr. rer. nat. Tom Trapphoff, Dr. phil. Petra Thorn, Dr. med. Mascha Petersen, and PD Dr. med. Birgit Wetzka. Thanks are also due to the fertility centers that, as previous training centers, have hosted the practical day marking the conclusion of the continuing education program.

Prof. Dr. med. Monika Bals-Pratsch M.Sc.
Prof. Dr. med. Stefan Dieterle
Prof. Dr. med. Frank Nawroth

Contents

List of Authors

Prof. Dr. med. Monika Bals-Pratsch
KinderwunschWissen, Regensburg, Germany

Prof. Dr. med. Stefan Dieterle
Überörtliche Berufsausübungsgemeinschaft Kinderwunsch Dortmund, Siegen, Dorsten, Wuppertal GbR, Dortmund, Germany

Prof. Dr. med. Frank Nawroth
Facharzt-Zentrum für Kinderwunsch, Pränatale Medizin, Endokrinologie und Osteologie, amedes MVZ Hamburg, Hamburg, Germany

Abbreviations

AFC	antral follicle count		GDM	Gestational diabetes
AGS	adrenogenital syndrome		GOÄ	Private Medicinal Fee Schedule for Physicians
AID	Artificial insemination with donor		GKV	Statutory health insurance
AMG	Medicinal Products Act		GnRH	Gonadotropin-releasing hormone
AMH	Anti-Müllerian hormone			
AMWHV	Ordinance on the Manufacture of Medicinal Products and Active Substances		GV	Sexual intercourse
			hCG	human chorionic gonadotropin
ART	Assisted reproduction or fertilization		HyCoSy	Hysterosalpingo-contrast sonography
AZF	Azoospermia factor		ICSI	intracytoplasmic sperm injection
BÄK	German Medical Association		i. d. R.	as a rule
BGB	Civil Code		IUI	intrauterine insemination
BMI	Body Mass Index		IVF	In vitro fertilization
CBAVD	congenital bilateral aplasia of the vas deferens		IT	Information technology
COC	Cumulus-oocyte complex		KBV	National Association of Statutory Health Insurance Physicians
COS	controlled ovarian stimulation			
			LBR	Live birth rate
DERI	German Register for Insemination		LH	luteinizing hormone
D·I·R	German IVF Registry e.V.		MAR-Test	Mixed antiglobulin reaction test
DNA	Deoxyribonucleic acids		MESA	microsurgical epididymal sperm aspiration
DPO	Data Protection Officer			
GDPR	General Data Protection Regulation		MII	Metaphase II
			Mill	Millions
d. h.	that is		min	Minutes
EBM	Uniform Fee Schedule for statutory health insurance physicians		ml	Milliliter
			OHSS	ovarian hyperstimulation syndrome
EDV	electronic data processing		PN	Pronucleus
EDD	expected (calculated) due date		PCOS	polycystic ovary syndrome
			PEI	federal Paul Ehrlich Institute
ESchG	Embryo Protection Act			
ET	Embryo transfer		PICSI	physiological ICSI
EP	Ectopic pregnancy		PID	Preimplantation genetic diagnosis
TTTS	twin-to-twin transfusion syndrome			
			PKV	private health insurance
FSH	follicle-stimulating hormone		p.c.	post conception
			p.m.	post menstruationem
GB-A	Federal Joint Committee		QM	Quality management

QSReproMed	Working Group on Quality Assurance in Reproductive Medicine
QuaDeGA	Quality control of the German Society of Andrology
SaRegG	Sperm Donor Registry Act
SEC	Single European Code
SGB V	Social Code Book V - Statutory Health Insurance
SRY	sex determining region of Y
SSR	Pregnancy rate
SSW	Week of pregnancy
TESE	Testicular sperm extraction
TFG	Transfusion Act
TPG	Transplantation Act
TPG-GewV	TPG Tissue Ordinance
TPO-Ab	Thyroid peroxidase antibodies
TRAb	TSH receptor antibodies
TRH	Thyrotropin-releasing hormone
TSH	Thyroid-stimulating hormone
s. o.	see above
s. u.	see below
WHO	World Health Organization
z. B.	for example

Legal Foundations

Contents

Supplementary Information The online version contains supplementary material available at ▶ https://doi.org/10.1007/978-3-662-73035-5_1.

1

Development of Reproductive Medicine and Regulatory Frameworks

Louise Brown was born in 1978 in Oldham, England, as the world's first test-tube baby. This groundbreaking success was the result of the collaboration between Patrick Steptoe (gynecologist) and Robert Edwards (physiologist). Robert Edwards was awarded the Nobel Prize in Medicine in 2010 for his life's work. Through close clinical and scientific cooperation with the English team, university centers for **in vitro fertilization (IVF)** were established in Erlangen under the direction of Siegfried Trotnow, in Lübeck under Dieter Krebs, and in Kiel under Lieselotte Mettler. Germany's first IVF child was born in Erlangen in 1982, followed by IVF children in Lübeck and Kiel the following year. In 1991, another milestone in reproductive medicine was achieved with the introduction of **intracytoplasmic sperm injection (ICSI)**. In this technique, a single motile sperm is injected directly into the egg cell. This method is used when the quality of the sperm is insufficient for a sperm cell to penetrate an egg cell during IVF treatment.

As early as 1985, the German Medical Association issued **Guidelines for the Implementation of In Vitro Fertilization (IVF) and Embryo Transfer (ET)** as a treatment method for human infertility. It was not until five years later that the **Embryo Protection Act (ESchG)** was enacted (Appendix 1.1). Comparable regulatory frameworks for reproductive medicine did not exist in other countries at that time. The principles of these regulations remain essentially valid. However, many additions, clarifications, and additional national and European laws have since been introduced. For treating physicians and patients seeking fertility treatment, the complex legal and professional regulations today provide the framework for the retrieval, fertilization, and transfer of human gametes in the context of assisted reproduction.

At the beginning of every fertility treatment, a treatment contract is concluded between the physician as the service provider and the patient as the recipient of services, in accordance with § 630a of the **German Civil Code (BGB)**. The physician promises to provide a service according to recognized professional standards, and the patient undertakes to pay the fee, unless another payer is obliged to cover the costs.

Fertility therapy involving artificial insemination is carried out within a comprehensive legal framework. Since there is no specific law on reproductive medicine, the regulatory framework encompasses numerous different laws (◘ Fig. 1.1). Billing

	SGB V	Social Code Book V		ESchG	Embryo Protection Act
Gemeinsamer Bundesausschuss	GBA	Federal Joint Committee		GewebeG	Tissue Act
E B M	EBM	Uniform Fee Schedule for statutory health insurance		GenDG	Genetic Diagnostics Act
GOÄ	GOÄ	Private Medicinal Fee Schedule for Physicians		SaRegG	Sperm Donor Registry Act

◘ **Fig. 1.1**   Legal frameworks for artificial insemination

regulations for assisted reproduction are complex and subject to irregular, sometimes significant, changes. Since the **Statutory Health Modernization Act (GMG)** came into force in January 2004, couples with statutory health insurance must cover half of both the treatment and medication costs for artificial insemination. In no other area of statutory health insurance (GKV) are insured persons so heavily burdened financially for medical treatments as in reproductive medicine.

Statutory Health Insurance Funds and Billing of Services

Benefits for artificial insemination are regulated for statutory health insurance (GKV) in **§ 27a – Social Code Book V (SGB V)**. This paragraph stipulates that, since 2004, the health insurance fund only covers 50% of the costs (see above). The costs must first be approved by the health insurance fund on the treatment plan. The treatment must be carried out in a fertility center that has authorization to perform artificial insemination according to **§ 121a SGB V**. These **authorizations to perform artificial insemination** under § 121a SGB V are granted as needed in the federal states by the state medical associations or a state authority. The competent authority grants authorization to physicians who best meet the requirements (§ 27a para. 1) for the appropriate, efficient, and economical implementation of measures to achieve pregnancy, taking public interests into account. When applying, the necessary personnel, equipment, and spatial requirements for the granting of authorization must be met (◘ Table 1.1). In addition, a permit under the Tissue Act must be obtained (see below).

This regulatory framework is supplemented by the "Guidelines on Artificial Insemination" (see ► Chap. 10) and the "Guideline on Cryopreservation of Oocytes or Sperm or Germ Cell Tissue and Corresponding Medical Measures Due to Germ Cell-Damaging Therapy – Cryo-RL" (see ► Chap. 8) of the **Federal Joint Committee (GB-A)**. This body, consisting of representatives from the National Association of Statutory Health Insurance Physicians (KBV), the health insurance funds, and the hospital association, regulates the medical details regarding **requirements**, **methods**, and medical **indications**. For example, couples must be married and age limits must not be under- or exceeded. There must be a

◘ Table 1.1   Requirements for Authorization § 121a

Subfield	Equipment	Personnel
Reproductive Endocrinology	Hormone laboratory	Gynecologist specializing in gynecological endocrinology and reproductive medicine
Gynecological Sonography	Equipment for ultrasound diagnostics	Gynecologist with specialization
Operative Gynecology	Procedure room for oocyte retrieval, anesthesia	Gynecologist with specialization
Reproductive Biology, Focus on in vitro culture	Laboratory for in vitro fertilization, in vitro culture, microinjection, cryopreservation	Certified reproductive biologist, e.g., of the Working Group for Reproductive Biology of Humans (AGRBM)
Andrology in the context of IVF	Laboratory for sperm diagnostics and preparation	Gynecologist with specialization
Regular cooperation with a human geneticist, a physician with additional training in "andrology," and a medical or psychological psychotherapist		

1

reasonable prospect of success. The catalog of methods includes inseminations (IUI), in vitro fertilization (IVF) with embryo transfer (ET), and intracytoplasmic sperm injection (ICSI). The number of treatment cycles is limited. Treatments with donor sperm and embryo donation are **exclusion criteria**. There must be a medical indication for assisted reproduction. These include reduced sperm quality, tubal disease, but also unexplained (idiopathic) infertility.

Billing for reproductive medicine services is carried out in accordance with the **Fee Schedule for Physicians (GOÄ)** and, within statutory health insurance, according to the **Uniform Value Scale (EMB)** (see ▶ Chap. 10).

Quality of Care, Treatment- and Legal Certainty through the German Medical Association (BÄK) Guideline

The Tissue Act is supplemented by the updated **Guideline on the Retrieval and Transfer of Human Gametes or Germ Cell Tissue in the Context of Assisted Reproduction** of the **German Medical Association (BÄK)** from 2022. This professional, medical-scientific guideline was first adopted in 2018 in agreement with the Paul Ehrlich Institute (PEI) as the responsible federal authority (Transplantation Act TPG § 16b). The aim of this regulatory framework is to guarantee the quality of care and treatment safety in assisted reproduction and to provide the necessary legal certainty for all parties involved. The BÄK reviews the guideline for currency at least every two years. The guideline has already been supplemented, as in 2019 the cryopreservation of gametes and germ cell tissue prior to germ cell-damaging therapy was added to SGB V.

Embryo Protection Act (ESchG)

The most important law is the **Embryo Protection Act (ESchG)** (Appendix 1.1). Reproductive medicine has rapidly advanced due to new findings and methods. As a result, the content of the ESchG is being re-evaluated in light of current knowledge. Today, an **embryo** is understood to mean only those fertilized, cultured egg cells that are capable of development and from which a child can arise. **Court decisions** have provided legal certainty.

The Embryo Protection Act is anchored in the **Criminal Code** (StGB). Violations are punishable by a fine or imprisonment of up to three years. According to ESchG § 11, only a physician may perform artificial insemination, preimplantation genetic diagnosis, and cryopreservation or transfer an embryo (**physician requirement**). Biologists, medical assistants (MFA) and medical staff, medical-technical assistants (MTA), and other non-physician personnel may only carry out these procedures on the instructions of or under the supervision of a physician.

The ESchG was enacted 12 years after the world's first birth following IVF. Its purpose was to prevent the **abusive application** of the new methods. From a medical perspective, the ESchG also provides protection for affected couples and children conceived via IVF from the risks of new technologies (see below). The aim of the law is to achieve pregnancy in the woman from whom the egg cell originates. Since 1990, knowledge in reproductive medicine and gametes, fertilization, and the development of the fertilized egg cell to the embryo have advanced rapidly. However, laws are formulated in such a way that other circumstances, such as blastocyst transfer, lead to different legal assessments. This interpretation, **adapted to new circumstances**, has been confirmed by court decisions. Against this background, the ESchG is an old law, but with the updated interpretation, it enables the **best possible IVF treatment** at an **international level in Germany**. Society has also changed. Only **egg donation** and **surrogacy** are **prohibited**. Patients remain exempt from punishment for undergoing these procedures abroad.

Case Study: Prosecution of a Counseling Professional for Egg Donation Abroad

A 39-year-old patient sought further treatment after three unsuccessful ICSI cycles. The cause of the lack of treatment success was diminished ovarian reserve. Only two to four oocytes were retrieved in each cycle, of which a maximum of two could be fertilized. After two to three days of oocyte culture, two-cell stage embryos were transferred twice and a four-cell stage embryo once. Due to the poor prognosis for further treatment, the patient opted for treatment abroad with egg donation. Prior to this, she received psychosocial counseling on the specific issues following donation, such as how to address the circumstances of conception. Because the counseling also included information about facilities for fertility treatment abroad, the counseling professional was prosecuted, but not the patient. However, the patient had to testify as a witness in the trial. The proceedings were dropped after ten years.

The most important regulations for everyday practice in fertility centers are summarized in ◘ Table 1.2.

The prohibition of egg donation is set out in paragraph 1, section 1, numbers 1 and 2 (§ 1 para. 1 nos. 1 and 2) (Appendix 1.1). Since **egg donation** is now **socially desired**, the previous federal government appointed an expert commission on reproductive self-determination and reproductive medicine, which in 2024 submitted a report to prepare a legislative initiative in the Bundestag (Federal Government 2024). There has not yet been a subsequent legislative initiative.

The **transfer** of **more than 3 embryos** is **prohibited**. From today's perspective, this regulation in § 1 para. 1 no. 3 protects the **health** of women and children. It reduces the **risk** of higher-order **multiple pregnancies**. The goal of IVF treatment is a singleton pregnancy resulting in the birth of a healthy child.

The **stockpiling** of embryos is prohibited under § 1 para. 1 no. 2. This is also not the goal of IVF treatment. Therefore, only as many eggs should be fertilized as are needed to achieve a pregnancy in the treatment cycle. For the transfer, one, or at most three embryos, should be created according

◘ **Table 1.2** Embryo Protection Act and Court Decisions

Procedure	Prohibitions	ESchG, Court Rulings
Egg donation	Yes	§ 1 para. 1 nos. 1 and 2
Transfer > 3 embryos	Yes	§ 1 para. 1 no. 3
Stockpiling of embryos	Yes	§ 1 para. 1 no. 2
Preimplantation genetic diagnosis (PGD)	Yes, but exceptions	§ 3a para. 2
Fertilization with sperm from a deceased person	Yes	§ 4 para. 1 no. 3
Donation of pronuclear stage cells (PN cells)	Yes	§ 1 para. 1 no. 2, Bavarian Supreme Regional Court (BayObLG) 2020, Ref. 206 StRR 1461/19
Donation of embryos	No (not punishable)	§ 8 para. 1, Bavarian Supreme Regional Court (BayObLG) 2020, Ref. 206 StRR 1461/19

to the couple's decision. If a couple wishes to transfer a single embryo, then according to the **individual prognostic criteria**, as many pronuclear stage cells (PN cells) should be cultured (usually **culture of** 3–6 **PN cells**) as are needed to ensure that one embryo can be transferred. Prognostic criteria for embryo development include, above all, the woman's age, the number of previous treatments, and the quality of eggs and sperm. Since the **natural factor** does not allow for a precise prediction of the actual number of embryos produced, after culturing the PN cells, there may be either too many ("**unintended**") or too few or no **embryos** available for transfer. Any additional, but permissible, embryos developed in this process can be cryopreserved for later transfer.

Preimplantation genetic diagnosis (PGD) remains prohibited. However, with the introduction of § 3a para. 2 in 2011, an exception was created for couples with a known **hereditary disease** or for couples with evidence of a **chromosomal disorder** (see ▶ Chap. 9). Chromosomes are carriers of genetic information and consist mainly of DNA (deoxyribonucleic acids). PGD may be performed if there is a high risk of a serious hereditary disease in the offspring or if a serious impairment of the embryo is expected that is highly likely to result in stillbirth or miscarriage. In 2014, the federal government issued a regulation on the implementation of preimplantation genetic diagnosis (**Preimplantation Genetic Diagnosis Regulation – PIDV**). Only in this regulation was the implementation of § 3a para. 2 in everyday practice defined. PGD may only be performed after a positive vote by an **ethics committee for preimplantation genetic diagnosis** in centers authorized for this purpose. **Human genetics centers** may cooperate with several reproductive medicine centers. The **federal government** prepares a **report** every four years on the experiences and results of PGD treatments, most recently the third report in 2024. Currently, about 500 PGD treatments are per-

formed per year. Since Bavaria has the most authorized human genetics sites and the fees of the Bavarian Ethics Committee for Preimplantation Genetic Diagnosis are relatively low at €100 to €500, most PGD treatments are performed in Bavaria. The number of **rejected PGD applications** is now very low. This is because **administrative courts** in Regensburg (2019) and Leipzig (2020) have established criteria for determining a serious hereditary disease that must result in a positive vote. For example, a previous pregnancy termination due to the diagnosis of the hereditary disease in a fetus requires a positive vote. Psychological, social, and ethical aspects of the individual case must be taken into account. Thus, the **discretion** of the PGD committees in determining a serious hereditary disease is limited, and a negative vote is now only justifiable in exceptional cases (see ▶ Chap. 9).

Fertilization may only be performed if the woman whose egg is to be fertilized and the man whose sperm is to be used for **fertilization** have given their consent. This **consent** is no longer possible after the man's death. For this reason, fertilization with the sperm of a man after his **death** is prohibited under § 4 para. 1 no. 3.

The donation of **pronuclear stage cells** (PN cells, impregnated oocytes) is prohibited according to the ruling of the Bavarian Supreme Regional Court (BayObLG) from 2020. The judge based her decision on § 1 para. 1 no. 2 by equating an unfertilized oocyte with an impregnated oocyte at the PN stage. ▣ Fig. 1.2 shows an unfertilized oocyte after follicular puncture. During the so-called "PN check" (fertilization control) 16 to 20 hours after injection of a sperm cell or insemination, the two pronuclei in the oocyte can be seen as a sign of a regular **fertilization process** (▣ Fig. 1.2). These dissolve about 24 hours after insemination or injection of the oocytes. This stage is already considered an **embryo** under the ESchG, which, if development proceeds normally, will develop into a blastocyst by

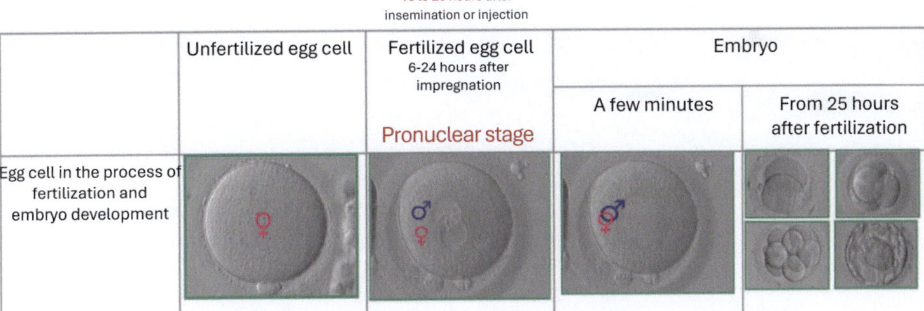

Fig. 1.2　Development of an unfertilized oocyte to an embryo

day five. The obvious **legal inequality** between altruistic **egg donation** and the **donation of cryopreserved pronuclear stage cells** was something the federal government, in accordance with its 2021 coalition agreement, intended to correct: "We will clarify that **embryo donation at the pronuclear stage is legal**…" (Kentenich et al. 2022). The federal government's expert commission on reproductive self-determination and reproductive medicine also expressed this view in its 2024 report (see above).

In its aforementioned ruling, the BayObLG also determined that the **donation of embryos is not punishable**. The judge justified her decision by stating that in embryo donation, the cryopreserved cells are already fertilized and have developed into an embryo as defined in § 8 para. 1.

Tissue Act (GewebeG)

The procedures of oocyte and sperm retrieval, fertilization, oocyte culture, embryo transfer, and cryopreservation with cell storage fall under the **Tissue Act (GewebeG)** of 2007 (Appendix 1.2). This law implements Directive 2004/23 of the European Community on the handling of tissues and cells into German law. Human germ cells (oocytes and sperm cells), but not embryos, are considered tissue within the meaning of the law.

The Tissue Act has led to changes and additions in the Medicinal Products Act (AMG) with the Medicinal Products and Active Substances Manufacturing Ordinance (AMWHV) and the Good Manufacturing Practices (GMP) Guideline Annex 1, in the Transplantation Act (TPG) with the TPG Tissue Ordinance (TPG-GewV), and in the Transfusion Act (TFG). Violations of AMG § 63i, § 97 para. 3, TPG § 18, and TFG §§ 31–32 are punishable by law (fines up to €25,000, imprisonment up to five years).

The **Medicinal Products Act (AMG)** is intended to ensure the safety of the handling of medicinal products, in particular the quality, efficacy, and safety of medicinal products. Only if the competent state authority has granted a **permit** (license) according to **AMG § 20b** and **§ 20c** may a fertility center perform treatments with **intrauterine insemination (IUI)** or IVF and **ICSI**. Sole hormonal stimulation without assisted reproduction procedures does not fall under this law.

The **license** according to **§ 20b** (1) for the fertility center as a **retrieval facility** is only granted if, in addition to the qualified **responsible person** with professional experience as per § 15, there is also other qualified and demonstrably regularly **trained staff** involved (■ Table 1.3). **Cooperating retrieval facilities** for the surgical retrieval of testicular tissue,

Table 1.3   Requirements for Granting/Revoking Permit AMG 20b, 20c

Inspection content	Requirements	Tissue Act (relevant laws and ordinances)
Qualified and responsible person; senior medical qualified person	University degree of at least 4 years, at least 2 years of professional experience; medical license	AMG § 15, §§ 20b, 20c; TFG § 4
Involved staff	Qualification through regular training according to a program including hygiene and medical devices, organizational chart	AMG §§ 20b, 20c; AMWHV § 4, § 34; TFG § 4
Facilities for tissue retrieval	Type, size, number, and equipment suitable for the intended purposes, adequate lighting, suitable climatic conditions, hygiene measures	AMG §§ 20b, 20c; AMWHV §§ 5–6, § 36; TFG § 4
Ensuring the state of medical science and technology	Regular assessment of whether test procedures are still valid, revalidation if necessary	AMG § 20b
QM system	Compliance with the principles of Good Manufacturing Practice (including up-to-date job descriptions)	AMG § 20c; AMWHV § 33
Tissue donor laboratory	If applicable, under contractual agreement, quality assurance for anti-HIV-1, 2, HBsAg, anti-HBc, anti-HCV-Ab	TPG §§ 8d; TPG-GewV Annex 4
Donor suitability	Blood samples up to 3 months before retrieval, checks within 24 months for the same partnership, release by a physician, traceability, handling of infectiousness	TPG §§ 8d; TFG §§ 4, 19

ovarian tissue, or for conducting laboratory tests do not require their own license under § 20b (2) if they operate under a **contractual agreement**. For the permit under **§ 20c** (**processing** or **handling, preservation, testing, storage**, or **placing on the market** of tissue or tissue preparations), the same requirements as above apply as for the license under § 20b (1). In addition, it must be demonstrated that the processing or handling, including **labeling**, preservation, and storage, is carried out according to the **state** of **science** and **technology**, and that a **QM system** according to the principles of **Good Manufacturing Practice (GMP)** has been established and is kept up to date. The requirements for implementing GMP are set out in the ordinance (**AMWHV** §§ 32–41). These include the determination of **donor suitability** by a physician and the necessary **laboratory tests** (human immunodeficiency virus (HIV), hepatitis B, and hepatitis C) in a **tissue donor laboratory**. This laboratory must have a permit according to the provisions of the AMG (see below). A licensed fertility center is listed in the **EU register** of approved tissue establishments.

According to **AMG § 63i, serious incidents** such as incorrect identification of tissues or **serious adverse reactions** such as malformations in a donor child or severe ovarian hyperstimulation syndrome (OHSS) must be reported to the Paul Ehrlich Institute (PEI) as the federal supervisory authority without delay (but no later than within 15 days of becoming known) (see ▶ Chap. 6). This also applies to suspected cases. **§ 64** regulates **inspection**. Licensed centers are monitored by the competent authority. This authority checks compliance with the regulations of the principles and guidelines of GMP, including the relevant sections of the TPG and TFG. The inspection should take place at least **every three years**.

Fertility centers are **tissue establishments** within the meaning of the **Transplantation Act (TPG)**. This law applies to the donation, retrieval, and transfer of tissues, including the preparation of these procedures. The **tissue donor laboratory** must have a permit under the provisions of the AMG for infection diagnostics (§ 8e). **Blood samples** must be taken within three months **before donation**, and **checks** within the same partnership must be performed no later than after 24 months. For the **release** of tissue for processing, handling, preservation, or storage, a **medical assessment** of the donor is required. The donor must be medically and, based on the laboratory results, suitable (§ 8d). Further requirements for the quality and safety of tissue retrieval and transfer, as well as documentation, are set out in the ordinance with Annexes 3–4 (TPG-GewV).

The **TPG prohibits** according to § 1 (2) the **trade in human germ cells**.

According to the **Transfusion Act (TFG)**, a qualified senior medical person must be appointed (TGP § 4). Donor suitability is regulated in § 5. § 19 regulates the **traceability** of tissue and the procedures in case of suspicion and confirmation of infection prior to tissue donation.

Genetic Diagnostics Act (GenDG)

In genetic diagnostics prior to artificial fertilization, the **Genetic Diagnostics Act (GenDG)** of 2010 must be observed.

The GenDG must be observed in genetic testing of the couple as part of pre-diagnostic procedures before assisted reproduction and in the case of PGD. In pre-diagnostics, blood samples for chromosome analysis or for genetic diagnostics in the case of clinical suspicion of a hereditary disease may only be forwarded to a human genetics laboratory after medical counseling. In contrast to such **"diagnostic" genetic diagnostics**, in so-called **"predictive" genetic testing** the **quality requirements** for the responsible **medical professional** providing counseling must be met (specialist with additional qualification in "Medical Genetics," specialist with "qualification for subject-specific genetic counseling," or specialist in human genetics). For example, testing for **cystic fibrosis** in a clinically healthy man with suspected **obstructive azoospermia** is **diagnostic**. If a pathogenic gene mutation for cystic fibrosis is detected, the recommended subsequent **testing** of the **healthy partner** is, however, **predictive**. Specialist counseling should also include the consequences of a positive test. If a mutation is detected in the healthy partner, the risk of having a child with cystic fibrosis is 25%. Due to this **high genetic risk**, a couple affected would in principle have the option of **preimplantation genetic diagnosis (PGD)**.

Sperm Donor Registry Act (SaRegG)

Since 2018, the **Sperm Donor Registry Act (SaRegG)** has been in effect. Since then, the fundamental right of donor children to know their origins has been ensured (see ► Chap. 6). Prior to the legislation, donor children had sued some reproductive medicine specialists and sperm banks for the release of information about their genetic fathers. These were ordered to provide information in several court cases. A **donor child** can now obtain information about the data of the sperm donor stored in the sperm donor registry. Before reaching the age of 16, the claim can already be asserted by the legal representative.

The law was also enacted to exempt **donors** from the risk of claims such as maintenance payments from donor children. Because of these risks, donations were previously mostly anonymous. Sperm donors are now especially exempt from claims in the areas of custody, maintenance, and inheritance law, as their paternity is excluded. This required a supplementary regulation in the German Civil Code (BGB).

🏠 Learning objectives

- Expertise regarding the regulations of statutory health insurance for artificial fertilization
- Specialist knowledge of practice-relevant content of the Embryo Protection Act for the culture of fertilized oocytes
- Classify legal regulations in the Tissue Act
- Application of the Genetic Diagnostics Act in everyday practice

Reproductive medicine services are provided in a "jungle" of complex legal regulations and guidelines that must be observed by fertility centers. In vitro fertilization (IVF) was first successfully performed in England in 1978 with the birth of Louise Brown. In Germany, the first "test-tube baby" was born in 1982. Statutory health insurance funds contribute to IVF costs. However, access is restricted by eligibility requirements. Thus, treatment is only possible in fertility centers that have been approved by the relevant state authority. This approval is granted according to needs-based principles, provided that the permit from the competent government authority for the handling and processing of oocytes and sperm cells and of ovarian and testicular tissue is available. To ensure the quality of care and treatment safety in IVF treatment, the German Medical Association has issued a guideline. Orders for genetic analysis of blood samples are subject to the Genetic Diagnostics Act, for which patients must first be counseled by a qualified physician. For donor sperm treatments, the Sperm Donor Registry Act has applied since 2018. This ensures, on the one hand, the fundamental right of donor children to know their origins and, on the other hand, protects the donor from claims in the areas of custody, maintenance, and inheritance law.

Below is the link to the electronic supplementary material.

References

Bundesärztekammer (2022) Richtlinie zur Entnahme und Übertragung von menschlichen Keimzellen oder Keimzellgewebe im Rahmen der assistierten Reproduktion. ► https://www.bundesaerztekammer.de/fileadmin/user_upload/BAEK/Themen/Medizin_und_Ethik/RiLi-ass-Reproduktion.pdf. Zuletzt 11.06.2025

Bundesregierung (2024) Dritter Bericht der Bundesregierung über die Erfahrungen mit der Präimplantationsdiagnostik. ► https://dserver.bundestag.de/btd/20/100/2010060.pdf. Zuletzt 17.06.2025

Bundesregierung (2024) Bericht der Kommission zur reproduktiven Selbstbestimmung und Fortpflanzungsmedizin. Kurzbericht Drucksache 20/11530 ► https://dserver.bundestag.de/btd/20/115/2011530.pdf. Zuletzt 17.06.2025

Kentenich H, Taupitz J, Hilland U (2022) Der Koalitionsvertrag der Bundesregierung: Was sich in der Reproduktionsmedizin verändern soll. J Reproduktionsmed Endokrinol 19–90

Physiology of Spontaneous Conception

Contents

© The Author(s), under exclusive license to Springer-Verlag GmbH, DE, part of Springer Nature 2026
M. Bals-Pratsch et al., *Workplace: Fertility Clinic*, https://doi.org/10.1007/978-3-662-73035-5_2

Introduction

Conception is the result of the interplay of the natural bodily functions of both woman and man. At the center is the fertilization of the egg cell by a sperm. After six days, the developed fertilized egg cell, now a blastocyst, implants itself into the uterine lining. From the inner cell mass of the blastocyst, the bilaminar embryonic disc forms, from which the embryo continues to develop. The **embryonic period** ends at the beginning of the eighth week of development, or, calculated from the first day of the last menstrual period, at the 10th week of pregnancy. The embryo then develops into a fetus, marking the beginning of the **fetal period**.

Sexual Organs and Gonads

The Müllerian duct and the Wolffian duct are the embryonic precursors. From these, starting in the seventh week of development, the internal and external female and male sexual organs develop, respectively (◨ Fig. 2.1). The sex chromosomes X and Y determine the differentiation. If two X chromosomes are present, the **Müllerian ducts** develop into the **female sexual organs**; if one Y chromosome and one X chromosome are present, the **Wolffian ducts** develop into the **male sexual organs**. As early as the eighth week of embryonic development, testicular tissue has developed in a male embryo and produces the male

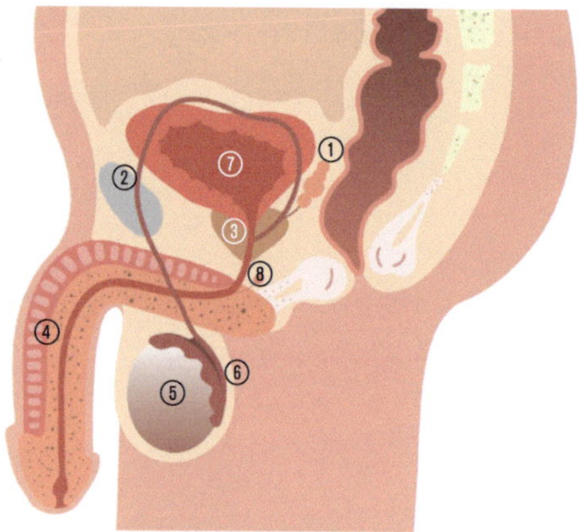
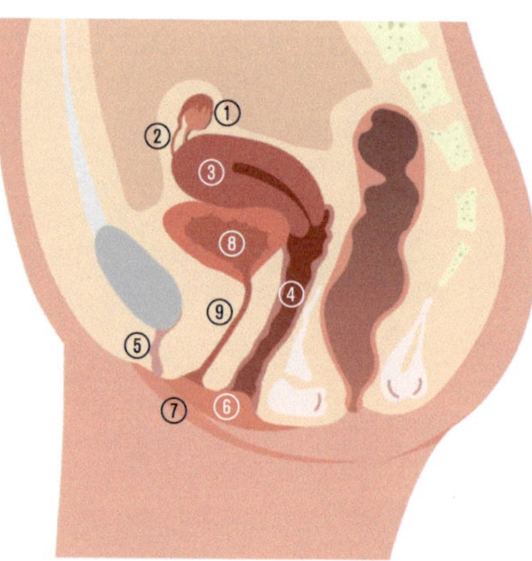

① **Seminal vesicles**
② **Vas deferens**
③ **Prostate gland**
④ **Penis**
⑤ **Testicle**
⑥ **Epididymis**
⑦ **Urinary bladder**
⑧ **Urethra**

① **Ovary**
② **Fallopian tube (tuba uterina)**
③ **Uterus**
④ **Vagina**
⑤ **Clitoris**
⑥ **Vestibule of the vagina (Vestibulum vaginae)**
⑦ **Labia**
⑧ **Bladder**
⑨ **Urethra**

◨ **Fig. 2.1** Female and male sexual organs (longitudinal section)

hormone **testosterone**. This initiates the sex-specific differentiation toward the **male** shape (**phenotype**). By the fourth month of pregnancy, this process is largely complete. In the absence of the Y chromosome, a female phenotype develops.

The **internal female sexual organs** include the ovary, fallopian tube (Tuba uterina), uterus, and vagina, while the **external** sexual organs include the vestibule of the vagina (Vestibulum vaginae), labia, and clitoris (◘ Fig. 2.1). **The internal male sexual organs** are the vas deferens (Ductus deferens), prostate gland, and seminal vesicles (Vesicula seminalis), and the **external** sexual organs are the testes, epididymis, and penis. Ovaries and testes are referred to as gonads, also known as germ glands.

Prenatal Germ Cell Development

The **primordial germ cells** migrate to the genital ridge as early as the fourth week of development. Once there, they proliferate through mitotic divisions. In the female embryo, the primordial germ cells become **oogonia**, and in the male embryo, they become **spermatogonia**. The maturation of egg and sperm cells from stem cells into fertilizable cells is called **oogenesis** and **spermatogenesis**, respectively. The development of these stem cells in oogenesis and spermatogenesis occurs separately from the rest of the body cells. From the sixth week of development, the oogonia and spermatogonia, together with supporting and connective tissue, form the primary **germ cords**. At this stage, the gonadal primordia are indifferent, meaning that female and male embryos are not yet distinguishable. The oogonia and spermatogonia, like somatic cells, still carry two sex chromosomes, XX or XY. From the gonadal primordia (**gonadal anla-**

gen), the **ovary** and **testis** differentiate starting in the seventh week of development. The decisive factor for differentiation into a female or male embryo is the absence or presence of the Y chromosome.

In the ovary, egg cells mature beneath the cortex, while in the testis, sperm cells develop in the seminiferous tubules. The **meiotic divisions (meiosis)** of egg and sperm cells are necessary because the cells must each have only a single set of 23 chromosomes for fertilization. After fertilization, the cells of an embryo again have 46 chromosomes. A key difference between egg and sperm cell maturation is that only one **egg cell** arises from an oogonium, whereas four **sperm cells** develop from a spermatogonium (◘ Fig. 2.2). The egg cell is the largest cell in the human body and more than 20 times larger than a sperm cell. It is highly sensitive to the microenvironment both within the female body and under laboratory conditions.

Other significant **differences** between the maturation of egg and sperm cells include the proliferation of oogonia and spermatogonia by mitotic divisions, the timing with resting phases for meiosis, the **consumption of egg cells** already **prenatally** through programmed cell death (apoptosis), and the duration and efficiency of egg and sperm maturation (◘ Table 2.1). Oogonia divide by mitosis until the fifth month of pregnancy and then degenerate. At **birth**, **no oogonia** remain.

As early as the third month of pregnancy, the **primary oocytes** differentiate from the oogonia. The maturation phase of the egg cells begins from the third to the seventh month of pregnancy. The primary oocytes enter the first meiotic division. However, at the beginning (prophase) of meiosis, a halt occurs. The primary oocytes

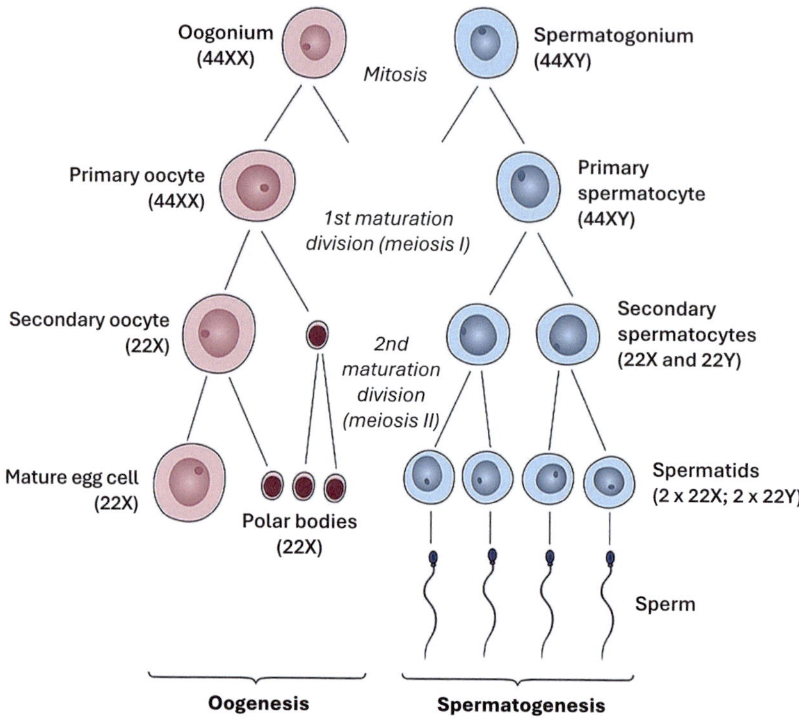

Fig. 2.2 Meiotic divisions during oogenesis and spermatogenesis

are transferred into a resting stage known as the **dictyotene** stage. Flat epithelial cells surround the primary oocytes (**Fig. 2.3**). The unit consisting of the follicular epithelial cells and the primary oocyte is called a **primordial follicle**. The follicular epithelial cells that surround the primary oocyte are later called granulosa cells during the maturation process. A woman has the highest number of egg cells as an embryo in the seventh month of pregnancy. Even prenatally, the number of her egg cells continuously decreases. This process continues until menopause at around age 50. Only about 400 of these cells will mature and ovulate before then. The primordial follicles are almost completely lost by the end of the reproductive phase.

■ Table 2.1 Sex differences in germ cell maturation

	Egg cell (oocyte)	Sperm cell (spermatozoon)
Size*	110 µm (0.11 mm)	5 µm (0.005 mm)
Proliferation by mitosis	Oogonia divide until approx. 5th month after fertilization	Spermatogonia initially divide, resting phase until puberty
Differentiation	Prenatal primary oocytes, 3rd–7th month after fertilization, atresia of oogonia	Postnatal (only after birth): spermatogenesis begins at puberty
Meiosis I	Prenatal, 3rd–7th month after fertilization with arrest in prophase, completion after puberty at ovulation	Postnatal from onset of puberty
Meiosis II	At ovulation until sperm entry	After completion of meiosis I with a delay of 22 days
Duration of maturation from puberty	12 months from completion of meiosis I to ovulation	3 months (64–74 days) including maturation in the epididymis
Germ cell resources	Before birth approx. 7 million egg cells in the 5th month after fertilization, then atresia, at menopause about 10,000 egg cells remain	From puberty into old age, as spermatogonia can continue to proliferate
Production of mature germ cells	Approx. 400 mature egg cells (ovulations) during the reproductive phase	Approx. 40–100 million mature sperm cells per day in a young, healthy man

*Sperm head

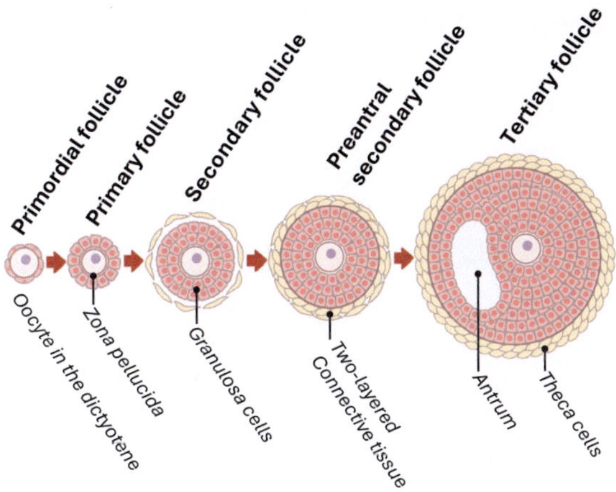

■ Fig. 2.3 Egg cell maturation from primordial follicle to tertiary follicle

Oogenesis and Follicle Growth from Puberty Onward

The development of primordial follicles into the mature **preovulatory follicle** begins at puberty and takes almost **one** full **year** (◘ Fig. 2.4). First, the growth of the primordial follicles must be initiated. Groups of 15–20 primordial follicles are regularly recruited to mature. This process takes more than five months. Primordial follicles have a diameter of 0.14 mm, while a mature follicle has a diameter of 20 mm (◘ Table 2.2). Only one from a group (cohort) of egg cells that begin to grow matures into an ovulation-ready follicle. All

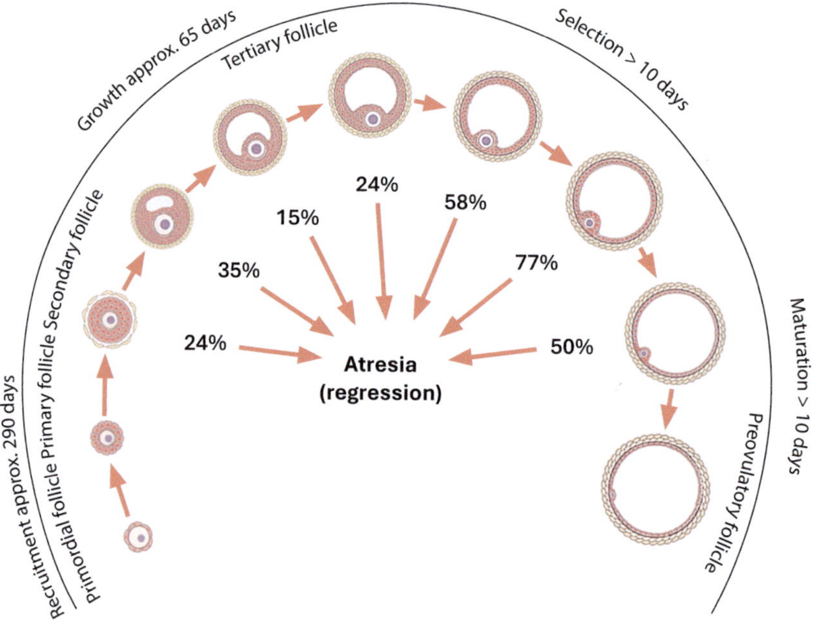

◘ **Fig. 2.4** Timeline of egg cell maturation over one year: development of an egg cell from a cohort of primordial follicles to the ovulation-ready follicle

◘ **Table 2.2** Egg cell maturation from primordial follicle to preovulatory tertiary follicle over 1 year

Developmental stages	Oocyte-granulosa cell complex	Atresia (%) during folliculogenesis	Duration in number of menstrual cycles
Primordial follicle	0.14 mm		5
Primary follicle	0.17 mm	24	2
Secondary follicle	0.23 mm	35	1
Small tertiary follicle	0.31–2 mm	15–28	2
Medium and large tertiary follicle	5–16 mm	50–77	0.3 (10 days)
Preovulatory tertiary follicle	20 mm		0.3 (10 days)

other follicles regress. This process is called **atresia**. Depending on the stage of maturation, 15 to 77% of developmental stages become atretic. The primary oocyte itself is only 0.1 mm in size and does not increase in size during maturation. Initially, it is surrounded by flat follicular epithelial cells (■ Fig. 2.3). Then the epithelial cells become cuboidal, so that the complex of the primary oocyte and follicular epithelial cells increases to 0.17 mm. The **zona pellucida** (the shell around the egg cell) forms, and the **primary follicle** develops. This process takes about two months. In the following month, the follicular epithelial layer continues to grow and becomes multilayered. **Secondary follicles** with a diameter of 0.23 mm are formed. A cavity (antrum) forms between the follicular epithelial cells, now called granulosa cells. These "antral" follicles are called **tertiary follicles** and are classified as small, medium, large, and preovulatory according to the size of the antrum. The granulosa cells surrounding the egg cell are called cumulus cells. Around the tertiary follicles, the connective tissue forms two layers: the inner theca interna (facing the secondary oocyte) and the outer theca externa (facing the interior of the ovary). Development up to the secondary follicle is slow and independent of the **regulatory hormones LH** and **FSH**. However, these hormones influence the subsequent accelerated growth of the tertiary follicles up to ovulation. The dominant follicle is selected from the cohort of medium antral follicles, which have a diameter of 5 to 10 mm.

The **secondary oocyte**, together with the theca interna, theca externa, and granulosa cells, forms an **endocrine unit**. Under the influence of the regulatory hormones LH and FSH, this unit produces the steroid hormones (**androgens, estrogens**, and **progesterone**).

Thus, the development from primordial follicle to dominant follicle resumes only at the onset of puberty, 12 to 50 years after the start of meiosis, which began prenatally in the third to seventh month of pregnancy and halted at the dictyotene stage. The **meiotic division** of the primary oocyte (44, XX) in the primordial follicle occurs in two steps (■ Fig. 2.2, see ▶ Chap. 9): in the first step (**meiosis I**), the chromosome set is halved. The meiosis I, which began prenatally, is continued. The paired homologous double-stranded chromosomes are distributed to two daughter cells. The secondary oocyte (23, X) is formed. This first step is completed at the **time** of **ovulation**. As a result, the mature, fertilizable egg cell is produced. However, only one mature egg cell arises from a primary oocyte. The three "daughter cells" consist only of fragments of the cell nucleus and degenerate in the further course. These "by-products" of meiosis are called **polar bodies**. In the second step (**meiosis II**), the two strands (chromatids) of each chromosome are distributed to two further daughter cells. Entry into meiosis II begins during ovulation, which is initiated by the regulatory hormone LH. The secondary oocyte pauses in meiosis II (MII oocyte) until the onset of **fertilization** (entry of a sperm into the egg cell).

Spermatogenesis and Spermiogenesis

Sperm cells can mature into old age, because unlike the oogonia in the ovary, the stem cells of sperm maturation (spermatogonia) are still present in the testicular tissue and, from the time of **puberty** onward, begin to proliferate again (■ Fig. 2.5, ■ Table 2.1). In contrast to the egg cell reserve, the **pool** of **spermatogonia** is not depleted but is **continuously renewed**. From puberty onward, the formation of sperm

2

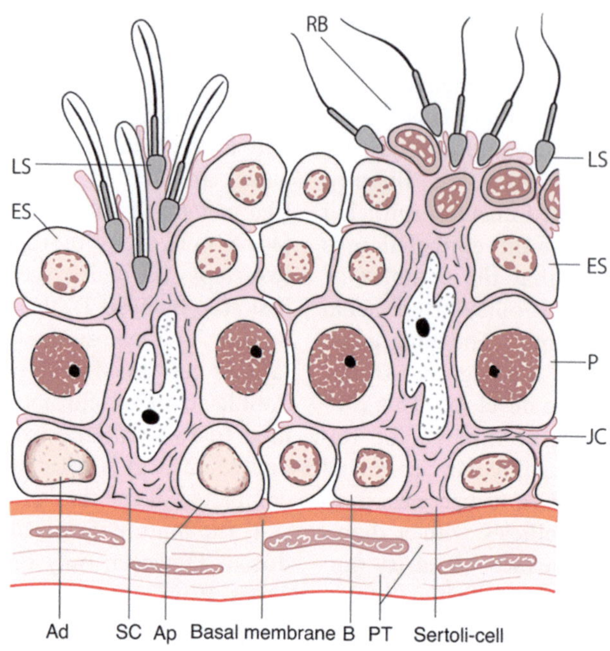

◘ **Fig. 2.5**   Spermatogenesis and spermiogenesis; section of a seminiferous tubule (tubulus). Reproduced with permission from: Nieschlag E, Behre HM, Kliesch S et al. (2023)

Tubule wall consisting of peritubular cells (PT) and a basal membrane, RB = residual body (remnants of cytoplasm during spermiogenesis), LS = elongated spermatids, ES = round spermatids, P = spermatocytes, Ad = testicular stem cells (dark spermatogonia), Ap = spermatogonia (pale spermatogonia), B = precursors of spermatocytes, SZ = Sertoli cells, JC = tight junctions, which together with Sertoli cells form the blood-testis barrier (SC)

cells (**spermatogenesis**) also begins in the seminiferous tubules (tubuli seminiferi). The total length of all seminiferous tubules in an adult man is more than 300 to 700 m. Spermatogenesis takes **64 to 74 days**. The spermatogonia, which are located at the wall of the seminiferous tubules, begin to divide and develop into primary spermatocytes (44,XY). These cells begin the meiotic division, first becoming secondary spermatocytes (2x 22,X and 2x 22,Y). In this first division step (**meiosis I**), there is also a delay in prophase, as with primary oocytes. However, in sperm cells, this delay lasts only 22 days, not several decades as in egg cells. In the second step (**meiosis II**), spermatids are formed. In contrast to oogenesis, four spermatids arise from one primary spermatocyte, not just one (◘ Fig. 2.2). As

with egg cell maturation, the maturation of sperm cells is controlled by the regulatory hormones LH and FSH. The **Leydig cells** between the seminiferous tubules produce the male hormone testosterone under the influence of LH. The function of the **Sertoli cells** as nourishing and protective supporting cells for the maturing sperm cells in the tubules is dependent on FSH and testosterone. The **blood-testis barrier** is formed by the interconnected Sertoli cells (◘ Fig. 2.5). As long as this barrier is intact, the immune system cannot form harmful antibodies against sperm cells. Sperm cells are foreign to the immune system because they are only produced after birth.

The maturation of spermatids into mature sperm (spermatozoa) is called **spermiogenesis**. The initially round spermatids become elongated, develop an acrosome cap, and a tail. After completion of spermiogenesis, the sperm cells consist of a **head**, **midpiece**, and **tail**. While the spermatogonia are located at the wall of the tubules (basal zone), the subsequent developmental stages from primary spermatocytes to mature sperm cells are arranged inward toward the central cavity (lumen) (◘ Fig. 2.5). In summary, the maturation of sperm cells proceeds from the outside in. The mature sperm cells are released into the lumen. From there, they are transported to the epididymis, where they acquire motility. In a healthy young man, 40–100 million sperm are produced daily.

Fertilization

Fertilization refers to the "**fusion**" of the **egg cell** with a **sperm cell**. Of the 200–300 million sperm ejaculated into the vaginal vault during intercourse, only one percent reach the cervix (cervix uteri). Usually, only 300–500 sperm reach the site of fertilization at the bulbously widened end of the fallopian tube (ampulla). Sperm can survive for many hours and days in the cervix. Depending on the phase of the cycle, they reach the ampulla within 30 minutes to six days. At the time of ovulation, sperm motility is particularly high. Upon contact of the sperm cells with the epithelium of the fallopian tubes, proteins detach from the sperm surface, enabling them to become capable of fertilization. This process takes about seven hours and is called **capacitation**.

At the time of ovulation, the follicle ready to rupture first bulges outward. The egg cell is already arrested in metaphase II ("**MII oocyte**"). Through contractions of smooth muscle cells in the wall of the ovary, it is released together with surrounding granulosa cells (**oocyte-cumulus complex**, abbreviated as **COC**) and, after rupture of the follicle wall, is expelled from the ovary along with follicular fluid. Shortly before ovulation, the fimbrial funnel covers the surface of the ovary, and the released egg cell is swept into the fallopian tube by sweeping movements. The egg cell is capable of being fertilized for about 10 hours. The inner granulosa cells, which are arranged radially around the zona pellucida, are called the **corona radiata**.

Only capacitated sperm can penetrate the corona radiata and come into contact with the zona pellucida (◘ Fig. 2.6). The latter triggers the **acrosome reaction**. The enzymes released from the acrosome ("head cap") locally dissolve the zona pellucida, allowing the sperm to enter the egg cell. First, the zona pellucida is penetrated, then the **fusion** of the cell membranes of the **sperm** and **egg cell** occurs. Only the sperm envelope remains on the surface of the egg cell membrane. The sperm nucleus and tail enter the egg cell (**impregnation**). The egg cell is activated and completes the second meiotic division with the extrusion of the second polar body. The cell nucleus transforms into the **female pronucleus**. The sperm continues to move closer to the female pronucleus. The nucleus and tail separate, the tail dissolves, and the nucleus swells to form the **male pronucleus** (◘ Fig. 1.2). The nuclear membranes of the female and male pronuclei dissolve. Both pronuclei replicate their genetic material (DNA), so that each chromosome again consists of two sister chromatids. The replicated chromosomes align on the mitotic spindle for the first **cleavage**. The sister chromatids migrate to opposite poles. A **2-cell stage** is formed. Egg cells fertilized by a sperm carrying an X chromosome result in a female embryo, and egg cells fertilized by a sperm carrying a Y chromosome result in a male embryo.

The entry of additional sperm into the egg cell is prevented by the **zona pellucida reaction**. This is triggered instantaneously by

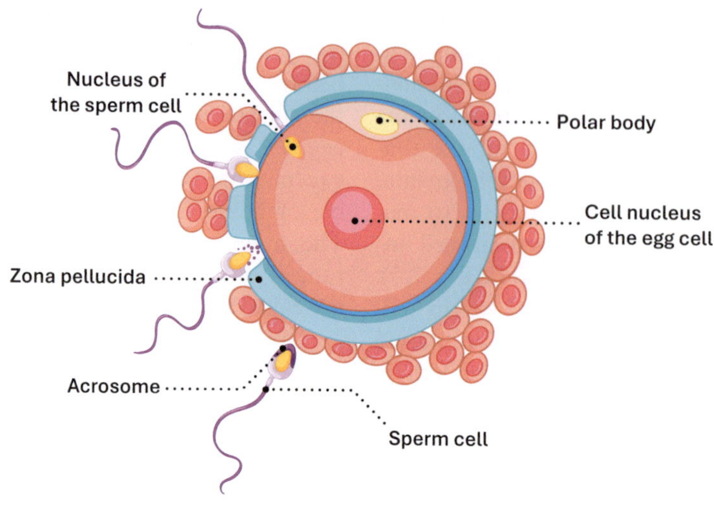

Fig. 2.6 Phases of fertilization

the egg cell upon contact with the sperm. Due to changes in the zona pellucida, further sperm can no longer enter the egg cell. This prevents irregular fertilization with multiple sperm (polyspermy).

Early Embryonic Development and Implantation

After fertilization at the end of the fallopian tube, **egg transport** begins. The cumulus cells detach from the zona pellucida. The five-day transport to the uterus occurs through rhythmic contractions of the wall of the fallopian tube, which is a muscular tube. The embryonic cells continue to develop during transport through successive cleavages, which are still controlled by the egg cell. With normal development, a **4-cell stage** is reached after two days, an **8-cell stage** after three days, and after four days, a morula stage (**morula**) with about 16 cells. Then, cell contacts are established within the previously loose cell cluster, a process called **compaction**. This condensation makes the cell boundaries indistinct. From the time of compaction, further develop-

ment is also influenced by paternal genes, and the embryo begins its own metabolism. From the fifth day of development, the outer cells differentiate into **trophoblast** cells and the inner cells into **embryoblast** cells. The latter are also referred to as the inner cell mass. The trophoblast cells are important for implantation, and the embryoblast cells will later form the child. A cavity forms within the embryo. This developmental stage is called the **blastocyst**. At this stage, the trophoblast cells and the inner cell mass are already microscopically visible. During transport through the fallopian tube, the embryo is protected by the zona pellucida. An **embryo hatches** from the zona pellucida only after reaching the uterus. This "hatching" is also referred to as "hatching." Implantation of the embryo begins about six days after fertilization.

A hatched, developmentally competent blastocyst first makes contact with the uterine lining from day six after fertilization. The trophoblast cells then actively invade the layer of endometrium that cyclically builds up and sheds (functionalis). This invasion is called **implantation**. The blastocyst implants at the pole where the embryoblast is located. After implantation, early placental development begins: the *trophoblast cells* differentiate into two components: the **outer syncytiotrophoblast cells** and the inner cytotrophoblast cells. The syncytiotrophoblast produces human chorionic gonadotropin (**hCG**). As a result, the drop in progesterone and estradiol and thus menstruation are prevented. The endometrium also responds to implantation. The cells of the functionalis become the cytoplasm-rich *decidua*, which is rich in vital nutrients for the embryo. Sometimes, at the time of the expected menstrual period, bleeding can occur from the implantation site (**implantation bleeding**). By day 12, the embryo is fully embedded in the mucosa and the implantation site is sealed with a coagulum. The embryoblast develops into a two-layered **germ disc**, consisting of the *epiblast* and *hypoblast* (see ▶ Chap. 7). From the spaces between the epiblast and the trophoblast cells, the **amniotic cavity** forms. This is lined with flat cells (amnioblasts) derived from the epiblast. The hypoblast provides the epithelium (exocoelomic membrane) that lines the blastocyst cavity, and the extraembryonic mesoderm, which fills the space to the trophoblast. It produces additional cells that migrate along the inner side of the exocoelomic membrane (Heuser's membrane), proliferate and grow, and form a new, smaller cavity called the **yolk sac**. Its main function is nutrition and blood formation during the early embryonic period. Later, a cavity forms in the extraembryonic mesoderm, the **chorionic cavity** (gestational sac). The outer wall, together with the trophoblast, forms the chorion. Between the inner and outer wall of the chorionic cavity, a connecting stalk remains, which from the fourth week becomes the early **umbilical cord**. The chorion is the embryonic part of the placenta. When the young **placenta** takes over the function of the yolk sac after the 10th week of pregnancy, the yolk sac regresses. The epiblast of the germ disc contributes only minimally to the extraembryonic mesoderm. However, the epithelium lining the amniotic cavity, which forms dorsally above it, is derived from the epiblast. The amniotic cavity will later increasingly fill with amniotic fluid (amniotic sac). It enlarges at the expense of the chorionic cavity and envelops the embryo, so that the chorionic cavity becomes obliterated after the 10th week of pregnancy.

🏠 Learning Objectives
- Understanding the embryonic development of female and male reproductive organs
- Understanding the physiology of reproduction

Egg and sperm cells are at the center of reproductive medicine. Egg cells require about a year to mature, while sperm cells need only about 70 days. Oogonia and spermatogonia, the stem cells for egg and sperm cells, can proliferate through mitotic divisions. In contrast, oogenesis and spermatogenesis produce, through meiotic divisions, one egg cell from an oogonium and four sperm cells from a spermatogonium. Egg cells begin meiosis before birth but complete it only at fertilization. Since no oogonia remain at birth, the pool of egg cells is limited. The supply of spermatogonia, however, is maintained and renewed through mitotic divisions. From these cells, sperm mature from puberty onward. Fertilization takes place in the fallopian tube and begins when a mature egg cell (metaphase II) fuses with the membrane of a sperm cell. The sperm nucleus and tail enter the egg cell (impregnation). This activates the egg cell and completes the second meiotic division. The female and

2

male pronuclei are formed. When the pronuclei dissolve, the cell immediately divides into a two-cell stage. Implantation in the uterus usually occurs six days after ovulation. This is followed by the development of the early placenta, formation of the chorionic cavity (gestational sac) with the yolk sac, and the establishment of the basic body plan of the embryo. The sex chromosomes X and Y determine the development of a female or male phenotype.

Reference

Nieschlag E, Behre H, Kliesch S, Nieschlag S (eds) (2023) Andrology. Male Reproductive Health and Dysfunction, 4rd edn. Springer, Heidelberg, p. 18.

Epidemiology of Unfulfilled Desire for Children

Contents

3

Background

Most couples wish to have their own children at some point in their lives. They want to experience the development of a child together from the very beginning of pregnancy and become a mother and father. In the general population, becoming pregnant is perceived as the most natural thing in the world. Before the desire to have children is realized, reliable contraception is usually practiced for years. The possibility of one's own body failing to achieve pregnancy is not anticipated. All the more affected are many couples when pregnancy does not occur as expected.

The **natural conception rate** per cycle across all age groups averages 27 to 30%. When couples wish to have children, pregnancy usually occurs within the first three cycles. In natural family planning (NFP), pregnancy was reported in 80% of cases after six cycles (Gnoth et al. 2005). Of the remaining 20%, half can expect to become pregnant in the following six months (■ Table 3.1). Even after 12 unsuccessful cycles, 50% will become pregnant within the next 36 months. After a total of 48 cycles without pregnancy, spontaneous conceptions are only observed sporadically. This also applies to couples undergoing fertility treatment. In this group, spontaneous conception still occurs in about 5% of cases. Prospective studies of pregnancy and birth rates, such as the relationship and family panel "parfam," which annually surveys childless women about their current desire for children, show a pronounced age dependency (Trappe and Köppen 2021). While 40% of women aged 30 to 34 had become pregnant or had a child within five years of the survey, only 18% of women in the older age group of 35 to 47 years had a successful pregnancy. Among younger women aged 16 to 29, only 18% became pregnant after five years as well. However, other factors play a role here, such as relationship conflicts and partner changes.

In summary, the most important **prognostic factor** for pregnancy success is the **age** of the **woman**. Knowledge about the age-dependent decline in fertility is lacking in the general population. In fact, 40% and 14% of respondents believe that becoming pregnant only becomes more difficult at age 40 or 45, respectively (Allensbacher Berichte 2007). The reason for declining fertility is the limited supply of oocytes, which is determined two to three months before birth and is not replenished by division of oogonia. The depletion of oocytes begins even before birth. In addition, oocytes age until ovulation, as they are as old as the woman herself, since their maturation began during the fetal period. Meiosis is arrested at the beginning in prophase. The oocytes then enter a resting phase known as dictyotene. The maturation of oocytes is usually not completed until several decades later, when ovulation occurs during the reproductive phase.

■ **Table 3.1**   Natural conception rate (according to Gnoth et al. (2005))

Time (months)	Frequency	Chance of subsequent spontaneous conception
6 cycles without pregnancy	20%	50% in the following 6 cycles
12 cycles without pregnancy	10%	50% in the following 36 cycles
48 cycles without pregnancy	5%	Sporadic in subsequent cycles

Definition of Unfulfilled Desire for Children

According to the definition of the **World Health Organization (WHO)**, those who do not achieve pregnancy **after 12 months** of regular unprotected intercourse are diagnosed as infertile.

The frequency, causes, and consequences of an unfulfilled desire for children depend on various factors such as age, education, migration, conflicts, wars, and economic resources. If infertility is diagnosed, further evaluation should be performed and the possibility of fertility treatment considered. Basic diagnostics include cycle assessment and a semen analysis; in the presence of risk factors, early evaluation of tubal patency is also indicated (see ▶ Chaps. 4 and 5). In women aged 35 and older, age becomes increasingly important, as the "biological clock" starts ticking. Fertility treatment should then be initiated promptly, as the success rate decreases with increasing age.

Since **infertility** is not a matter of lifestyle but is a **recognized medical condition**, private health insurers are required, depending on the policy, to cover the necessary treatment. Statutory health insurance (GKV) usually covers 50% of the treatment and medication costs for assisted reproduction, provided the legal requirements are met. In addition, statutory health insurers may provide further subsidies as so-called statutory benefits (see ▶ Chap. 10).

Same-sex couples are, by nature, unable to have biological children together and therefore do not fall under the WHO definition of infertility or sterility. However, lesbian couples have the legal option to fulfill their desire for children with donor sperm. In contrast, gay male couples can only have children through a combination of egg donation and surrogacy. This is prohibited in Germany.

Couples with unsuccessful pregnancies (**miscarriages** and **stillbirths**) are not included in the WHO definition. This includes pregnancy losses without signs of life with a birth weight under 500 g and/or births before the 24th week of pregnancy. About 20% of pregnancies end in early miscarriage, which is often unnoticed and perceived as a delayed menstrual period. Miscarriages between the 13th and 24th week of pregnancy are rare. These are referred to as **late miscarriages**. According to the Federal Statistical Office, the hospital statistics for 2023 show an increase in the miscarriage rate. However, it must be emphasized that reliable or official data on the frequency of miscarriages are lacking, and care for patients with uncomplicated miscarriages is very often provided on an outpatient rather than inpatient basis.

Miscarriages: Pregnancy losses without signs of life with a birth weight under 500 g and/or pregnancy losses before the 24th week of pregnancy. **Late miscarriages**: Miscarriages between the 13th and 24th week of pregnancy.

Prevalence

The WHO estimates the **infertility rate** over a woman's lifetime in Europe at 16.5% for the period 1990 to 2021, while the global infertility rate was estimated to be slightly higher at 17.5%. This means that worldwide, **one in six women is infertile** (World Health Organization 2023).

In Germany, one in five women is now childless. However, this high childlessness rate of 20% varies considerably when analyzed by new and old federal states, migration status, and educational level. For example, the **childlessness rate** is only 11% among women with a low level of education, but 21% and 23% among those with medium and high educational levels, respectively (Kuhnt and Trappe 2024). There are also significant differences in childlessness rates between the old and new federal states, such as Thuringia and Hamburg (13% and 29%), and additionally between rural and urban regions. However, the childlessness rate includes not only women who are involuntarily childless, but also **presumably** fertile women who are **voluntarily childless** or **do not have a partner**.

The proportion of childless women increased until 2012 and has remained at a high level since then. Childlessness has now become a life plan that is more accepted by society. In this context, the term "childfree" appears to be ideologically charged, and babies are even regarded as an environmental sin of the parents (Brunschweiger 2019).

In summary, the frequency of involuntary childlessness cannot be measured directly and precisely, as reliable statistics are lacking and analyses can only be conducted indirectly. Reliable data on the frequency of involuntary childlessness among men are not available. In principle, a couple's **fertility** is also **mutually linked** to the **fertility** of both **woman** and **man**. Thus, a couple may still conceive spontaneously if there is reduced oocyte quality but good semen quality, or vice versa, good oocyte quality and reduced semen quality.

Causes

In most cases, the causes of infertility are initially unknown. According to the results of fertility diagnostics, **female** and **male factors** are diagnosed, each accounting for 25 to 30% of cases. In the remaining cases, there is combined female and male infertility, or the causes remain unclear. In the latter case, this is referred to as unexplained or idiopathic infertility. In women, the most common causes are functional disorders of the ovaries, but also organic changes in the uterus and fallopian tubes, such as after tubal infections or in endometriosis. **Oocytes** cannot **naturally** be **directly examined**, so maturation disorders are only detected **in the context of artificial fertilization**. **Sperm cells**, on the other hand, can be **directly examined** during semen analysis. In men, impaired semen quality is the most common cause of infertility. In most cases, the cause is unknown (**idiopathic**). In men of reproductive age, testicular tumors are also a recurring cause of impaired semen quality. Therefore, in cases of unfulfilled desire for children, every man should undergo a physical examination by a urologist or andrologist.

The **age** of the **woman** plays a central role in unfulfilled desire for children. It is a natural factor that, in modern society, has taken on a new dimension due to social change, as birth statistics show that women are increasingly older at the birth of their first child. Men are, on average, three years older than women when starting a family (Kuhnt and Trappe 2024), although this observation does not have a direct biological consequence for male fertility (◘ Fig. 3.1). Until 2003, most women gave birth to their first child between the ages of 25 and 29, but since 2004, most women have their first child at age 30 to 34. These figures show that, in recent decades, women have increasingly postponed their desire for children. This trend began before reunification, in the early 1970s in West Germany and from the mid-1980s in East Germany (Bujard and Diabat'e 2016). In 1989, East German women were just under 23 years old at the birth of their first child, about four years younger than West German women. However, the **age at first birth** has not yet fully converged since reunification. In 2018, the age at first birth was 30 years in the old

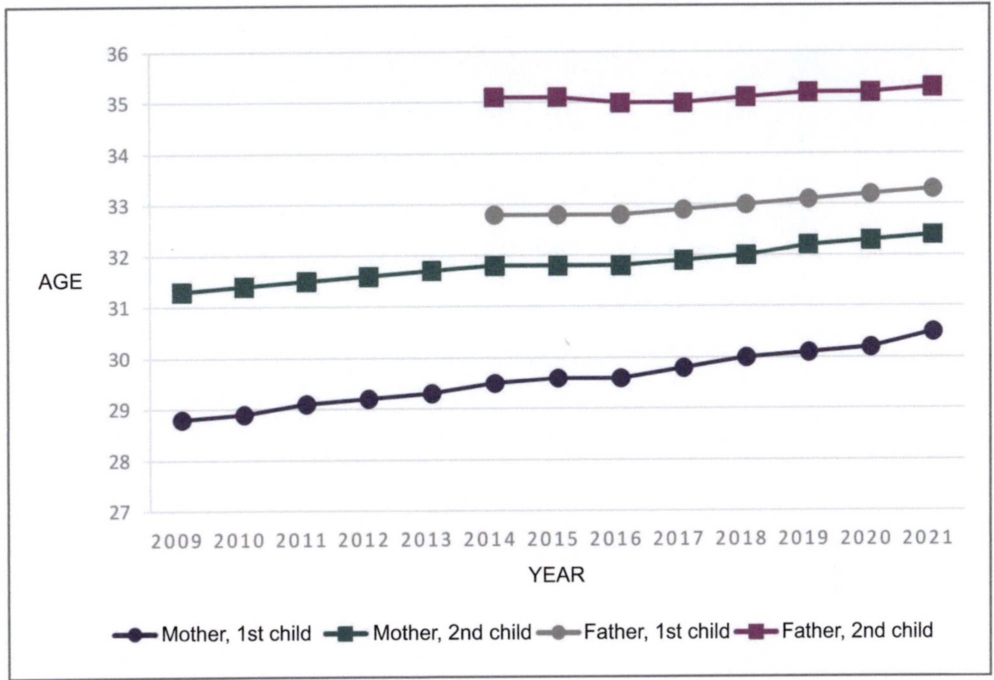

☐ Fig. 3.1 Average age of parents at the birth of the mother's first and second child. (With kind permission from: Kuhnt and Trappe (2024))

federal states and 29.2 years in the new federal states (bpb 2020). The shift in the age at first birth to older ages has occurred at the expense of women aged 20 to 24 and 25 to 29 (☐ Fig. 3.2). Noteworthy is the increase in first births among women aged 35 to 39 to 16%, and especially the rise in first births among women aged 40 and older to 3%. In the early 1990s, late first births at age 40 and above were still an exception.

Reasons for postponing the desire for children, in addition to economic, partnership-related, and cultural factors, are primarily professional qualification and career. In addition, social acceptance of childlessness and societal expectations of parenthood have increased. The timing of fulfilling the desire for children is coordinated with professional and other life plans. With appropriate financial resources, women today also have the option of freezing oocytes for postponed childbearing (**social freezing**). Apple and Facebook have offered their female employees support of up to $20,000 for this since 2014. Sperm cells have been successfully frozen for fertility preservation for decades.

These developments have led to a shift in the concentration of births to women aged 30 to 34 as the age at first birth increases, and, naturally, the intervals between subsequent births have shortened for those wishing to have more children. In family research, the term **"rush hour of life"** has been coined for this compression of the reproductive phases.

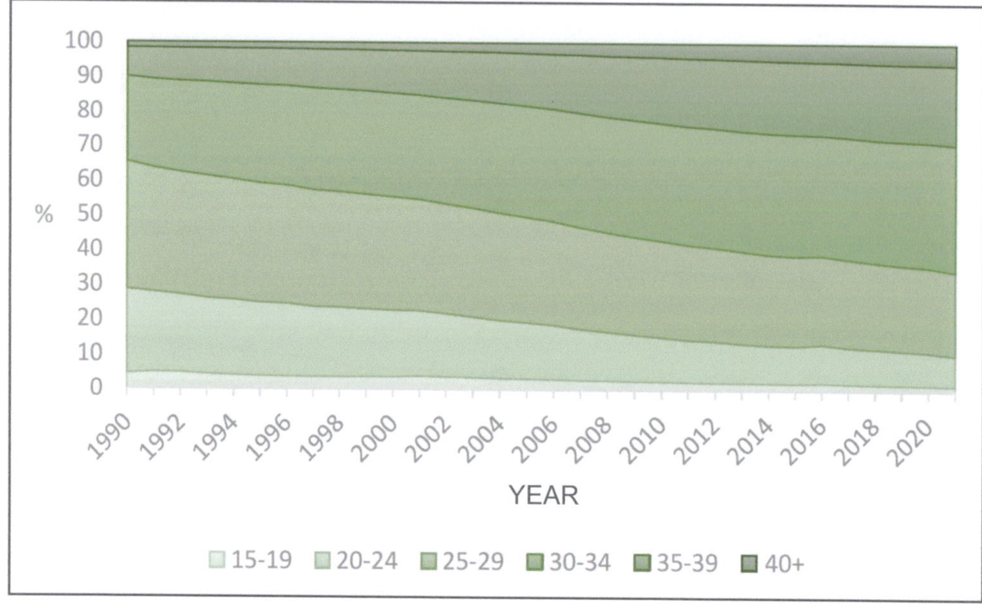

Fig. 3.2   Birth rates by age group, 1990–2021. (With kind permission from Kuhnt and Trappe (2024))

Treatment Prognosis

Fertility treatment increases the chances of pregnancy. Today, most infertile couples can be successfully treated in fertility centers with the **options** of **artificial fertilization** (assisted reproduction). However, there is no guarantee of success. The treatment method is selected individually after medical consultation, based on the results of preliminary diagnostics and the chances of success. However, it is always the woman or the couple who decides whether to proceed with the recommended fertility treatment. Not all couples take advantage of these options. Often, limited financial resources are a factor, as are difficulties in reconciling multiple appointments during the treatment cycle with everyday life, as well as personal reasons. These also include relationship conflicts or ethical concerns.

Many affected women have not yet considered the possibility of fertility treatment. Others use alternative methods such as cycle and nutrition apps or traditional Chinese medicine (TCM) techniques to increase their chances of conception. They want to give nature another chance. Only at the end of their thirties, when the "**clock is ticking**," do they increasingly turn to IVF treatment as the **ultima ratio**. According to the Federal Ministry for Family Affairs, Senior Citizens, Women and Youth (BMFSFJ) (2021), 17% and 18% of women aged 20 to 29 and 30 to 39, respectively, used medical fertility treatment, while this proportion jumped to 31% among women aged 40 to 50.

The simplest method of assisted reproduction is intrauterine insemination (**IUI**). Fertilization takes place in the fallopian tube ("in vivo fertilization"). At the time of ovulation, sperm and oocytes are brought closer together in the woman's body. This technique is mainly used in cases of moderately reduced semen quality (see ▶ Chap. 6). However, **pregnancy rates** are **disappointingly low** at a maximum of 11.1% for women under 30 (Hammel et al. 2024). IUI alone or in combination with clomiphene stimulation is no more effective than no therapy (Bhattacharya et al. 2008). Only the combination of IUI with hormonal stimulation using FSH or hMG injections leads to acceptable pregnancy rates (Gregoriou et al. 2008).

Since couples have already been waiting many months for a child and want to achieve pregnancy as soon as possible with fertility treatment, **in vitro fertilization (IVF)** has become established as the **most common treatment method**. Fertilization outside the woman's body, also known as "extracorporeal fertilization," is much more successful compared to IUI. **Pregnancy rates** for women under 30 are **cumulative** at **75%** after 3 embryo transfers (D·I·R 2024). IVF treatment led to the first pregnancy and birth in England in 1978. Robert Edwards was the scientist who, together with gynecologist Patrick Steptoe, achieved the groundbreaking success that led to the birth of Louise Brown. Edwards was awarded the Nobel Prize in Medicine in 2010 for his life's work.

In 2023, approximately 130,000 IVF cycles were documented in Germany among almost 70,000 women (D·I·R 2024). Each fertility patient underwent nearly two treatment cycles. This includes all initiated IVF cycles (oocyte retrieval and cryocycles, including discontinued cycles). The **German IVF Registry (D·I·R)** has documented treatment cycles since 1982, when the first German IVF baby was born in Erlangen (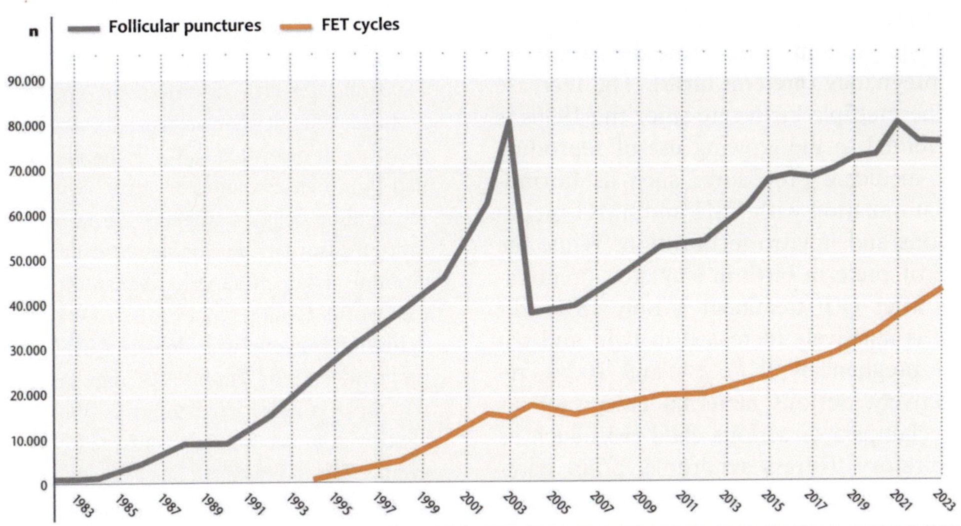 Fig. 3.3). The initiative came from the five exclusively **university IVF centers** that existed at the time. The number of participating centers has now grown to 141. There are still 22 university centers, most of which perform only a few treatment cycles. Many of the predominantly **private centers** have been restructured into medical care centers (MVZ) and sold to **investors** over the past 10 to 20 years.

In the past 20 years, **cryopreservation** has become increasingly important. This is mainly due to improvements in freezing techniques. With the introduction of vitri-

Fig. 3.3 German IVF Registry D·I·R: Number of follicle punctures, frozen embryo transfer (FET) cycles 1982–2023. (With kind permission from D·I·R (2024) Annual Report 2023)

fication ("glassification") into routine IVF laboratory practice, thawing rates have improved significantly and pregnancy rates have increased. Currently, one third of transfer cycles are performed with frozen cells (D·I·R 2024). **Pregnancy** and **birth rates** are comparable at about 31% and 22%, respectively, both for transfer after oocyte retrieval and after thawing. As expected, **younger women up to age 34** have a **higher success rate**. The D·I·R Annual Report 2023 reports pregnancy and birth rates of 39.3% and 31.2% for women aged 30 to 34, while success rates for women aged 41 to 44 are low at 17.4% and 8.4%. More than half of pregnancies in this age group end in **miscarriage**. The frequency of miscarriages in women aged 38 and older is already higher than the frequency of births. Ectopic pregnancies account for about 2% and play a minor role, provided there is no tubal damage.

The most important **complications** of IVF treatment include **multiple pregnancies**. The probability of multiples in spontaneous conception is only 1.2%. The risk for twins is 1:85, for triplets 1:7200. Risks of multiples include especially premature labor and preterm birth before the 38th week of pregnancy (**preterm birth**). The increase in the multiple birth rate since the 1990s is attributed to the growing use of reproductive medicine procedures such as hormonal stimulation with FSH and hMG preparations and in vitro fertilization. While the rate of preterm birth in singleton pregnancies after IVF treatment is only 18%, this rate is massively increased in twin and triplet pregnancies at 86.2% and 100%, respectively. Serious **maternal risks** such as preeclampsia or serious **child risks** such as respiratory distress syndrome, brain damage, and necrotizing enterocolitis (NEC) are the result.

To avoid multiples, it is recommended from the outset of fertility treatment with IVF to **transfer** only **one embryo**. The multiple birth rate is closely related to the number of embryos transferred. According to D·I·R analyses, an average of 2.56 embryos were transferred in 1997 (D·I·R 2024). This led to an unacceptable multiple birth rate of 25.2%. As the transfer of only one or two embryos ("single" or "double" embryo transfer, abbreviated SET or DET) has become more common and, in 2022, an average of only 1.46 embryos were transferred, the multiple birth rate dropped to 12%. Fortunately, this means it has more than halved. The transfer of only one or at most two embryos, with even improved pregnancy outcomes, is also related to the implementation of blastocyst culture, which can be performed in compliance with the German Embryo Protection Act (ESchG). Only developmentally competent fertilized oocytes are selected for embryo transfer after extended culture.

Learning Objectives

- Knowledge of natural fertility
- Frequency and causes of unfulfilled desire for children
- Treatment prognosis for unfulfilled desire for children

Detecting fertility disorders in women is more difficult than in men, as oocyte maturation disorders can only be identified by direct examination after surgical retrieval of oocytes, whereas sperm maturation disorders can be detected by examining a semen sample. According to the World Health Organization (WHO) definition, anyone who does not achieve pregnancy after 12 months of regular intercourse is considered infertile. Worldwide, one in six women is affected. The average age at first birth has risen significantly over the past 30 years. Today, first-time mothers are already 30 years old, whereas in 1989, women in the new federal states were only 23 years old at first birth. Reasons for this shift include professional qualification and career for both women and men. In addition, social acceptance of childlessness has increased. The most important prognostic factor for pregnancy is the woman's age. Even though the biological clock is already "ticking" after age 40, many still wait, hoping to give nature another chance. Ultimately, IVF treatment is used as the ultima ratio. Thus, the proportion of women aged 40 to 50 seeking medical treatment has risen sharply.

References

Allensbacher Berichte (2007) Unfreiwillige Kinderlosigkeit. Allensbacher Archiv 11. Institut für Demoskopie Allensbach, 78472 Allensbach am Bodensee. ► https://www.ifd-allensbach.de/fileadmin/kurzberichte_dokumentationen/prd_0711.pdf. Zuletzt 19.1.2025

Bhattacharya S, Harrild K, Mollison J et al (2008) Clomifene citrate or unstimulated intrauterine insemination compared with expectant management for unexplained infertility: pragmatic randomised controlled trial. BMJ 337:a716. ► https://doi.org/10.1136/bmj.a716. Zuletzt 22.1.2025

Brunschweiger V (2019) Kinderfrei statt kinderlos – ein Manifest. Büchner-Verlag, Marburg.

Bundesministerium für Familie, Senioren, Frauen und Jugend BMFSFJ (2021) Ungewollte Kinderlosigkeit 2020. ► https://www.bmfsfj.de/resource/blob/161018/b36a36635c77e98bcf7b4089cd1e562e/ungewollte-kinderlosigkeit-2020-data.pdf. Zuletzt 22.1.2025

bpb Bundeszentrale für politische Bildung (2020) Alter der Mütter bei der Geburt ihrer Kinder. ► https://www.bpb.de/kurz-knapp/zahlen-undfakten/soziale-situation-in-deutschland/61556/alter-der-muetter-bei-der-geburt-ihrer-kinder. Zuletzt 23.1.2025

Bujard M, Diabat'e S (2016) Wie stark nehmen Kinderlosigkeit und späte Geburten zu? Neue demografische Trends und ihre Ursachen. Der Gynäkologe 5:393–404.

D·I·R (2024) Jahrbuch 2023. J Reproduktionsmed Endokrinol 21 (Sonderheft 4), 1–64.

Gnoth C, Godehard E, Frank-Hermann P et al (2005) Definition and prevalence of subfertility and infertility. Hum Reprod 20:1144–1147. ► https://doi.org/10.1093/humrep/deh870

Gnoth C (2019) Definition und Prävalenz von Subfertilität – ein Update und mehr. J Reproduktionsmed Endokrinol 16:221–226.

Gregoriou MD, Nikos F, Vlahos MD et al (2008) Randomized controlled trial comparing superovulation with letrozole versus recombinant follicle-stimulating hormone combined with intrauterine insemination for couples with unexplained infertility who had failed clomiphene citrate stimulation and intrauterine insemination. Fertil Steril 90:678–683. ► https://doi.org/10.1016/j.fertnstert.2007.06.099. Zuletzt 22.1.2025

Hammel H, Bleichrodt C, Thorn P et al (2024) DERI Deutsches Register für Insemination. In: D·I·R (ed) Jahrbuch 2023. Reproduktionsmed Endokrinol 21:49–51.

Kuhnt AK, Trappe H (2024) Demografische Perspektive auf den Kinderwunsch und die Inanspruchnahme reproduktionsmedizinischer Assistenz in Deutschland – Herausforderungen für die Zukunft. J Reproduktionsmed Endokrinol 21:6–14.

Trappe H, Köppen K (2021) Sozialdemografische Ursachen und Folgen des Aufschubs des Erstgebäralters von Frauen. In: Kupka M (ed) Reproduktionsmedizin. Zahlen und Fakten für die Beratung. Elsevier GmbH, München, 95–102.

Statistische Bundesamt (2023) Krankenhausstatistik: Diagnosedaten der Patienten und Patientinnen in Krankenhäusern. ► https://www.bundestag.de/resource/blob/966288/a08e859af024345cc8b-87420d61acfcf/WD-9-054-23-pdf-data.pdf. Zuletzt 19.1.2025

World Health Organization (2023) Infertility prevalence estimates, 1990–2021. Geneva. Licence: CC BY-NC-SA 3.0 IGO. ► https://www.who.int/publications/i/item/978920068315. Zuletzt 19.1.2024

Basics and Diagnostics of Female Reproduction

Contents

© The Author(s), under exclusive license to Springer-Verlag GmbH, DE, part of Springer Nature 2026
M. Bals-Pratsch et al., *Workplace: Fertility Clinic*, https://doi.org/10.1007/978-3-662-73035-5_4

Anatomy of Female Reproduction

The reproductive organs are the uterus, the fallopian tubes (also called salpinges), and the ovaries (Fig. 2.1, longitudinal-section).

Uterus

The uterus is divided into the cervix (**cervix**) and the uterine body (**corpus**). The lower part of the cervix protrudes as a "cone" into the posterior portion of the upper third of the vagina. For cervical screening, cells are collected from both the external and internal cervix. The uterus is a muscular hollow organ. The uterine musculature is called the myometrium (Fig. 4.1, cross-section). The cavity of the uterus is the **cavum**, which is lined with the endometrium. The endometrium has two layers. The lower layer (**basalis**) borders the myometrium and is constant, while the upper layer (**functionalis**) builds up and breaks down according to the phase of the cycle. This layer becomes thicker during the cycle. If pregnancy does not occur, it is shed at the end of the cycle during menstruation. With the start of a new cycle, the endometrium is rebuilt.

The lining (**endometrium**) must be receptive for the implantation of an embryo at the blastocyst stage. Only then can an embryo, after hatching from the zona pellucida, attach to and invade the endometrium. If the endometrium is not receptive, implantation in the uterus will not be successful, and pregnancy will not occur even with a developmentally competent embryo. Barriers to implantation can also have organic causes. These include **malformations**, but especially benign **tumors** of the uterus such as myomas of the musculature or polyps of the endometrium.

Ovaries

The paired ovaries are important both for the maturation of oocytes and for hormone production. Female hormones (**estrogens**) are produced in the **granulosa cells**. These surround the oocytes. As the oocyte matures, the granulosa cells are also referred to as cumulus cells (Fig. 2.3). At this stage, the connective tissue around the oocyte differentiates into two layers of **theca cells**: the inner theca interna faces the oocyte, and the outer theca externa faces the interior of the ovary. The theca cells produce

- Vagina
- Uterus
    - Cervix
    - uterine body (corpus)
      with mucous membrane (endometrium)
      and muscle layer (myometrium)
- Fallopian tubes
- Ovaries

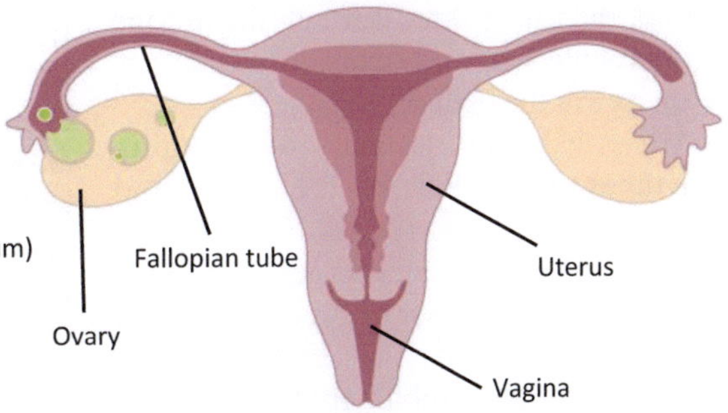

Abb. 4.1 Schematic overview of female genital organs (cross-section)

male hormones (**androgens**). Granulosa and theca cells nourish the maturing oocyte. The oocyte and granulosa cells together form a functional unit: the **follicle**. About three months before ovulation, the theca cells are also considered part of the follicle. After ovulation, the **corpus luteum** forms in the former follicular cavity. This develops from both granulosa cells and theca interna cells, which migrate into the cavity and differentiate into **granulosa lutein** and **theca lutein cells**. The corpus luteum gets its yellow color from fat deposits. The granulosa and theca lutein cells primarily produce **progesterone**, which transforms the endometrium and makes it receptive. The ability of the endometrium to support implantation (**receptivity**) is a prerequisite for implantation and a successful pregnancy.

Fallopian Tubes (Tuba uterina or Salpinx)

The fallopian tubes, like the ovaries, are paired organs. They are muscular tubes 10 to 15 cm long and consist of four sections. The end of the tube closest to the ovary is called the infundibulum (**infundibulum**). It is equipped with 20 to 30 fimbriae, each 1 to 2 mm long. The infundibulum is followed by the approximately 7 cm long **ampulla**, which then narrows to a 2 to 3 cm long constriction called the **isthmus**. After that, the tube passes through the uterine wall (**pars uterina**) and opens into the uterine cavity via the ostium.

After ovulation, the tasks of the fallopian tubes are to pick up the oocyte and **transport** it to the uterus (◘ Fig. 4.2). After ovulation, the tube picks up the oocyte from the ovary through sweeping movements. For transport, the tubes are lined with surface cells (tubal epithelium) that bear **cilia**. Oocyte transport is further supported by **muscle cells** in the wall of the

tubes. Fertilization (**fertilization**) takes place in the ampulla. The fertilized oocyte undergoes cell divisions (**cleavages**) and, from day four after fertilization, additional **differentiation** of the cells. At this point, the cells are at the morula stage. By day five, the cells have reached the **blastocyst stage**. After five days of transport, the blastocyst reaches the uterine cavity and begins to hatch from the zona pellucida. Implantation usually occurs on day six after ovulation.

The Cycle as an Interaction of the Reproductive Organs

Puberty

With puberty, oocyte maturation begins in the follicles, marking the start of the **reproductive phase**. In the ovary, the first group of primordial follicles completes the dictyate stage and begins developing into primary and secondary follicles (◘ Figs. 2.3 and 2.4). The complete process of oocyte maturation takes about one year (see ▶ Chap. 2). This is completed with the maturation to the preovulatory follicle and the completion of the first meiotic division at the time of ovulation. At the onset of puberty, around age 10, breast development (thelarche) occurs, followed by the development of pubic hair (pubarche). If there are no signs of puberty by age 13, delayed pubertal development is present. The first menstrual period usually occurs at age 13 and is called the **menarche**. The cycle is often still irregular in the following months. If no menstruation has occurred by age 16, a gynecological-endocrinological evaluation is advisable. If there are no signs of puberty or if pubertal development is not complete after five years or has stalled for 18 months, this is termed **delayed puberty (*pubertas tarda*)**. *Primary amenorrhea* is present if menarche does not occur despite normal pubertal development and normal linear growth.

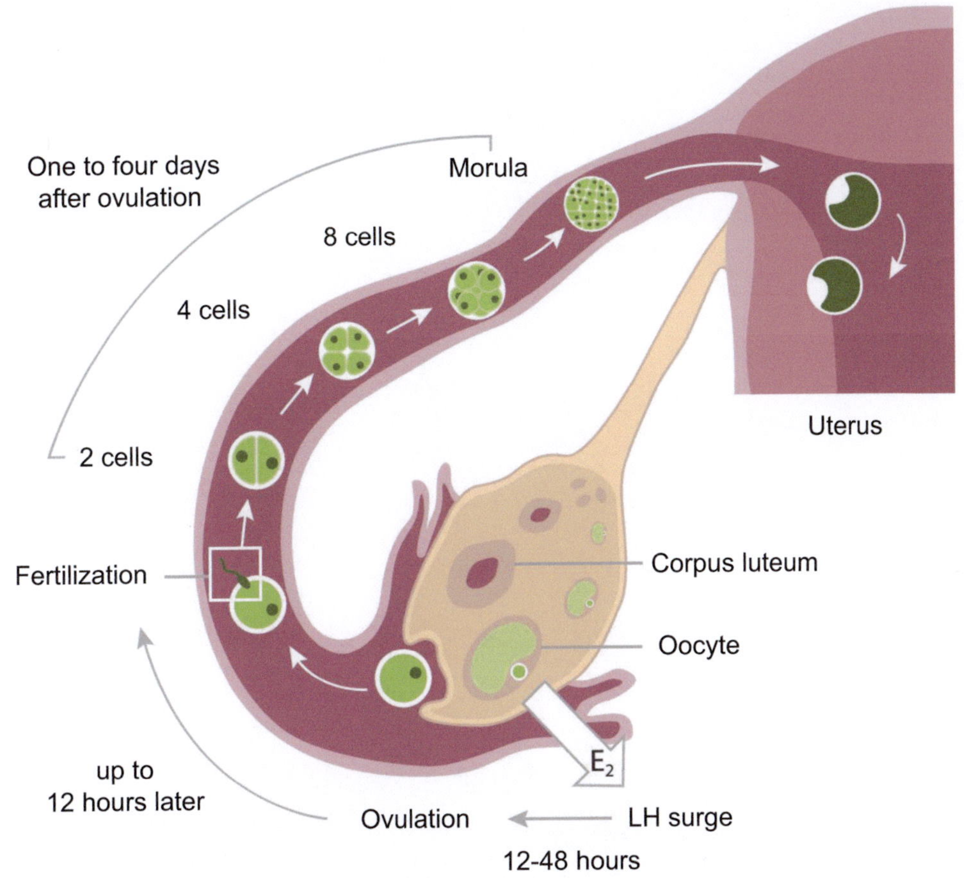

Abb. 4.2 Ovulation, fertilization, oocyte transport, and implantation. E2 (estradiol) = estrogen, h (hour) = hours

Cycle Function

Cycle function during the reproductive phase is a hormonal interplay between the **ovaries** and **uterus** with the goal of achieving pregnancy. Estradiol and progesterone are the female **sex hormones** produced in the follicle and, after ovulation, in the corpus luteum. Hormone production in the maturing follicle and after ovulation in the corpus luteum is regulated by the follicle-stimulating hormone **FSH** and the luteinizing hormone **LH**. The **regulatory hormones** are produced in the pituitary gland (**hypophysis**). Estradiol and progesterone are important for the develop-ment and **receptivity** of the endometrium (**Fig. 4.3**). A cycle lasts about **28 days** and consists of three phases: the **follicular phase**, the **ovulatory phase**, and the corpus luteum phase (**luteal phase**). The main hormone in the follicular phase is **estradiol**, and in the luteal phase, it is **progesterone**. The "switch" in hormone production is triggered by LH, which induces ovulation. In the follicular phase, a group of follicles grows, one of which becomes the leading, dominant follicle. In the ovulatory phase, the dominant **follicle** reaches its maximum size. Ovulation occurs around **day 14 of the cycle**. This is initiated about two days earlier by the regulatory hor-

4

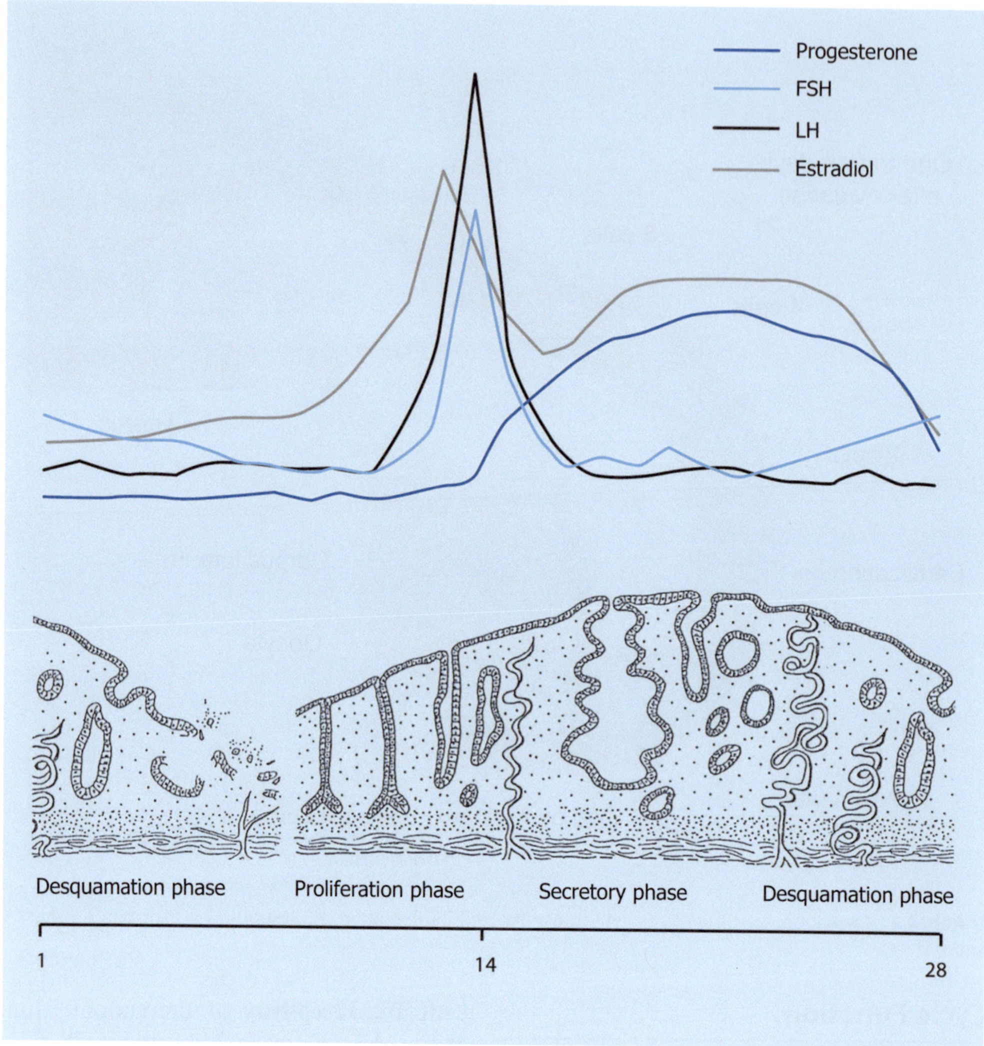

▫ Abb. 4.3   Hormone levels and cycle phase-dependent build-up and breakdown of the endometrium during the cycle (days 1 to 28). (Reproduced with permission from: Sonntag, B (2016))

mone LH. The ovulatory phase transitions into the luteal phase about two days after ovulation, during which the endometrium (**endometrium**) reaches its maximum thickness. The corpus luteum hormone progesterone rises until about seven days after ovulation. It not only promotes further development of the endometrium but also calms the uterine musculature. In this way, progesterone supports the establishment of pregnancy. If pregnancy occurs, the endometrial thickness continues to increase. If pregnancy does not occur, the luteal phase ends about 14 days after ovulation. With the onset of menstruation, a new cycle begins.

Cycle Phases and Hormone Profiles

The **cycle phases** are characterized by the typical **hormone profiles** for estradiol and progesterone (◼ Fig. 4.3). These are coupled with follicular maturation and functional changes in the endometrium. At the beginning of the **follicular phase**, a rise in **FSH** leads to the growth of a cohort of small antral **follicles** and an increase in **estradiol**. The FSH rise begins at the end of the preceding cycle. Follicular growth leads to increasing estrogen levels. In the **ovulatory phase** (around day 14), the maturation of the dominant follicle and the steep rise in estrogen levels trigger the preovulatory LH surge, known as the "**LH** peak." This is accompanied by a concurrent FSH rise. The LH peak induces ovulation and a sharp drop in estrogen levels. This is followed by the **luteal phase** with the development of the corpus luteum. This forms as granulosa and theca cells migrate into the follicular cavity, differentiate, and mainly produce **progesterone** in increasing concentrations. The remaining follicles also continue to produce estradiol in addition to the corpus luteum, so estradiol levels also rise again under the influence of LH and FSH. If a blastocyst implants, the **syncytiotrophoblast** soon secretes the pregnancy hormone **hCG** and stimulates the production of progesterone and estradiol. If pregnancy does not occur, the corpus luteum "regresses" and estrogen and progesterone levels drop sharply. The hormone cycle then starts anew.

Cycle-Dependent Changes in the Endometrium

Because the build-up and breakdown of the endometrium are coupled with the cyclic hormone profile, if pregnancy does not occur, the endometrium is first shed, followed by menstruation (◼ Fig. 4.3). The breakdown of the functional zone of the endometrium is also called the **desquamation phase**. Rising estrogens produced in the growing follicles lead to hemostasis and cessation of menstruation. The **proliferative phase** begins with the rebuilding of the endometrium, and the endometrial thickness increases. After ovulation, the **secretory phase** begins. Under the influence of rising progesterone levels and the renewed increase in estrogen after ovulation, the endometrium continues to grow. It must be receptive six days after ovulation for an embryo to implant. If implantation does not occur, a new desquamation phase begins.

Reproductive Phase

The reproductive phase is linked to the **oocyte reserve** in the ovary. The supply of oocytes is limited and can be measured by determining the **anti-Müllerian hormone (AMH)**. However, the prognostic value should not be overestimated. AMH regulates the growth of primordial follicles (◼ Fig. 2.4). Recruitment of primordial follicles is likely accelerated at low AMH levels, so depletion of the oocyte pool progresses more rapidly (Rebhan and Bachmann 2021). The term "**burn-out**" of the ovarian reserve has become established for this. Unlike FSH measurement, the AMH value can generally be determined independently of the cycle. However, AMH levels can fluctuate by about 20% within a cycle. Both an increased BMI and the use of ovulation inhibitors negatively affect the AMH value. Two months after discontinuing contraceptives, the AMH value returns to normal.

Menopause

Cycle function usually ceases at around age 51. **Menopause** is defined as the last spontaneous menstrual period in the reproductive

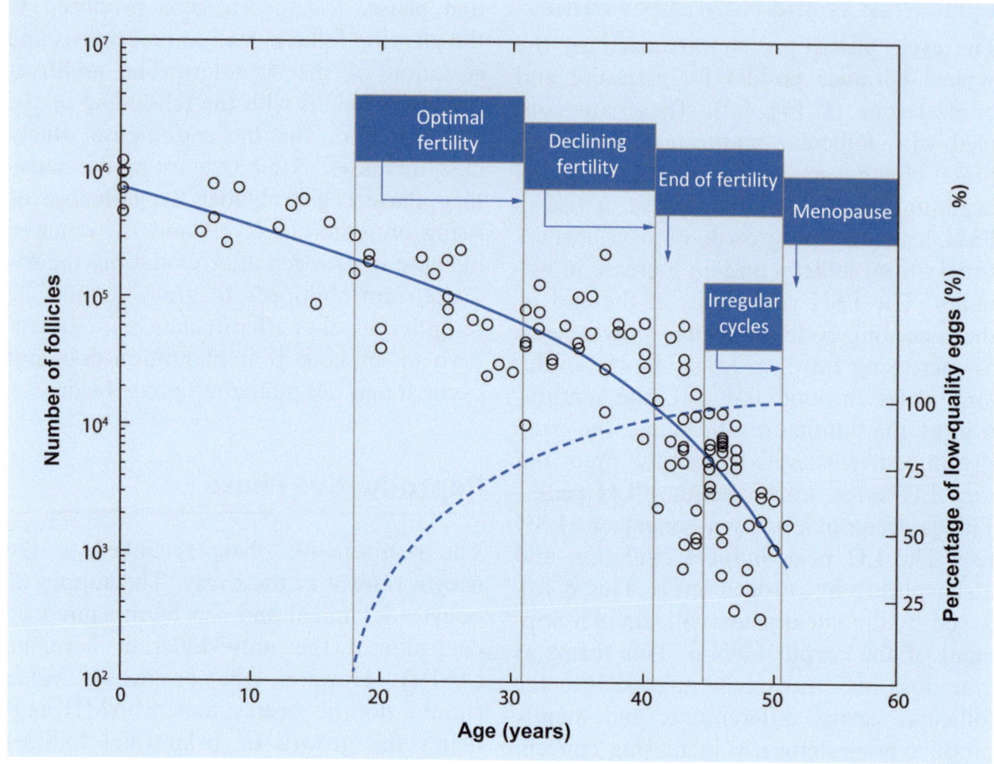

◘ Abb. 4.4 Follicle reserve and oocyte quality up to menopause. (Reproduced with permission from: Sonntag, B., Segerer, S. Keck (2019))

phase, provided no further spontaneous bleeding occurs in the following 12 months. The reason for the cessation of ovarian function is the **loss** of **primordial follicles**, which begins even before birth (◘ Fig. 4.4). At menopause, about 10,000 oocytes remain in the ovaries, but they can no longer mature. These are as old as the woman's chronological age. As age increases, the oocytes become less developmentally competent. At the end of the reproductive phase, oocytes no longer mature due to limited quality. The natural loss of oocytes is independent of the number of ovulations in a woman's lifetime. Without the use of ovulation inhibitors, there are only about 400 ovulations during the reproductive phase.

Central Regulation of Cycle Function

Cycle function is regulated by the **brain structures** of the pituitary gland (hypophysis) and the diencephalon (◘ Fig. 4.5). The **hypothalamus** is the region of the diencephalon that secretes gonadotropin-releasing hormone (**GnRH**). This travels via the pituitary stalk to the **pituitary gland**, which is located at the base of the skull. There, the hormones **LH** and **FSH** are released, which regulate the **ovary**. These stimulate granulosa and theca cells in the follicles during the follicular phase to produce estradiol and androgens. In addition to this basic regulatory principle of the **hypothalamic-pi-**

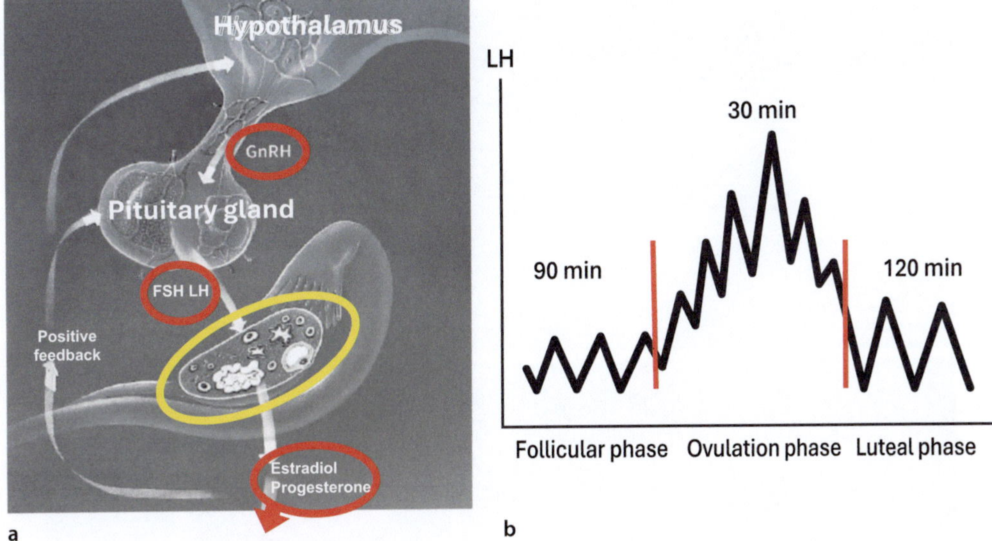

Abb. 4.5 Hypothalamic-pituitary-ovarian axis. **a**: Feedback control hypothalamus-pituitary-ovary with the regulatory hormones GnRH, LH, and FSH, as well as the hormones estradiol and progesterone produced by the ovary **b**: LH pulse pattern

tuitary-ovarian axis, there is also "fine-tuning." A rapid rise in estrogen at mid-cycle sensitizes the pituitary, resulting in a massive release of LH. This naturally triggers ovulation. After ovulation, granulosa and theca lutein cells in the corpus luteum, which forms in the follicular cavity after ovulation, mainly produce **progesterone** .

The hypothalamic-pituitary-ovarian axis functions as a **regulatory circuit**. Both the hypothalamus and the pituitary secrete GnRH and the regulatory hormones LH and FSH depending on estrogen levels. Progesterone is also involved in **central regulation**. When estrogen and estrogen/progesterone levels are low, more GnRH is released from the hypothalamus and more LH and FSH from the pituitary. Conversely, when estrogen or estrogen/progesterone levels are high, only small amounts of GnRH, LH, and FSH are secreted. This regulatory mechanism is called positive or negative "**feedback**." It is important to note that GnRH is always secreted in pulses,

which in turn leads to pulsatile LH release (**Fig. 4.5). If GnRH were secreted continuously, the pituitary would no longer release LH and FSH in response to the GnRH signal, and follicular development in the ovary would not occur. The **GnRH pulse pattern** varies in different phases of the cycle. In the follicular phase, there is an LH pulse every 90 minutes, while in the luteal phase, the pulse interval is extended to 120 minutes. In the ovulatory phase, both the pulse interval and amplitude increase. Understanding the **hypothalamic "pulse generator"** is important in fertility treatment for women with dysfunction of the hypothalamic-pituitary-ovarian axis.

Diagnostics of Cycle Function

In **cycle monitoring**, follicular growth is assessed by ultrasound (**Fig. 4.6) and by measuring hormone levels of estradiol, progesterone, LH, and FSH. More precisely, by measuring the diameter of the follicu-

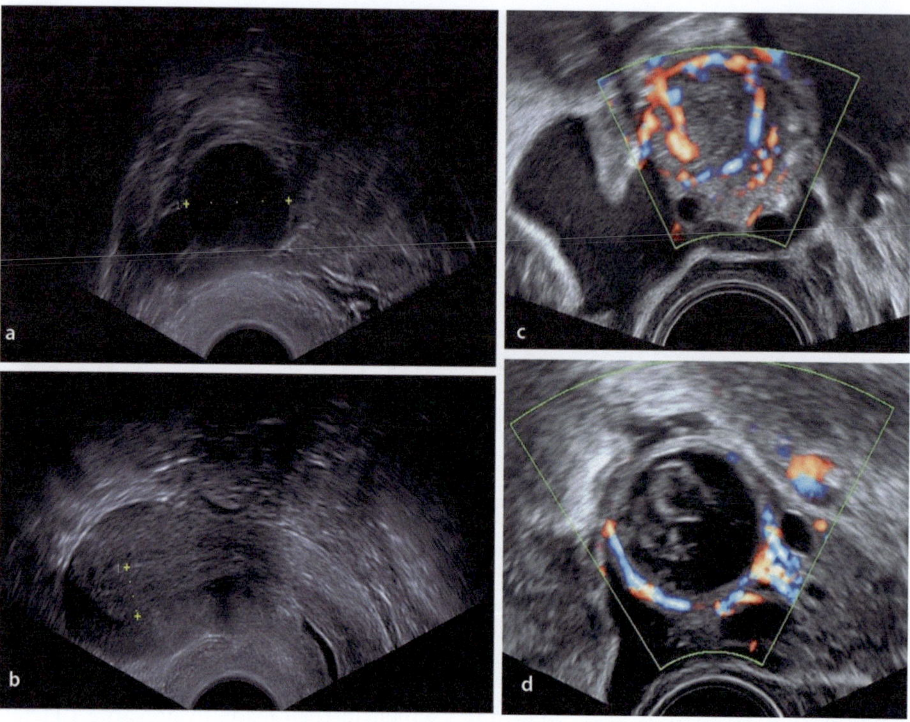

Abb. 4.6   Sonographic cycle monitoring. **a**: Follicle 23.5 mm; **b**: Endometrial thickness 9.7 mm; **c**: Corpus luteum, shown with color Doppler as "ring of fire," fluid in the abdominal cavity between rectum and uterus; **d**: hemorrhagic corpus luteum, recognizable by echogenic irregular diffuse structures inside

lar cavity and the hormone production, the **functional unit** of the **oocyte** with the **surrounding granulosa cells** is tested. Estradiol is produced by granulosa cells in the follicles. Rising estrogen levels reflect the growth of follicular diameter. Ultrasound is also used to measure the **thickness** of the **endometrium**, which becomes thicker or thinner in response to rising or falling estrogen levels. Towards mid-cycle, the **dominant follicle** is selected, which then grows 1–2 mm per day and leads to a **steep rise in estrogen** (■ Fig. 4.3). Usually, when the follicle reaches about 20 mm, there is an **LH surge** and **ovulation** is triggered. Shortly after ovulation, fluid can often be seen by ultrasound between the bowel and uterus (Douglas pouch) in addition to the ovary. Two days after the LH surge, the dominant follicle is no longer visible and estrogen levels have dropped. At the same time, **progesterone** production begins. The endometrium continues to grow due to the rapidly rising progesterone. The **corpus luteum** forms from granulosa and theca cells in the follicular cavity. This can also be visualized by ultrasound using color Doppler due to its increasing and massive blood supply (vascularization) (■ Fig. 4.6). The corpus luteum is the **most highly vascularized endocrine gland** in the female body. On ultrasound, it shows the characteristic appearance of a ring of fire ("**ring of fire**"). This allows the corpus luteum to be distinguished particularly well from the rest of the ovary. In about half of cases, the ruptured follicle bleeds into itself in the hours after ovulation. This results in a **corpus luteum cyst** with echogenic or diffuse structures inside. The color Doppler method is also helpful in cases of cycle disorders or suspected premature ovulation to quickly **determine the cycle phase**. Ultimately, the determination or confirmation of the cycle phase is made by measuring the hormones **estradiol** and **progesterone**.

Self-Monitoring

Many women wishing to conceive now use **cycle apps** and **cycle trackers** such as ovulation rings or cycle bracelets to better understand their bodies and become pregnant as quickly as possible. These applications can be used not only to document menstrual periods, but also to record body temperature upon waking (**basal temperature**) or continuous measurement, and to observe **cervical mucus**. This is produced in greater amounts before ovulation. The **LH surge** is detected with urine test strips. Cervical mucus is highly stretchable before the LH peak and exhibits the "fern phenomenon." The app then calculates the fertile days from the temperature, cervical mucus, and LH test results. This cycle **self-monitoring** can be further optimized by additionally testing for **estradiol in urine**.

Terminology of Bleeding Disorders (Tempo and Type Anomalies)

A regular cycle means that menstruation occurs every 21 to 35 days ("**eumenorrhea**"). Normally, menstruation lasts a maximum of 7 days and blood loss ranges between 25 and 150 ml. Preceding and subsequent spotting is not counted as part of menstruation. Many women with infertility experience cycle disorders. Shortened or prolonged bleeding intervals (**tempo anomalies**) are referred to as **polymenorrhea** or **oligomenorrhea**. The term **amenorrhea** means that menarche is delayed or menstruation

has been absent for at least 3 months. If menarche does not occur, this is called **primary amenorrhea**. If menstruation ceases for more than three months after menarche, this disorder is referred to as **secondary amenorrhea**. **Type anomalies** refer to bleeding with increased or decreased blood loss (**hyper-** or **hypomenorrhea**) as well as heavy bleeding with prolonged duration or intermenstrual bleeding. These are referred to as **menorrhagia** or **metrorrhagia**. **Menometrorrhagia** refers to the combination of irregular, heavy, and prolonged bleeding with additional intermenstrual bleeding.

Female Causes of Infertility

Infertility can have organic and functional causes involving the uterus, ovaries, and fallopian tubes. These may be congenital or acquired over the course of life. This includes malformations, but especially surgical interventions on the ovaries or uterus. In addition, inflammation of the fallopian tubes or chemo- and radiotherapy for previous tumor diseases can damage the reproductive organs. Affected patients often also report symptoms such as cycle disorders or lower abdominal pain.

Functional Disorders of the Ovaries

In cases of infertility, it is primarily **functional disorders** of the ovaries that lead to cycle disturbances. In adolescents, these can already result in the absence of menarche. A very common functional cause during the reproductive phase is the so-called **polycystic ovary syndrome (PCOS)**. About 15% of women in the reproductive phase have PCOS, but not all affected women are infertile. In infertility cohorts, the percentage is significantly higher if the diagnosis is consistently checked in every infertility patient.

4

> The **diagnosis** of PCOS is made based on the three Rotterdam criteria from 2004 (Fig. 4.7). At least two of the **three criteria** must be met. The cycle, ovarian sonography (alternatively AMH level), and signs of androgenization are assessed.

The first criterion states that the **cycle is longer than 35 days or ovulation does not occur**. According to the **ultrasound criterion**, at least 12 antral follicles smaller than 10 mm must be counted in at least one ovary. The follicles are often arranged like a string of pearls under the ovarian capsule. The term "string of pearls sign" is used for this. The third criterion checks whether **androgens** (free testosterone, DHEAS) are **elevated** in the follicular phase and/or whether there is **androgenization**. The clinical **symptoms** of increased action of male hormones are acne, hirsutism (increased growth of coarse hair especially on the upper lip, chin, chest, navel, inner thighs), and androgenetic alopecia (a frontal hairline remains).

Not all PCOS patients meet the ultrasound criterion, which requires documentation of at least 12 antral follicles < 10 mm in at least one ovary. If follicular or corpus luteum cysts are present in the ovary, the diagnostic ultrasound for PCOS should be repeated after the cysts have resolved. Women with androgenization and/or hyperandrogenemia and anovulation or a cycle length > 35 days also have PCOS according to the Rotterdam criteria, even if the ultrasound criterion is not met. According to a study of PCOS patients, only 21.6% of women met all three Rotterdam criteria (Merk 2019, Table 4.1). Instead of the ultrasound criterion, determination of the **AMH level** can also be used for the diagnosis of PCOS (Teede et al. 2023). However, a

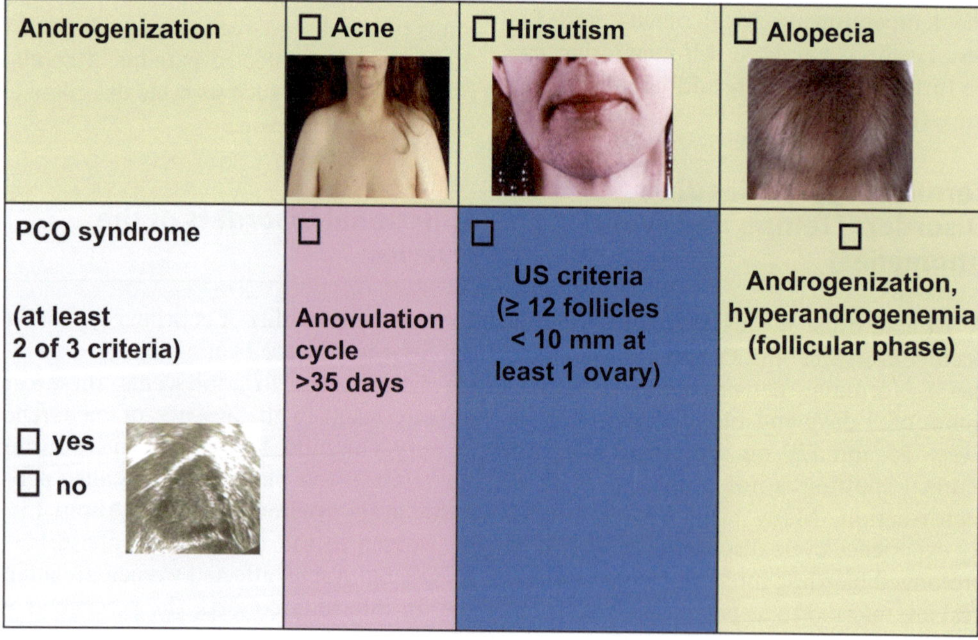

Fig. 4.7 Diagnostic criteria for PCOS (Rotterdam criteria)

Table 4.1 PCOS criteria in the study cohort (n = 153), presented in a cross-table for the three criteria and showing the percentage of patients who meet one or more criteria

PCOS criterion met	Cycle > 35 days, anovulation	Androgenization, hyperandrogenemia	Polycystic ovaries
Cycle > 35 days, anovulation	38.6%	27.5%	32.7%
Androgenization, hyperandrogenemia	–	88.9%	83.0%
Polycystic ovaries	–	–	94.1
All 3 criteria met	21.6%		

uniform cut-off value is not known. More often, the diagnosis of PCOS can already be made based on the medical history. This is the case, for example, when a young patient develops amenorrhea after stopping the pill and complains of acne and hirsutism.

The exact **causes** of PCOS are **not fully understood**. A familial clustering is observed. PCOS is usually associated with glucose metabolism disorders and insulin resistance (Merk 2019). It is the most common **metabolic disorder** in the reproductive phase. Elevated levels of dehydroepiandrosterone sulfate (DHEAS), which is produced in the adrenal gland, may also be measured. In assisted reproduction, it is notable that **oocytes** in women with PCOS often have **poorer quality** and are less capable of development. The theca cells in the many antral follicles produce increased amounts of androgens, which are only converted into estrogens by granulosa cells during follicle growth. In the case of an irregular cycle with infrequent or absent ovulation, this conversion to estrogens does not occur. The high androgen concentrations also have a negative effect on the hormonal regulation of ovulation. There is an imbalance of LH and FSH with elevated LH levels, which also disrupts oocyte maturation and ovulation. The antral follicles cannot mature and regress. This disturbance of follicle maturation is called **follicular atresia**.

Hypothalamic-Pituitary Functional Disorder

A functional cycle disorder can also be hypothalamic-pituitary in origin. Disorders at this higher level of the diencephalon and pituitary gland are rare but should not be overlooked. If there is a **failure of the hypothalamic-pituitary-ovarian axis**, menstruation ceases (secondary amenorrhea). Due to the lack of natural LH and FSH stimulation of the ovaries, they enter a state of functional rest. This clinical picture, characterized by a deficiency of LH and FSH, is referred to as **hypogonadotropic hypogonadism**. This central disorder can also occur before or during puberty. In this case, menarche does not occur (primary amenorrhea). This central disorder may be at the level of the **hypothalamus**. The GnRH pulse generator in the diencephalon (hypothalamus) fails, and the pituitary gland is no longer stimulated. As a result, the regulatory hormones LH and FSH are no longer secreted. The disorder can also be at the level of the **pituitary gland**, so that the release of LH and FSH into the bloodstream does not occur.

Hyperprolactinemia and Prolactinoma

Excessively high prolactin levels (**hyperprolactinemia**) also disrupt the hypothalamic-pituitary-ovarian axis. Women with hyperprolactinemia often complain of **galactorrhea** (milk discharge). Therefore, prolactin measurement is part of the basic diagnostic workup for infertility. Hyperprolactinemia is often functional and not due to a prolactin-producing tumor (prolactinoma). Prolactin secretion from the pituitary gland is under the control of the hypothalamus. The most important hypothalamic messenger for prolactin control is **dopamine.** It inhibits prolactin secretion. A hypothalamic messenger that increases prolactin secretion is **thyrotropin-releasing hormone (TRH)**. Therefore, when measuring prolactin, **thyroid-stimulating hormone (TSH)** must always be determined, as hyperprolactinemia can be mimicked by pronounced **hypothyroidism**. In this case, interdisciplinary treatment by internal medicine endocrinologists or radiologists is necessary. Elevated prolactin levels disrupt the GnRH pulse generator, so that at high levels, oocyte maturation disorders may occur. Very high prolactin levels lead to secondary **amenorrhea**.

Interfering Factors in Prolactin Measurement

Prolactin measurement can be influenced by **interfering factors**. For example, a **breast examination** stimulates prolactin secretion. Therefore, blood sampling for prolactin should always be performed before a breast examination. Prolactin secretion shows a circadian rhythm with higher nighttime values, triggered by melatonin. Therefore, when **drawing blood** for prolactin measurement, a sufficient time interval from morning **awakening** should be observed (at least two hours). When prolactin levels are elevated, the use of **medications** that can increase prolactin to tumor levels must always be ruled out. These include especially neuroleptics and antidepressants. Estrogens also increase prolactin levels. For this reason, **cycle-dependent** prolactin levels rise at mid-cycle and return to baseline at the beginning of the cycle. Prolactin levels should therefore be measured at the start of the cycle.

Micro- and Macroprolactinomas

Markedly elevated prolactin levels > 50–60 ng/ml (> 1200 mIU/l) may indicate a prolactinoma. These pituitary tumors are generally benign. Fortunately, diagnosis is now usually made at an early stage, as early diagnostics are now possible with prolactin measurement and targeted CT or MRI **examination** of the **skull**. Effective **pharmacological therapy** with dopamine agonists is also available, often treating hyperprolactinemia before a tumor is detected. Prolactinomas are only rarely operated on. **Pituitary surgery** is performed by specialized neurosurgeons through the nose. According to tumor size, a distinction is made between **micro-** (< 1 cm) and **macroprolactinomas** (≥ 1 cm). If a tumor is detected, further interdisciplinary evaluation is indicated (internal medicine endocrinologists, radiologists, ophthalmologists, possibly neurosurgery) to confirm the diagnosis and initiate the necessary conservative therapy with dopamine agonists (bromocriptine or cabergoline) or surgical treatment.

Thyroid Diseases and Cycle Function

Thyroid diseases are also a risk factor for infertility. However, the significance of especially latent ("hidden") functional disorders is often overestimated (Bals-Pratsch et al. 1997). The natural **cycle-dependent fluctuations** of TSH are often not considered. Like prolactin, TSH levels also rise at mid-cycle and return to baseline at the start of the cycle. Like prolactin levels, TSH levels fluctuate throughout the day, with higher values at night and lower values in the early evening. For fertility consultations, **hyperthyroidism**, **hypothyroidism**, and autoimmune diseases such as autoimmune thyroiditis (AIT) are relevant. **Hashimoto's thyroiditis** is a common chronic autoimmune disease of the thyroid. It is mainly diagnosed in women, especially in cases of infertility. Over time, the inflammatory processes in the thyroid tissue subside. The inflammation "burns out." The result is often hypothyroidism, which should be treated interdisciplinarily with thyroid specialists (internal medicine endocrinologists, radiologists). In principle, thyroid diagnostics should include, in addition to blood values such as TSH (thyroid-stimulating hormone), determination of **thyroid peroxidase antibodies (TPO-Ab)** and, if hyperthyroidism of the Graves' type is suspected, determination of **TSH receptor antibodies (TRAb)**. **Thyroid sonography** with determination of thyroid volume is always part of the assessment of thyroid function. Thyroid enlargement (**goiter**) is present if thyroid volume in women exceeds 18 ml. This is often already visible as a widened neck silhouette and can lead to swallowing difficulties. Thyroid cysts and nodules should not be overlooked. Such **focal findings** can also develop carcinomas. The indication for further investigations such as thyroid scintigraphy or biopsy is made by the treating **thyroid specialists**. Drug therapy with thyroid hormone for hypothyroidism or with antithyroid drugs for hyperthyroidism is always carried out according to the guidelines of the professional societies.

Organic Causes of Infertility

The cause of infertility can be organic, such as congenital or acquired changes of the vagina, uterus, tubes, and ovaries. **Organic causes** may be due to malformations (e.g., Mayer-Rokitansky-Küster-Hauser syndrome) or genetic factors (e.g., Ullrich-Turner syndrome).

Ovarian Changes

Due to the increasing postponement of childbearing beyond the fourth decade of life, more and more women at the end of their reproductive phase are seeking fertility treatment. These women may still have a regular cycle. In the phase before menopause (premenopause), the **follicle reserve** in the ovary is largely **depleted** and the onset of **menopause** is foreseeable. Due to the lack of follicle reserve in the ovary, there is an estrogen deficiency. Women in this phase of life typically complain of hot flashes and sleep disturbances. There are cultural differences in the perception of such menopausal symptoms. If the oocyte reserve is prematurely depleted, as in genetically determined Ullrich-Turner syndrome (UTS), this is referred to as **premature ovarian insufficiency** (POI). The term "premature ovarian failure" (POF) is also used. This diagnosis applies to women who have **not yet reached the age of 40**. POF occurs with a frequency of one to two percent. Further interdisciplinary diagnostics involving human genetics are always indicated if there is no ovarian damage due to surgery or gonadotoxic treatments such as chemo- or radiotherapy. The **differentiation** between **menopause** ("change of life") and **premature ovarian insufficiency** is important not only clinically but also psychologically for affected women. In premature ovarian insufficiency, as long as occasional menstruation occurs as an expression of **residual function** of the ovaries, about five percent of women may still become pregnant. These women should be informed about donation options and psychosocial counseling services.

Changes in the Fallopian Tubes

Another common cause of infertility is damage to the **fallopian tubes** due to previous bacterial infections. The inflammatory process often also involves the ovaries. This combined infection is referred to as **adnexitis**. Most often, these are infections with chlamydia, which are sexually transmitted. Women under 25 years of age are often affected. For this reason, statutory health insurance offers annual **chlamydia screening** for women up to 25 years of age. A significant risk factor is also changing sexual partners. Consequences of salpingitis or adnexitis are severe scarring and **adhesions** with neighboring organs as well as chronic **lower abdominal pain**. There is a high risk of impaired egg transport with subsequent infertility. In addition to loss of function, the fallopian tubes may also become occluded. A **sactosalpinx** (scarred fallopian tube wall) and a **hydrosalpinx** (distended, fluid-filled, scarred fallopian tube) may result. On ultrasound, a hydrosalpinx is often mistaken for ovarian cysts. Pregnancies outside the uterine cavity—referred to as **extrauterine pregnancies** or ectopic pregnancies (EP)—occur more frequently. Most often, an EP implants in the fallopian tube. An initially unrecognized tubal pregnancy repeatedly leads to serious **emergencies** when rupture with bleeding into the abdominal cavity occurs.

Adhesions of the fallopian tubes with neighboring organs can also occur after inflammatory processes in the abdomen, such as appendicitis or inflammatory bowel diseases like **Crohn's disease** or **ulcerative colitis**. Similarly, surgical interventions in the lower abdomen often lead to adhesions. Ovarian drilling in PCOS can also result in adhesions and thus fallopian tube problems.

Changes in the Uterus (Myomas and Polyps)

Acquired changes in the uterus can also individually be a reason for infertility. These include benign muscle nodules in the uterine wall, known as **myomas**, which occur in 50% of women, usually between the ages of 45 and 50. However, younger women, espe-

cially Black women, are also affected. The muscle nodules are usually smaller than 3 to 5 cm. Heavy menstrual bleeding can lead to anemia. With larger myomas, patients often complain of a feeling of pressure on the bladder and bowel. Myomas can be located beneath the endometrium (**submucosal**), within the uterine muscle (**intramural**), and beneath the peritoneal covering (perimetrium) of the uterus (**subserosal**). Even if several myomas are diagnosed, this finding does not necessarily cause infertility. Submucosal myomas are suspected to be an infertility factor in cases of implantation failure. The main indication for surgical therapy is the **symptom profile** of the patient, rather than infertility itself.

Benign endometrial growths, known as **polyps**, can also occur in the uterine cavity. Polyps can cause bleeding disorders and may interfere with implantation. In some cases, surgical removal should be considered, which can be performed during a hysteroscopy (**hysteroscopy**). In this procedure, the hysteroscope is advanced into the uterine cavity for further evaluation, including polyps (◘ Fig. 4.9). The procedure is usually performed under short anesthesia. It is important to remember that all surgical procedures on and in the uterus can cause permanent damage and result in a serious **Asherman syndrome**. This refers to adhesions (synechiae) in the uterine cavity caused by injury to the basal layer of the endometrium, which can lead to secondary amenorrhea and thus permanent sterility.

Endometriosis as a Factor in Infertility

Endometriosis is one of the most common gynecological diseases. It is estimated that **one in four women with endometriosis** is affected by **infertility**. There are explanatory models for the development of endometriosis, but the cause is not sufficiently understood. Endometriosis is often diagnosed only after several years. The leading symptoms are cycle-dependent **chronic lower abdominal pain** and pronounced **dysmenorrhea**, which often leads to inability to work. However, the symptom profile can vary greatly between individuals. Absence of pain is not an exclusion criterion for endometriosis. The disease progresses insidiously and often begins as early as age 20. Endometriosis is **tissue** similar to the endometrium and is associated with chronic inflammation. The tissue settles **outside the uterine cavity**. Endometriosis tissue can be found on the fallopian tubes and ovaries, in the abdominal and pelvic cavity, in the vagina, on the bowel, and on the peritoneum. It can also occur outside the abdominal cavity, e.g., in the lungs. Endometriosis foci can also grow in the **uterine wall**. This is referred to as **adenomyosis** (adenomyosis uteri). The suspicion of adenomyosis can be confirmed with high probability based on the often typical clinical symptoms and ultrasound assessment of the uterus. On the one hand, laparoscopy is performed to confirm the diagnosis and, on the other hand, to achieve the best possible treatment of endometriosis. There are endometriosis centers specializing in the treatment of endometriosis (▶ https://endometriose-sef.de). Whether surgical removal of endometriosis lesions improves the chances of pregnancy in women wishing to conceive is controversial today and must be decided individually depending on the extent of endometriosis. Even after endometriosis treatment, affected women often require intensified fertility treatment (e.g., IVF).

Endometriosis lesions in the ovary can be visualized sonographically as cysts of varying size with homogeneous internal echoes. **Endometriosis cysts** grow expansively and damage the ovarian tissue, thereby reducing the naturally limited reserve of follicles in the ovary. Endometriosis involvement of the fallopian tubes can lead to nodular scarring in the narrow (isthmic) portion of

the tube. Such changes are referred to as **salpingitis isthmica nodosa** (SIN).

Examination Methods and Application Examples

In fertility consultations, hormone measurements in blood and vaginal sonography are the most important examination methods. The hormones relevant for fertility diagnostics and therapy are produced in the pituitary and the ovaries (see above). These endocrine organs are also referred to as **glands**. The **hormones** communicate as **messenger substances** via the **bloodstream** with other hormone glands.

Hormone Measurements

When drawing blood for hormone determination, strict attention must be paid to patient identification to reliably avoid sample mix-ups. ▫ Table 4.2 provides an overview of the hormones relevant to reproduction and assigns diagnoses according to increased or decreased levels. This table refers to untreated women under 40 years of age. If a **pregnancy** occurs, the **syncytiotrophoblast** as an early precursor of the placenta produces the pregnancy hormone **hCG** shortly after successful implantation. Hormone measurements in blood are now performed automatically and with quality control. In clinical routine, hormone values are usually reported in conventional units, but regionally also in SI units (International System of Units). Therefore, it is absolutely necessary, especially with laboratory values brought in by patients, to check the specified **unit of measurement** for the **hormone values**. Hormones such as LH, estradiol, and hCG can also be tested in urine. These semi-quantitative tests generally do not play a role in fertility consultations. However, many women use these tests as a supplement to self-monitoring of their cycle.

▣ Table 4.2 Fertility-relevant hormones, endocrine organs, and suspected diagnoses according to hormone values in untreated, non-pregnant women under 40 years of age

Hormone	Endocrine Organ	Value increased	Value decreased
LH	Pituitary gland	LH pulse, ovulation, premature ovarian insufficiency (POI)	Central hormone deficiency
FSH	Pituitary gland	Ovulation, premature ovarian insufficiency (POI)	Central hormone deficiency
TSH	Pituitary gland	Hypothyroidism	Hyperthyroidism
Prolactin	Pituitary gland	Hyperprolactinemia	Central hormone deficiency
Estradiol	Ovary (follicle)	Ovulation	Hormone deficiency
Progesterone	Ovary (corpus luteum)	Luteal phase	Anovulation
Testosterone	Ovary	Hyperandrogenemia, e.g., PCOS	Hormone deficiency
DHEAS	Adrenal gland	Hyperandrogenemia	Adrenal insufficiency
AMH	Ovary (follicle)	PCOS	Premature ovarian insufficiency (POI)

Case Study

A 34-year-old patient has endometriosis, which was completely surgically treated. She presents together with her husband for an initial consultation, as she has had an unfulfilled desire for children for four years and her gynecologist therefore recommended fertility treatment with in vitro fertilization. She is healthy and has a regular cycle. As part of the stage II infertility workup (see below), the gynecologist had already measured the baseline hormone values throughout the cycle. ▣ Table 4.3 shows the hormone values in the follicular, ovulatory, and luteal phases. At first glance, the hormones are unremarkable, with lower values at the beginning of the cycle, a rise in estradiol during the ovulatory phase, and an initial increase in LH. In the luteal phase, the progesterone value has increased. However, the values for estradiol and progesterone are so high that it appears as if ovarian stimulation treatment had been performed. Upon inquiry, the patient reports that she has not received any stimulation medication so far. Upon closer examination of the laboratory report she brought with her, it is noticed that the measured values for estradiol and progesterone are given in SI units pmol/l and nmol/l. To convert SI units to conventional units pg/ml and ng/ml, the values are divided by the conversion factors for estradiol and progesterone (3.671 and 3.18, respectively). After conversion, the estradiol and progesterone values are consistent with a natural cycle.

◼ Table 4.3 Cycle phase hormone values in the natural cycle (measured values in conventional units, conversion factors for SI units)

Hormone (conventional unit)	Follicular phase	Ovulatory phase	Luteal phase	SI unit (conversion factor)
LH (IU/l)	6.2	22.4	5.2	–
Estradiol (pg/ml)	18	151	102	pmol/l (3.671)
Progesterone (ng/ml)	0.15	0.92	16.45	nmol/l (3.18)

Vaginal Sonography

Strict adherence to **hygiene regulations** is essential during vaginal sonography. The vaginal probe must be prepared for the examination by covering it with an ultrasound condom. Afterwards, cleaning and reprocessing with suitable disinfectants are necessary. The examination chair must also be prepared and cleaned before and after the procedure according to the practice hygiene plan.

Uterus

During vaginal sonography, the uterus, ovaries, and fallopian tubes are examined for abnormalities. For the uterus, both the size and the uterine wall and endometrium are assessed. The endometrium must be developed according to the phase of the cycle. If the endometrial lining is very thin, for example, there may be suspicion of adhesions in the uterine cavity (Asherman syndrome). A polyp appears as an echogenic (bright), well-defined **focal lesion** in the uterine cavity (◼ Fig. 4.8). Myomas are also well-defined but have an irregular, hypoechoic (dark) and hyperechoic internal structure. It is also important in vaginal sonography to detect uterine **malformations** (see ▶ Chap. 6). To avoid missing these, the uterus must be consistently scanned longitudinally from ovary to ovary, with the cavity visualized. If the cavity can be visualized twice, which

appears as the "cat's eye phenomenon" in the transverse view, there is either a double uterus (**uterus duplex**), a **uterus bicornis**, or a septum (partition) in the sense of a **uterus subseptus** or **uterus septus**. The cervix may be normal or duplicated in these cases, as uterus unicollis or uterus bicollis. Uterine malformations also frequently occur together with a vaginal septum. There is a wide variety of other unilateral or bilateral uterine malformations, which may also be associated with malformations of the tubes, ovaries, vagina, kidneys, and ureters. In **Mayer-Rokitansky-Küster-Hauser syndrome**, the uterus and vagina are completely absent. The ovaries, however, are normally developed, so puberty proceeds according to age.

Ovaries

Ultrasound diagnostics of the ovaries are essential not only for cycle monitoring but also for detecting abnormalities in the ovary and assessing the ovarian follicle reserve. The latter is determined by counting the antral follicles (< 10 mm) in both ovaries, preferably at the beginning of the cycle (around day 3), and then adding them together. An **antral follicle count** (AFC) of 10 to 15 in women aged 35 to 40 is considered normal. This value is a predictor of **pregnancy success** in assisted reproduction. Younger women have higher, older women lower AFC values. Although higher pregnancy rates are reported with higher AFC,

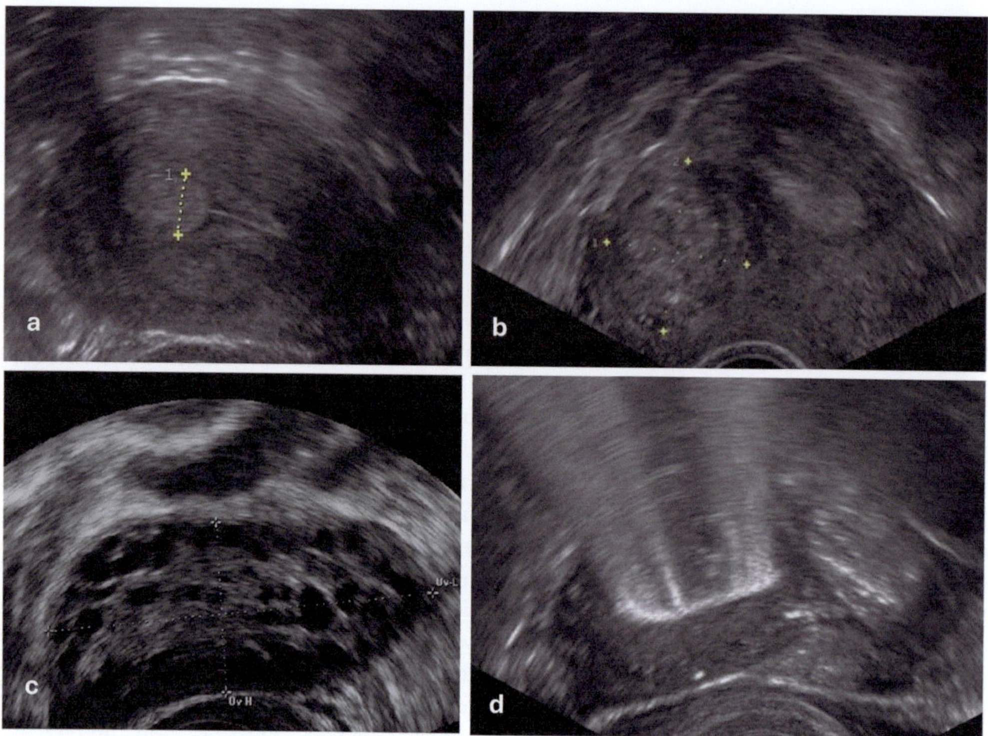

Abb. 4.8   Pathological findings on vaginal sonography and hysterosalpingo-contrast sonography. **a**: approx. 1 cm endometrial polyp, **b**: approx. 3 cm intramural myoma; **c**: polycystic ovary 5.5 × 2.2 cm; **d**: hysterosalpingo-contrast sonography. Contrast visualization of uterus and tubes

oocyte quality is not necessarily impaired with a lower AFC (Vrontikis et al. 2010). This means that women with a low AFC and good oocyte quality can have a comparable pregnancy prognosis to women with a normal AFC.

For the diagnosis of **PCOS**, the ultrasound criterion must be checked during vaginal sonography, and the number of antral follicles must be determined separately for each ovary (**Figs. 4.7 and 4.8**). Ovarian cysts in women with preserved cycle function are predominantly functional, resulting from the growth of follicles and the subsequent formation of corpora lutea. These **functional cysts** include preovulatory follicles, sometimes very large or hemorrhagic corpora lutea, or large follicular cysts if ovulation has not occurred. This may happen, for example, at the end of the reproductive phase when oocyte quality is no longer sufficient for maturation into a functional preovulatory follicle. Functional cysts usually regress after menstruation. Therefore, cysts with unclear findings should be monitored sonographically after menstruation. In rare cases, ovarian carcinomas can develop in cystically altered ovarian tissue even in young women. Other notable focal lesions include **endometriosis** and **dermoid cysts.** The latter may contain various tissues such as skin, hair, teeth, or fat. Such lesions should be treated surgically on an individual basis or at least closely monitored, as malignancy cannot be ruled out by ultrasound.

Fallopian Tube

The fallopian tubes are usually not visible on vaginal sonography. In pathologies such as **hydrosalpinx**, the tubes can be recognized as cystic lesions. A hydrosalpinx is a fluid-filled fallopian tube with a characteristic **post-horn-like** shape. Typically, a hydrosalpinx is particularly large in the luteal phase. At the time of menstruation, it may no longer be well visualized and can be missed. The large, irregular, usually elongated hydrosalpinges are often misinterpreted as ovarian cysts. The diagnosis of a hydrosalpinx confirms a tubal factor, and artificial fertilization is indicated.

The **patency** of the fallopian tubes is usually tested during a **laparoscopy** with dye test (chromopertubation) under general anesthesia. This examination must be performed under sterile conditions in an operating room. During this procedure, gas (usually carbon dioxide) is first introduced into the abdominal cavity via the so-called Veress needle (● Fig. 4.9). The needle is then replaced by a trocar (tube), through which the optics, the so-called **laparoscope**, is advanced. This allows examination of the uterus, fallopian tubes, and ovaries. During **chromopertubation**, a blue dye is injected through the uterine cavity into the fallopian tubes, which, if patent, can be seen exiting from the fimbrial ends. An operating room is usually not available in a fertility center, as for fertility treatment with artificial fertilization and other minor procedures via the vagina, a procedure room is sufficient. If the patient's history is unremarkable, tubal patency can alternatively be tested in the procedure room of the fertility center using **hysterosalpingo-contrast sonography** ("hystero-salpingo contrast sonography," HyCoSy) and without anesthesia (● Fig. 4.8). For this, a catheter is inserted into the uterus. The ultrasound contrast agent is injected into the uterus via the catheter, and with patent tubes, it flows into the abdominal cavity. The contrast agent makes the tubes visible. The flow of contrast through the tubes can also be documented by Doppler ultrasound. If there is an **increased risk** of tubal disease (e.g., after chlamydia infection or previous lower abdominal surgery), tubal patency testing by laparoscopy is preferable, as any tubal damage can be treated surgically if necessary.

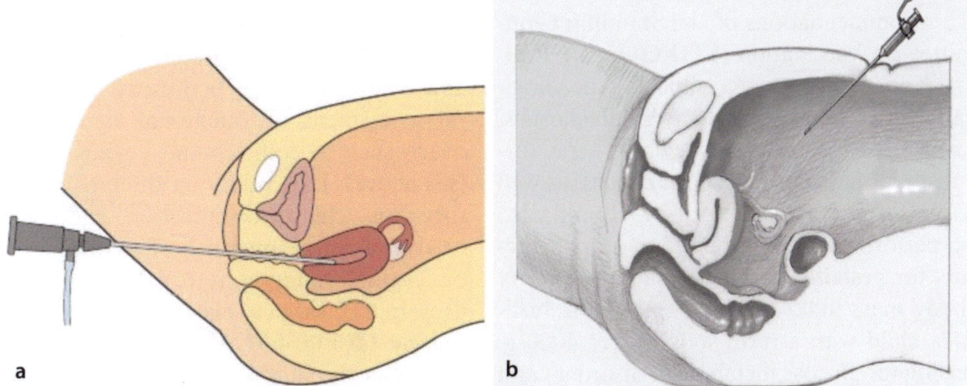

● **Abb. 4.9** Diagnostic hysteroscopy and laparoscopy. **a**: hysteroscopy, **b**: laparoscopy. (With kind permission from: Wallwiener M (2018) and Wallwiener D (2009))

Infertility Diagnostics

About 90% of women wishing to conceive become pregnant spontaneously within one year (see ▶ Chap. 3). Accordingly, during the first 12 months of trying to conceive, preparation for pregnancy is usually carried out according to stage I infertility diagnostics by the gynecologist. If pregnancy has not occurred after 12 months and the couple presents at a fertility center, stage II infertility diagnostics can be performed. Once this has been completed for both partners, the indication for fertility therapy can be established. Before starting fertility treatment, all preparations for pregnancy should be systematically completed, necessary vaccinations updated, and any required medical or surgical treatments initiated or performed.

Stage I Infertility Diagnostics

For women wishing to conceive, basic infertility diagnostics according to stage I include a preventive examination by the referring gynecologist and verification of **rubella-** and **varicella immunity**. If there is no vaccination protection, the recommended vaccinations should be updated according to the recommendations of the Standing Committee on Vaccination (STIKO) at the Robert Koch Institute. A clinical gynecological examination with **chlamydia diagnostics**, assessment for symptoms such as acne, hirsutism, or hair loss (**androgenization**), as well as galactorrhea (**galactorrhea**), should also be performed. In the presence of **risk factors** for **gestational diabetes** such as obesity (body mass index (BMI) > 30) or the birth of a child with a birth weight over 4000 g, testing for glucose metabolism disorders and insulin resistance is indicated. Risk factors for **tubal occlusion** include, for example, a previous chlamydia infection, chronic lower abdominal pain, complicated appendec-

tomy, lower abdominal surgery with adhesiolysis, or endometriosis. **Vaginal sonographic abnormalities** with suspected malformations or changes in the ovaries, fallopian tubes, or uterus are an indication for surgical clarification and, if necessary, therapy.

Stage II Infertility Diagnostics

In the case of a **conspicuous medical history** (such as previous chlamydia infection, endometriosis) or **clinical abnormalities** such as cycle disorders, as well as in **advanced maternal age** ($\geq$ 35 years), extended infertility diagnostics for both partners according to stage II should be carried out without delay. If the **desire for children** remains unfulfilled after **12 months**, extended fertility diagnostics (Bals-Pratsch and Eder 2023) are also indicated. This includes basic **hormone diagnostics** with determination of LH, FSH, estradiol, prolactin, TSH, and progesterone levels. In cases of androgenization, hormone diagnostics should be expanded to include the androgens testosterone and DHEAS. Most often, this is due to PCOS. Differential diagnosis should also consider the rare adrenogenital syndrome (AGS). If AGS is suspected, referral to internal medicine specialists in endocrinology and diabetology is usually indicated. **Vaginal sonography** of the uterus and ovaries must be performed with careful assessment of functional signs in the ovary such as follicles and corpus luteum (see above). Depending on the medical history (e.g., chlamydia infection, endometriosis) and in the presence of abnormalities on vaginal sonography (e.g., myomas, hydrosalpinx), **surgical clarification** by hysteroscopy (▪ Fig. 4.9) and laparoscopy with chromopertubation or hysterosalpingography (HyCoSy) may be necessary.

Abnormalities in women also include **overweight** and **obesity** (BMI $\geq$ 25 and $\geq$ 30 kg/m^2). In most cases, **insulin resistance** is present, and prediabetes is often already established (Bals-Pratsch et al. 2023). Overweight and obese women can benefit from weight reduction. Effective treatment with new anti-obesity medications such as semaglutide leads not only to significant weight loss but also to spontaneous pregnancies. The reduction in BMI improves glucose metabolism. This likely normalizes the microenvironment in the ovary, so that the sensitive oocytes may mature better. The most important diabetes medication worldwide, however, remains metformin, which is also frequently used in polycystic ovary syndrome (PCOS) to improve pregnancy outcomes. PCOS women also often have insulin resistance and glucose metabolism disorders. Metformin treatment improves insulin resistance and glucose metabolism. As a result, the spontaneous pregnancy rate can increase up to 22% (Fill Malfertheiner et al. 2017). In cases of infertility, overweight and obese patients should therefore be advised to optimize weight and metabolism with professional support.

◉ Learning Objectives

— Understanding the physiology of the female cycle, its changes over the course of life, and the causes of cycle disorders

— Providing knowledge about different diseases that affect fertility, as well as their diagnosis and therapy

Oocyte maturation is cyclical, while sperm maturation is a more constant process. Cycle function is regulated by various systems from the brain to the ovaries. For pregnancy to occur, oocyte maturation in the ovary, egg transport through the fallopian tube, and preparation of the endometrium for embryo implantation must be coordinated. Cycle disorders are often due to disturbed regulation of oocyte maturation. In some cases, such functional disorders can be treated with medication, as in polycystic ovary syndrome, prolactinoma, or thyroid diseases. The age-dependent reserve of oocytes in the ovary is crucial for pregnancy prognosis. If the oocyte reserve is depleted, pregnancy with one's own oocytes is no longer possible. Functional disorders of the ovaries can be detected by hormone measurements and vaginal ultrasound examination. In addition, fertility disorders can be caused by congenital and acquired changes in the female reproductive organs. These include genetic disorders and malformations, as well as damage to the ovaries, fallopian tubes, and uterus (e.g., endometriosis or myomas). It must then be decided on an individual basis whether a patient may benefit from surgical correction.

References

Bals-Pratsch, M Bachmann, A Sharma AM (2023) Adipositas und Kinderwunsch. cme-kurs ► https://www.cme-kurs.de/kurse/adipositas-undkinderwunsch/ Zuletzt 5.3.2025

Bals-Pratsch M, De Geyter Ch, Müller T et al (1997) Episodic variations of prolactin, TSH, LH, melatonin and cortisol and relationship to sleep stages in infertile women with subclinical hypothyroidism. Hum Reprod 12:896–904.

Bals-Pratsch, M Eder A (2023) Kinderwunsch. In: Seitz S (Hrsg) Gynäkologie und Geburtshilfe. Springer, Heidelberg, pp. 143–154.

Fill Malfertheiner S, Gutknecht D, Bals-Pratsch M (2017) Preconception Optimization of Glucose and Insulin Metabolism in Women Wanting to Conceive – High Rate of Spontaneous Conception Prior to Planned Assisted Reproduction. 77:1312–1319. ► https://doi.org/10.1055/s-0043-122279. Zuletzt 5.3.2025

Merk K (2019) Outcome der Assistierten Reproduktionstechnik bei Patientinnen mit polyzystischem Ovar-Syndrom mit versus ohne Insulinresistenz unter präkonzeptioneller Metformintherapie. Universität Regensburg. ► https://epub.uni-regensburg.de/40061/2/Dissertation%20PCOS%20Merk%202019%20online.pdf. Zuletzt 2.2.2025

Rebhan D, Bachmann A (2021) Update zur Einschätzung des Anti-Müller-Hormons (AMH) als Marker der ovariellen Reserve. Gynäkologische Endokrinologie 24,138–143.

Sonntag B (2016) Zyklusstörungen. Gynäkologe 49:357–372. ► https://doi.org/10.1007/s00129-016-3878-1

Sonntag B, Segerer S, Keck C (2019) Kinderwunsch: Beratung und Therapie in der gynäkologischen Praxis. Gynäkologe 52:217–228. ► https://doi.org/10.1007/s00129-018-4376-4

The Rotterdam ESHRE/ASRM-sponsored PCOS consensus workshop group (2004) Revised 2003 consensus on diagnostic criteria and long-term health risks related to polycystic ovary syndrome (PCOS). Hum Reprod 19:41–47. ► https://doi.org/10.1093/humrep/deh098

Teede HJ, Tay CT, Laven JJE et al (2023) International PCOS Network. Recommendations from the 2023 international evidence-based guideline for the assessment and management of polycystic ovary syndrome. Eur J Endocrinol 189:G43–G64. ► https://doi.org/10.1093/ejendo/lvad096

Vrontikis A, Chang PL, Kovacs P et al (2010) Antral follice counts (AFC) predict ovarian response and pregnancy outcomes in oocyte donation cycles. J Assist Reprod Genet 27:383–389. ► https://doi.org/10.1007/s10815-010-9421-8

Wallwiener D (2009) Laparoskopie. In: Wallwiener D, Jonat W, Kreienberg R et al (eds) Atlas der gynäkologischen Operationen 7th edn. Thieme-Verlag, Stuttgart, pp. 49–51.

Wallwiener M (2018) Diagnostische Hysteroskopie. In: Solomayer EF, Juhasz-Böss I (eds) Kursbuch Gynäkologische Endoskopie, Thieme Verlag, Stuttgart, pp. 70–72.

Basics and Diagnostics of Male Reproduction

Contents

Sexual Medicine Aspects

In fertility consultations, reproductive medicine is the main focus, rather than sexuality. However, there are couples with fertility desires in whom sexual medicine disorders play a significant role (e.g., in vaginismus and erectile dysfunction). These couples should be treated in cooperation with a physician specialized in sexual medicine (additional qualification). Due to **"reproductive stress,"** sexual dysfunctions such as erectile and ejaculatory disorders (■ Table 5.1) occur more frequently, as intercourse is often performed "on command" to increase the efficiency of conception. As a result, intercourse does not occur out of desire, but rather at ovulation. In addition to the **dimension of desire**, the satisfaction of psycho-emotional basic needs for security, acceptance, comfort, and closeness (**relationship dimension**) also loses significance.

During intercourse, the **orgasm** in women is triggered by stimulation of the clitoris by the glans, shaft, and root of the penis. The nerve fibers of this approximately 11 cm long organ, of which only the tip of the clitoris is visible, extend into the vagina and thighs. Orgasmic disorders can interfere with fertilization. For example, in the absence of orgasm, no sexual secretions are released into the vagina. These normally enhance lubrication and can improve sperm motility. In men, stimulation of the penile shaft and glans during penetration of the shaft into the vagina leads to orgasm and triggers **ejaculation**. Ejaculation before penetration is called premature ejaculation, absence of ejaculation is aspermia, and absence of orgasm is anorgasmia (■ Table 5.1). Retrograde ejaculation, like delayed ejaculation, anejaculation, or premature ejaculation, is among the ejaculatory disorders. The **boundaries** between **orgasmic** and **ejaculatory disorders** can be **fluid**. Common causes include prostate surgery, medications, chronic diseases, or trauma such as spinal cord injuries.

■ **Table 5.1**   Semen deposition in the female genital tract, organic and sexual disorders in men

Disorders of reproductive function (penile anomalies/sexual dysfunctions)	Term	Explanation
Penis	Hypospadias	Urethra ends on the underside
	Epispadias	Urethra ends on the upper side
	Phimosis	Narrowing of the foreskin
	Penile deviation	Bending of the penis
Erection	Erectile dysfunction (ED)	Inability to achieve an erection
	Priapism	Persistent erection
Orgasm	Anorgasmia	Absence of orgasm
	Aspermia	No semen despite orgasm
	Premature ejaculation	Premature orgasm
	Delayed ejaculation	Significantly delayed ejaculation
Ejaculation	Retrograde ejaculation	Ejaculation into the bladder
	Anejaculation	Loss of ejaculation (as in aspermia)

Anatomy of the Male Reproductive System

Sperm cells (spermatozoa) are produced in the **testes** and stored in the epididymis until ejaculation (◘ Fig. 2.1), a highly convoluted duct about 5 to 6 cm long that caps the testis.

Spermatogenesis and Spermiogenesis and Their Disorders

With the onset of **puberty**, the seminiferous tubules (**tubuli seminiferi**) develop, and the initiation of **spermatogenesis** leads to the growth of the previously small testes. Testicular volume is largely determined by the number of intact tubules in which sperm cells are produced (◘ Fig. 5.1). The tubules have a length of 300 to 700 m. Before puberty, the germinal epithelium in the tubules consists only of the stem cells of sperm maturation (**spermatogonia**) and the supporting cells (**Sertoli cells**). Between the tubules lie the **Leydig cells**, which are important for hormone production in the testis. From puberty onward, the spermatogonia enter meiosis, and from one spermatogonium, four spermatids are formed (◘ Fig. 2.2). This is followed by **spermiogenesis**. The initially early round spermatids develop into late elongated sperm cells (◘ Fig. 2.5). Morphologically mature sperm cells (spermatozoa) consist of a **head**, **midpiece**, and **tail**. The stem cells of sperm maturation (spermatogonia) are located on the outer wall of the tubules. The sperm cells formed during spermatogenesis are released into the lumen in the center of the seminiferous tubules after completion of spermiogenesis for further transport to the epididymis. A small testicular volume indicates impaired sperm maturation. A **spermatogenesis disorder** can vary in severity (◘ Fig. 5.2). The spectrum includes disorders with **arrest** at the level of the spermatocytes or spermiogenesis disorders at the level of the spermatids (e.g., round spermatids). More commonly, tubules with impaired spermatogenesis are **focally** distributed among tubules with intact spermatogenesis in the testicular tissue. The damage to the germinal epithelium can be so severe that only the supporting cells (Sertoli cells) remain in the seminiferous tubules. This severe damage is referred to as **Sertoli-cell-only syndrome (SCO syndrome)**.

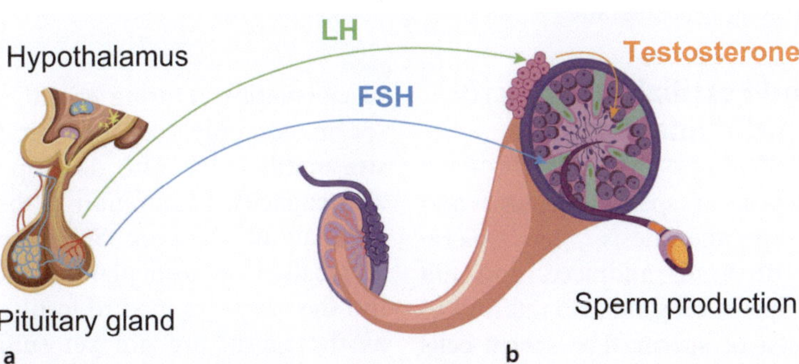

◘ **Fig. 5.1** Hypothalamic-pituitary-testicular axis and sperm production in the seminiferous tubule. **a**: Release of LH and FSH from the pituitary gland, **b**: Cross-section of a seminiferous tubule with Sertoli cells (green) inside and Leydig cells outside (schematic)

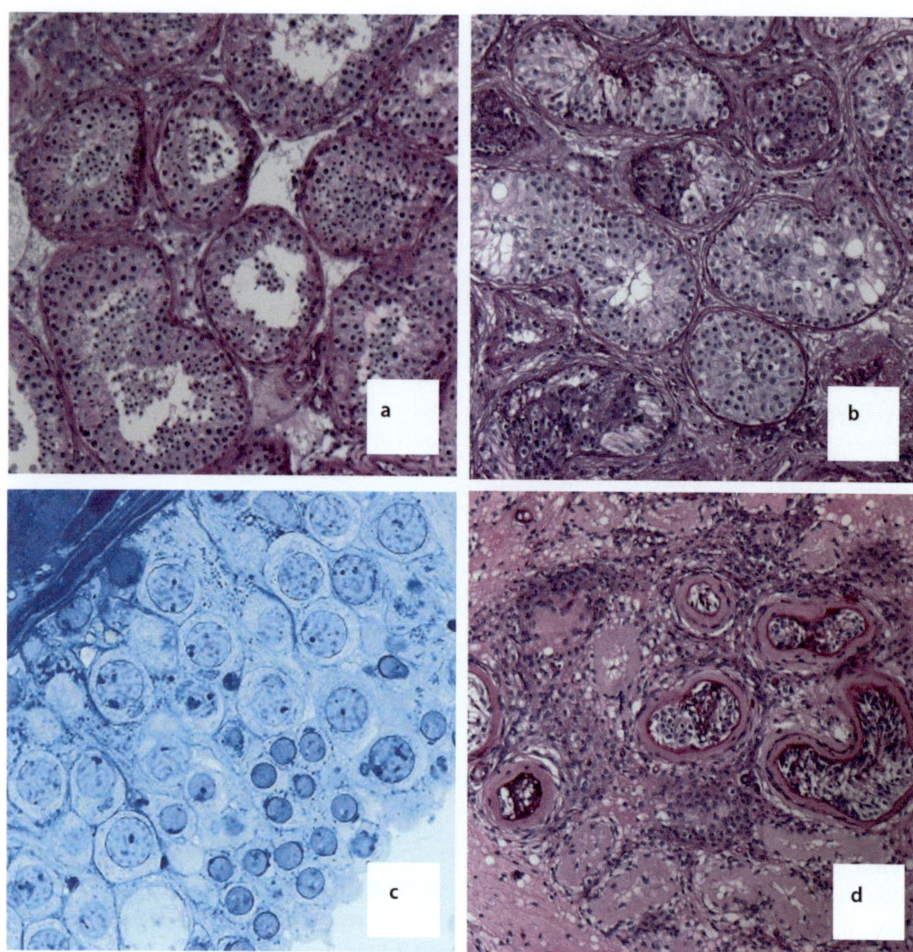

Fig. 5.2 Spermatogenesis and spermiogenesis disorders (semi-thin section histology). **a**: qualitatively intact spermatogenesis, **b**: spermatogenesis arrest at primary spermatocytes, **c**: spermiogenesis arrest at round spermatids, **d**: Sertoli-cell-only syndrome (SCO)

Motility and Fertilizing Capacity through Epididymal Passage

After completion of spermatogenesis and subsequent spermiogenesis, the **sperm cells** consist of head, midpiece, and tail (**Fig. 2.5**). Sperm cells are also referred to as spermatozoa or sperm. The sperm cells acquire their **motility** during passage and subsequent storage in the epididymis. In the **epididymis**, the sperm cells are stored un- til ejaculation. During epididymal passage, sperm not only acquire their full **progressive motility**, but also develop their **fertilizing capacity.** Maturation in the epididymis takes about one week. Sperm cells obtained surgically from testicular tissue cannot ferti- lize the oocyte in in vitro fertilization (IVF), as the sperm are not yet sufficiently mo- tile or capable of fertilization. Even sperm from the epididymis cannot fertilize in vitro, as fertilizing capacity is only fully achieved with capacitation in the female genital tract. For this reason, when fertilizing with sperm from testicular tissue or the epididymis, the method of intracytoplasmic sperm injection (ICSI) is required in addition to IVF.

Processes in Fertilization

The task of sperm is **fertilization** of the oocyte. Therefore, sperm cells must be able to move purposefully forward (progressively), recognize the oocyte, and bind to the oocyte membrane in order to then fuse with it (◘ Fig. 2.6). The sperm head consists of the nucleus, the acrosomal cap, which covers two-thirds of the sperm head, and the centriole at the posterior end of the sperm head. The **acrosome** contains enzymes to dissolve the zona pellucida and enable sperm binding to the oocyte membrane (oolemma). The sperm head and tail enter the oocyte. After penetration of the sperm cell into the oocyte, the sperm head approaches the female pronucleus and swells to form the **male pronucleus**. The pronuclear stage is formed (◘ Fig. 1.2). The **centriole**, located at the posterior end of the sperm head, is necessary for the formation of the **mitotic spindle** and subsequent embryonic development. If a functional centriole is missing, arrest occurs at the pronuclear stage and embryonic development fails to proceed. In normal fertilization, the two nuclei dissolve. This completes fertilization, and the oocyte begins to divide into a two-cell embryo.

Physiology of Male Reproduction

After intercourse, sperm cells must swim to the end of the fallopian tube to fertilize an oocyte. The important physiological prerequisites for successful fertilization are capacitation and the acrosome reaction of the sperm during passage through the female genital tract (see ▶ Chap. 2).

Testes, epididymis, seminal vesicles, and prostate contribute to the **semen** in varying proportions. Only five percent of the ejaculate volume comes from the testes and epididymis. To assess the function of the **epididymis**, **seminal vesicles**, and **prostate**, **functional markers** can be determined (◘ Table 5.2). For example, if alpha-glucosidase values as a marker for epididymal function are low, it must be assumed that there is a pathological obstruction at the level of the epididymis or vas deferens. Men after vasectomy also have reduced alpha-glucosidase values, as in this case the vas deferens have been surgically severed. The ejaculate volume is normal after vasectomy. The secretion of the seminal vesicles is alkaline and important for adjusting the pH value in the ejaculate, as an alkaline pH above 7.2 is optimal for sperm motility and buffers the acidic vaginal environment after intercourse. The prostatic secretion contains numerous substances that serve to liquefy the ejaculate.

◘ **Table 5.2** Functional markers for epididymis, seminal vesicles, and prostate

Glands	Function	Proportion of ejaculate volume	Marker
Testes/Epididymis	Provision of sperm cells, storage	5%	Alpha-glucosidase
Seminal vesicles	Adjustment of pH value	50–80%	Fructose
Prostate	Liquefaction of ejaculate	15–30%	Citrate, zinc

Hypothalamic-Pituitary-Testicular Axis

The male hormone **testosterone** is produced in the Leydig cells located between the tubules. Sufficient concentrations of testosterone are necessary for spermatogenesis. This hormone is also important for the function of the penis, epididymis, seminal vesicles, prostate, and for other bodily functions such as sexuality, hair growth, blood formation, muscle development, and bone metabolism.

The **hormonal regulation** of testicular function by the hypothalamus and the pituitary gland is essentially the same as in ovarian function (■ Fig. 4.5). The pituitary is stimulated by pulsatile secretion of gonadotropin-releasing hormone (GnRH) (hypothalamic-pituitary-testicular axis). However, in men, the GnRH pulses have a stable frequency of about 120/min. The pituitary responds to this signal by releasing luteinizing hormone (LH) and follicle-stimulating hormone (FSH). LH stimulates the Leydig cells to produce testosterone, and FSH stimulates the Sertoli cells in the seminiferous tubules to promote spermatogenesis.

However, there are significant **differences between men** and **women** in the regulation of the **hypothalamic-pituitary-gonadal axis**. Sperm maturation occurs continuously and not cyclically. Therefore, the GnRH signal does not change its pulse frequency or amplitude. The target organs for LH and FSH differ: the **testes** with Leydig and Sertoli cells, and the **ovaries** with the follicular apparatus (granulosa and theca cells). Accordingly, in men, feedback at the levels of the pituitary and hypothalamus operates via **testosterone** (■ Fig. 5.1). Therefore, anabolic steroid abuse or testosterone therapy leads to suppression of LH and FSH secretion and thus to suppression of spermatogenesis. Sperm maturation is no longer sufficiently stimulated by endogenous LH and FSH. For this reason, bodybuilders or fertility patients undergoing testosterone therapy often have reduced sperm concentrations, up to the absence of sperm in the ejaculate (azoospermia). Therefore, testosterone therapy is fundamentally contraindicated in men actively seeking to conceive. The hormone **inhibin** is produced by Leydig cells and also plays a role in the regulation of sperm maturation. If spermatogenesis in the seminiferous tubules is impaired, Leydig cells secrete less inhibin, leading to a compensatory increase in LH and FSH secretion. Elevated LH and FSH levels indicate a disorder of spermatogenesis. However, increased LH and FSH stimulation of the testes is generally ineffective in cases of severe damage to the germinal epithelium.

Fertility disorders at various anatomical and functional levels

Male infertility can have its cause at a functional and/or organic level. The disorders can be either congenital or acquired.

Impaired semen deposition

In rare cases, a couple's infertility may be due to impaired semen deposition in the vagina during intercourse (■ Table 5.1). This includes malformations or acquired **anomalies of the penile shaft**. If the urethra opens on the underside or upper side of the penile shaft, this is referred to as hypospadias or epispadias. In such cases, semen cannot be ejaculated into the posterior vaginal fornix. As a result, the entry of sperm into the cervix, which protrudes like a plug into the posterior fornix, is hindered. A phimosis can also be so pronounced that it interferes with sexual intercourse. Scarring of the penile shaft, as seen in rare connective tissue diseases (induratio penis plastica), can lead to penile curvature with pain during erection. **Erectile dysfunction** (ED) is more often due to psychological or hormonal causes, but can also be organic, for example after prostate surgery. It can also be caused by medications such as antidepressants, or by circulatory disorders associated with chronic diseases such as diabetes mellitus, hypertension, or neurological disorders. **Priapism** is defined as a persistent erection lasting more than two hours. This situation is a urological emergency. Causes are usually medications such as psychotropic drugs, alcohol and drugs, neurological diseases, but also intracavernous injection (ICI) for erectile dysfunction.

Testicular damage

In the case of testicular damage, the **FSH level** is usually elevated depending on the extent of the spermatogenesis disorder. To better assess the severity of impaired spermatogenesis, the **inhibin level** can also be measured (see above). Testicular damage is fundamentally not treatable.

Spermatogenesis can be impaired by congenital and acquired **organic changes** of the testes. Among the acquired changes, **varicocele** can be included. This is a varicose formation of the venous plexus in the scrotum (pampiniform plexus). About 30% of both infertile and fertile men have a varicocele. As a **factor of sterility**, it can lead to reduced blood flow and testicular volume, increased temperature, and fragmentation of genetic material (DNA). DNA fragmentation can impair embryo development and thus implantation. A varicocele can be treated surgically or by radiological interventions. If a varicocele does not cause clinical symptoms, there is generally no indication for surgical intervention. However, if there is an unfulfilled desire for children and a compromised semen analysis, treatment of the **varicocele** can be offered to the patient even in the absence of symptoms. However, an improved pregnancy rate after varicocele therapy has not been proven.

Infections of the male genital organs can also lead to infertility. The **mumps** infection before and after puberty, involving the testes and epididymis, is well known. After puberty, 20 to 30% of men develop mumps orchitis (Masarani et al. 2006). Testicular swelling (**orchitis**) occurs five to ten days after the onset of parotitis (inflammation of the parotid gland). In about 10 to 30% of cases, this is bilateral. In 30 to 50% of cases, the infection leads to shrinkage (atrophy) of the affected testis and consequently to infertility. If both testes are affected by mumps orchitis, 30 to 87% of affected men can be expected to have fertility disorders. Mumps vaccination is very effective in preventing mumps orchitis. **Sexually transmitted infections (STIs)** such as syphilis (lues) and gonorrhea, as well as chlamydia, can also frequently lead to infertility. These infections can spread within the male genital tract and often cause obstruction of the seminal pathways, but in some cases also lead to testicular atrophy.

Cryptorchidism (undescended testis) is the most common malformation of the urogenital tract. Up to three percent of male newborns are affected. Often, the testicular tissue is already congenitally damaged. The risk of azoospermia is increased by 25%. There is also a higher probability of developing testicular cancer later in life.

Acute febrile illnesses such as influenza-like infections can also damage testicular tissue. However, such infections usually only cause a **temporary disturbance** of spermatogenesis or damage to sperm cells in the seminiferous tubules and epididymis. ◘ Table 5.3 shows the course of sperm concentration and motility before and after a febrile illness with temperatures of 39 to 40 degrees Celsius over two days in sperm donors. Five weeks after the infection, **sperm concentration** and **progressive motility** as well as the **DNA fragmentation index (DFI)** had dropped sharply or increased into the range of infertility (see below). After more

Table 5.3 Course of semen quality over 6 months after febrile illness (after Sergerie M, Mieusset R, Croute F et al. (2007))

Day	0	15	37	58	79	> 180
Concentration (Mill/ml)	47.0	20.2	2.4	21.4	70.0	48.5
Progressive motility (a+b) %	60	35	15	60	40	45
DNA fragmentation index % (DFI)	9	24	31	15	8	9

Table 5.4 Environmental influences and semen quality

Influencing factors	Selection
Stimulants	Alcohol, tobacco, drugs
Pharmaceuticals	Cytostatics, antiandrogens, testosterone, anabolic steroids
Physical factors	Heat, ionizing radiation
Chemicals	Pesticides, herbicides, insecticides, heavy metals, solvents, plasticizers

than two months, all parameters had normalized again, as a new, undamaged generation of sperm cells had matured during this time. The duration of spermatogenesis is 64 to 74 days.

Spermatogenesis can also be damaged by **abuse** of alcohol, tobacco, and drugs, chemotherapy, hormone treatment with androgens or antiandrogens, or by other risk factors such as chemicals and radiation (**Table 5.4**).

Diagnostics of Male Fertility Disorders

In cases of involuntary childlessness, evaluation should follow a **stepwise diagnostic approach** that includes **both partners**. This is usually carried out by the gynecologist within the first 12 months (see ▶ Chap. 4). The diagnostics according to **Step I** begin with the medical history, which should also include the use of medications and an-

abolic steroids in the man as well as sexuality. If abnormalities are found in the woman, such as indications of a tubal occlusion or reduced ovarian reserve, and in cases of advanced reproductive age (> 34 years), extended diagnostics according to **Step II** should promptly be initiated, including examination of the man by a urologist, preferably an andrologist (see ▶ Chap. 4). This diagnostic workup should also be performed without delay if the man's medical history is notable. The examinations include, in addition to the clinical-andrological assessment, a basic semen analysis. The most important risk factors for infertility are a history of undescended testis in childhood, mumps infection, or chemotherapy. If both partners have an unremarkable history and the woman is young (age < 35 years), extended infertility diagnostics are only performed after infertility has been established for one year. Diagnostics for the man at a fertility center are generally limited to semen and hormone analysis.

Clinical-Andrological Examination

A specialist **clinical-andrological examination** includes inspection of the body with assessment of body hair and the external genitalia. In particular, it is checked whether a varicocele or breast enlargement (gynecomastia) is present. The penis and testes, including the epididymides, are inspected and palpated, and testicular volume is determined, for example, using an **orchidometer**. An orchidometer is a medical measuring instrument consisting of 12 numbered wooden beads with volumes ranging from 1 to 25 ml, strung on a chain. The palpable epididymides sit like a cap on the upper outer part of the testes. In addition, the vas deferens must be palpable to rule out malformations such as absence of the vas deferens. If one or both vas deferens are missing, this may indicate a **genital form** of **cystic fibrosis** with a genetic risk for the desired child. This malformation is referred to as congenital unilateral or bilateral absence of the vas deferens (**CUAVD** or **CBAVD**). To avoid missing a testicular tumor, the clinical-andrological examination is usually supplemented by a **scrotal ultrasound** with sonographic determination of testicular volume. An abnormal semen analysis can always be a sign of a **testicular tumor**. Testicular cancer is the most common tumor diagnosis in young men, with a peak incidence between 25 and 45 years of age. Early-stage tumors are now highly curable. Therefore, monthly self-examination is generally recommended.

Hormonal Diagnostics

The clinical-andrological examination is supplemented by **hormonal diagnostics**. In the basic assessment, the hormones **FSH** and **total testosterone** are measured; if abnormalities are found, **prolactin** and **inhibin** are also determined. Only the free, unbound fraction of testosterone—not bound to sex hormone-binding globulin (**SHBG**)—is clinically active. Either the free, **bioavailable testosterone** is calculated from the total testosterone and the SHBG value, or it is measured directly using a special test. In addition, testosterone levels exhibit **diurnal fluctuations**, with high values in the early morning and low values in the early evening. Therefore, testosterone measurement should always be performed in the early morning to avoid the misdiagnosis of testosterone deficiency. Such misdiagnosis repeatedly leads to the inappropriate initiation of testosterone therapy. The result is suppression of FSH secretion and a deterioration of semen quality up to azoospermia. If an elevated FSH level is found in the basic assessment, testicular damage is suspected.

Semen Analysis

The final step in the clinical-andrological diagnostics is the **semen analysis**, which is performed in a **standardized** and quality-controlled manner according to the current sixth edition of the **WHO Laboratory Manual** for the Examination and Processing of Human Semen from 2021 (Köhn and Schuppe 2022). The fifth edition of the manual was last published in German in 2012. The WHO first published the manual for standardized semen analysis in 1980 to enable worldwide comparison of semen findings. Since then, it has been possible to conduct and evaluate studies on male fertility worldwide. The German Society of Andrology (DGA) offers external quality control (**QuaDeGA**). This is required for quality assurance in semen analysis according to the guidelines of the German Medical Association, in addition to internal quality control. Semen analysis alone, without

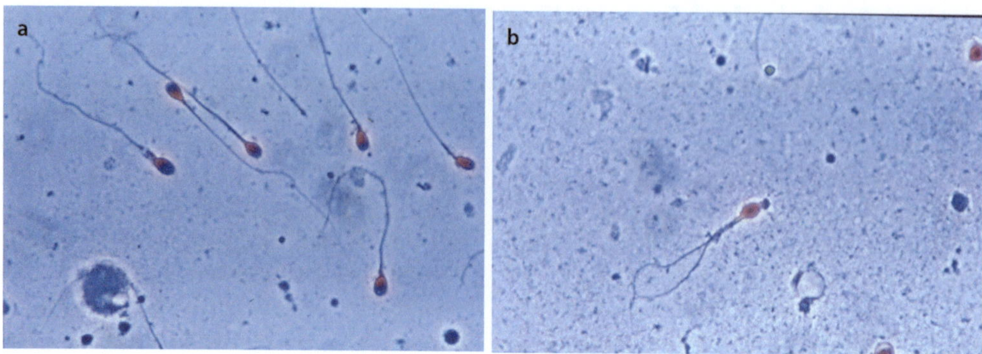

□ Abb. 5.3   Normal and abnormal sperm (Papanicolaou stain). **a**: Sperm with normal morphology, **b**: Sperm with double tail

evaluation of clinical-andrological findings and medical history, does not allow a reliable diagnosis of whether a man is fertile or infertile. Fundamentally, a semen analysis is a **snapshot**. In particular, sperm concentration values show significant fluctuations. Therefore, **two examinations** should always be performed at least two weeks apart.

Conducting Semen Analysis

According to the WHO Laboratory Manual, **abstinence** before semen analysis should be at least two days (**48 h**) and **no more than seven days**. The **semen collection container** must be cell culture-tested and should be provided by the andrology laboratory. Otherwise, contaminants from the container can damage the sperm cells, particularly affecting motility. The semen sample is obtained by masturbation. In exceptional cases, cell culture-tested special condoms may be used. Patients must **wash their hands** and **penis** before collection and thoroughly rinse off any harmful soap residues. This allows semen samples to be used for **microbiological examination** without significant contamination from bacteria on the penile skin. Collection of a semen sample at home is possible if the same procedures are followed as in the fertility center, the sample arrives at the laboratory within 60 minutes at body temperature, and patient identification is ensured. The semen should be incubated in an incubator at 37 degrees within 5 minutes after collection to allow liquefaction. Analysis begins 30 to 60 minutes later. The process starts with a **macroscopic examination** to assess color, volume, viscosity, and pH value. This is followed by preparation for the **microscopic examination**, determining motility, concentration, and morphology of the sperm cells. Sperm morphology is assessed after staining, for example, using the Papanicolaou method (**□** Fig. 5.3).

Semen Parameters

The most important semen parameters with **reference values**, clinical significance, and laboratory methods are summarized in **□** Table 5.5. There is a specific **nomenclature** for the evaluation of semen findings. **□** Table 5.6 contains the complete listing. If sperm concentration, motility, and morphology are each within the normal range, this is termed **normozoospermia**. If all three semen parameters are reduced, this is called **oligoasthenoteratozoospermia**. In the assessment of sperm density, according to the nomenclature, oligozoospermia is diagnosed if the sperm concentration (mill./ml) or, preferably, the total sperm count (mill./ejaculate) falls below the current reference val-

▣ Table 5.5 Semen parameters, clinical significance, reference values, and laboratory method (*WHO)

Parameter	Normal finding	Pathological	Method
Color	gray-opalescent	brown, red, suspicion of inflammation	macroscopic
Consistency	liquid	viscous, e.g., prostatic dysfunction	macroscopic
pH value	> 7.2	e.g., seminal vesicle dysfunction	pH paper 6–10
*Volume (ml)	1.4 (1.3–1.5)	e.g., ejaculatory disorder	e.g., weight (1 g/ml)
*Concentration (mill/ml)	16 (15–18)	Testicular damage suspected	pipette/counting chamber
*Total sperm count (mill/ejaculate)	39 (35–40)	Testicular damage suspected	calculation
*Progressive motility (%)	30 (29–31)	e.g., spermatogenesis disorder	manual cell counter
*Normal forms (%)	4 (3.9–4)	spermiogenesis disorder	e.g., Papanicolaou stain
MAR test (%)	< 50% (lab-dependent)	immunological infertility	IgG and IgA latex particles

▣ Table 5.6 Semen analysis findings, terminology according to WHO 2010

Term	Semen analysis finding
Normozoospermia	Sperm count, motility, and morphology within reference range
Oligozoospermia	Sperm count below reference range
Asthenozoospermia	Progressive motility below reference range
Teratozoospermia	Proportion of normal forms below reference range
Oligoasthenoteratozoospermia (OAT)	Combination as above
Azoospermia	No sperm detected in ejaculate
Aspermia	No ejaculate
Cryptozoospermia	Sperm detectable only after centrifugation
Haemospermia/Haematospermia	Erythrocytes in ejaculate
Necrozoospermia	Increased proportion of non-viable sperm in ejaculate

ues. The reference ranges published in the laboratory manual (World Health Organization 2021) were calculated from semen analysis results of men from all five continents whose partners became pregnant naturally within less than 12 months (5th percentile with 95% confidence interval). The reference values for semen parameters are no longer to be regarded as cut-off values that allow differentiation between fertile and infertile men. However, they provide the basis for recommendations regarding further diagnostics and therapy, as well as prognostic guidance.

Optional Tests

Optional tests are often performed to further assess sperm function. This includes testing for **antisperm antibodies** using the **MAR test** in the ejaculate. This examination is important because the antibodies are cytotoxic and immobilizing. They are often found in men after vasectomy, testicular injury, and infections. If the MAR test is positive, the sperm cells can no longer fertilize the egg normally in the fallopian tube or in vitro, making intracytoplasmic sperm injection (ICSI) necessary. Assessment of **DNA integrity** is gaining increasing importance in extended semen analysis. It is a prerequisite for normal embryo development, successful implantation, and pregnancy. Damaged genetic material, such as strand breaks, can lead to poor embryo quality, unsuccessful IVF treatments, or recurrent miscarriages. An increased rate of DNA fragmentation must be expected with exposure to **toxic substances**, as well as in **diabetes mellitus**, **obesity**, and **smoking**. The Sperm Chromatin Structure Assay (**SCSA test**) is one of the assays included in the current WHO Laboratory Manual for assessing sperm DNA integrity. The test result is reported as the DNA fragmentation index (DFI). A low value below 15% is normal; values above 25% indicate clinically significant DNA fragmentation.

Human Genetic Diagnostics

If no sperm or fewer than 5 to 10 million/ml sperm cells are found in the semen analysis, then—taking into account the medical history, clinical-andrological examination, and laboratory diagnostics—there is an indication for **human genetic evaluation**. After medical counseling, blood is drawn for chromosome analysis and/or molecular

genetic diagnostics, as affected patients are at high risk for Klinefelter syndrome, Y-chromosome microdeletions, or mutations in the cystic fibrosis gene. If **Klinefelter syndrome (karyotype 47,XXY)** is detected, azoospermia is usually present, and histological examination of testicular tissue typically reveals Sertoli cell-only syndrome (SCO syndrome). Thus, the chances of finding sperm for artificial fertilization with ICSI during a testicular biopsy are very low. A similarly poor prognosis for having a biological child exists for most men with significant deletions of gene regions on the Y chromosome essential for spermatogenesis (**azoospermia factor**, abbreviated **AZF**). If the gene deletions are less severe, ICSI treatment with sperm from the ejaculate or testicular tissue may still be possible. If a son is born, he will also have a fertility disorder later, as he inherits the father's gene deletion. If mutations in the cystic fibrosis gene are detected in a healthy man with azoospermia, **obstructive azoospermia** due to **aplasia** of the vas deferens (**CBAVD**) should be assumed. In this case, the healthy partner should also be counseled regarding mutations in the so-called cystic fibrosis transmembrane conductance regulator (CFTR) and, after consent, tested for carrier status for cystic fibrosis. The risk of CFTR carrier status is 1:35. If the partner is also a carrier, there is a **high risk** of 25% for a **child** with **cystic fibrosis**. This disease is a severe hereditary disorder. Affected couples must receive genetic counseling regarding the possibility of **preimplantation genetic diagnosis**. ICSI treatment is usually possible, as suitable sperm for fertilization can generally be found during testicular biopsy, since in the genital form of cystic fibrosis, azoospermia is usually due to absence of the vas deferens and/or epididymis and not to a spermatogenesis disorder.

Learning Objectives

- To impart knowledge of sexual medicine aspects of reproduction
- Understanding the physiology of male reproductive function and its disorders
- Knowledge of the significance and conduct of semen analysis according to WHO

A semen analysis alone is not sufficient for male fertility diagnostics, even though the semen findings are often decisive for fertility treatment. Every patient with a desire to have children should receive andrological care. The specialist examination also includes a physical examination. Testicular tumors, as a possible cause of impaired semen quality, can be diagnosed by scrotal ultrasound. Both anatomical changes and genetic factors can influence fertility. Risk factors for male infertility include undescended testis in childhood, mumps, or chemotherapy. Acute factors such as febrile infections can also temporarily impair semen quality. Mature sperm cells are stored in the epididymis, where they acquire motility. During passage through the female genital tract, the sperm undergo "capacitation" to become capable of fertilization. As with oocyte maturation, sperm maturation is hormonally regulated. However, hormonal disorders are rare, so hormonal treatment options for men are generally lacking. Semen analysis with determination of concentration, motility, and morphology is performed according to WHO standards and can be supplemented by additional tests such as microbiological examinations. Unfulfilled desire for children often also affects sexuality. "Reproductive stress" can lead to erectile and ejaculatory disorders.

References

Köhn F-M, Schuppe H-C (2022) Das WHO-Laborhandbuch zur Untersuchung und Aufarbeitung des menschlichen Ejakulates -Darstellung und Kommentierung der Unterschiede zwischen der 5. und 6. Auflage. J Reproduktionsmed Endokrinol 19:177–82

Masarani M, Wazait H, Dinneen M (2006) Mumps orchitis. J R Soc Med 11:573–575. ► https://doi.org/10.1177/014107680609901116. Zuletzt 3.03.2025

Sergerie M, Mieusset R, Croute F et al (2007) High risk of temporary alteration of semen parameters after recent acute febrile illness. Fertil Steril. ► https://doi.org/10.1016/j.fertnstert.2006.12.045. Epub 2007 Apr 16. PMID: 17434502

World Health Organization (2021) WHO laboratory manual for the examination and processing of human semen. Sixth edition Geneva, Licence: CC BY-NC-SA 3.0 IGO. ► https://www.who.int/publications/i/item/9789240030787. Zuletzt 5.07.2025

Basics of Fertility Treatment

Contents

Supplementary Information The online version contains supplementary material available at ▶ https://doi.org/10.1007/978-3-662-73035-5_6.

Surgical Therapy in Women

A **hysteroscopy (HSK)** and a **laparoscopy (LSK)** with chromopertubation to examine the uterine cavity and assess tubal patency are standard procedures in operative fertility assessment (see ▶ Chap. 4, ◘ Fig. 4.9). These minimally invasive diagnostic methods are also suitable for operative therapies, e.g., for submucosal fibroids or endometriotic cysts. For this purpose, small surgical instruments can be introduced through the hysteroscope or, in the case of LSK, through the abdominal wall. In rare cases, a laparotomy (abdominal incision) may be required for planned surgical management, such as in extensive endometriosis.

Tubal Surgery

Microsurgery may be indicated, for example, if **refertilization** is desired after sterilization. In the case of a **post-inflammatory tubal damage** with occlusion or adhesions, such as after chlamydia infections, in vitro fertilization is now indicated. It is more successful compared to tubal surgery. In the case of unilateral or bilateral **hydrosalpinx**, laparoscopic removal of the fallopian tube (salpingectomy) or proximal tubal occlusion is recommended before IVF treatment, as the leakage of fluid from a hydrosalpinx into the uterus could interfere with embryo implantation.

Uterine Malformations

The **indication for surgical correction** of uterine malformations is based on the **symptoms**, the available surgical **options**, the **complication** and **success rates**. In infertility diagnostics, it is important to identify uterine malformations and assess their impact on fertility. However, clear definitions for the differentiated diagnosis of uterine malformations are lacking, so the boundaries are fluid. Instead of objective criteria, the diagnosis is partly based on the subjective assessment of the examiner (AWMF guideline 2020). For uterine diagnostics, vaginal sonography and hysteroscopy are usually sufficient. In individual cases, diagnostics can be supplemented with three-dimensional ultrasound, magnetic resonance imaging (MRI), and laparoscopy. However, during hysteroscopic diagnostics, therapy is often already performed depending on the surgeon and the surgical equipment, e.g., hysteroscopic septum resection.

Depending on the timing of the developmental disorder, there are different manifestations of uterine malformations. The earlier the developmental disorder occurs, the more severe the manifestation. These affect either the **uterine cavity** or the **shape** of the uterus and the **cervix**. The assessment focuses mainly on the external and internal shape of the uterus, with attention to the presence of an external indentation in the middle of the uterine fundus and an internal bulge in the middle of the roof of the uterine cavity.

Symptoms of Uterine Malformations and Uterine Organ Development

Clinical symptoms of malformations include a tendency to **miscarriages** in the first and second trimesters, as well as increased risks of preterm labor and **preterm birth**. There are also known **fetal malpresentations**, **growth retardation**, and **birth complications**. Uterine malformations are due to a disturbed fusion of the two Müllerian ducts in the lower region (see ▶ Chap. 2). In the embryonic period, the upper part develops into the fallopian tubes, and the lower part forms the uterus and the upper two-thirds of the vagina. First, the two Müllerian ducts come together in the lower region and then fuse to form the uterovaginal canal. Initially, this canal is divided by the fused walls of the Müllerian ducts, forming a septum. This septum regresses from bottom to top.

Uterine Malformation with Cavity Separation by a Septum

A **uterus arcuatus** represents the mildest anomaly of the uterus (◘ Table 6.1). The external shape is unremarkable, and the internal shape shows a slight inward bulge of the fundus (uterine roof) in the form of a minimally developed septum (AWMF S2k Guideline Female Genital Malformations (2020)). Its significance for reproductive medicine is debated. On the one hand, a uterus arcuatus is considered a normal variant; on the other, it is seen as a minimal form of uterine malformation. The classification of the European Society of Human Reproduction and Embryology and the European Society for Gynaecological Endoscopy (Grimbizis et al. 2013) appears to be decisive for clinical evaluation, as a uterus arcuatus is no longer listed as a separate subgroup. The situation is different for a **uterus subseptus**, in which the uterine cavity is partially divided by a septum (◘ Fig. 6.1).

In a uterus subseptus, the uterus appears slightly broadened externally. In a **uterus septus**, the septum extends to the cervix, so the uterine cavity is completely divided into two horns. This malformation often occurs together with a vaginal septum.

Malformation with Duplication of the Uterus

In a **uterus bicornis**, the uterus consists of two uterine horns. Due to the external indentation at the fundus, it appears heart-shaped. Sonographically, two horns can be visualized, each with its own cavity ("cat's eye phenomenon"). This malformation is more often associated not only with a vaginal septum but also with a unilateral **renal malformation**. Usually, a uterus bicornis unicollis is present, meaning the duplicated uterine body has only one cervix. A variant is a **uterus unicornis**. A second horn is often only incompletely developed. This can lead to obstetric complications such as uterine rupture. A complete duplication of the uterus exists when each uterine horn also has its own cervix. The two horns are also completely separated externally. This

◘ Table 6.1   Uterine Malformations

Uterine Malformation	Diagnosis	Surgical Recommendation	Type of Surgery
Uterine septum, partial or complete separation of the cavity	Uterus arcuatus (clinical relevance controversial)	none	Septum resection, hysteroscopic for shallow endometrium
	Uterus subseptus	Infertility, recurrent miscarriage	
	Uterus septus	Infertility, recurrent miscarriage	
Duplication of the uterus (bicorporeal uterus), rudimentary horn (hemi-uterus)	Uterus bicornis unicollis	Recurrent miscarriage, preterm birth	Abdominal metroplasty, possibly combined vaginal and laparoscopic
	Uterus unicornis	Detection of rudimentary horn	Possibly resection of rudimentary horn
	Uterus bicornis bicollis	Recurrent miscarriage, preterm birth	Abdominal metroplasty, possibly combined vaginal and laparoscopic

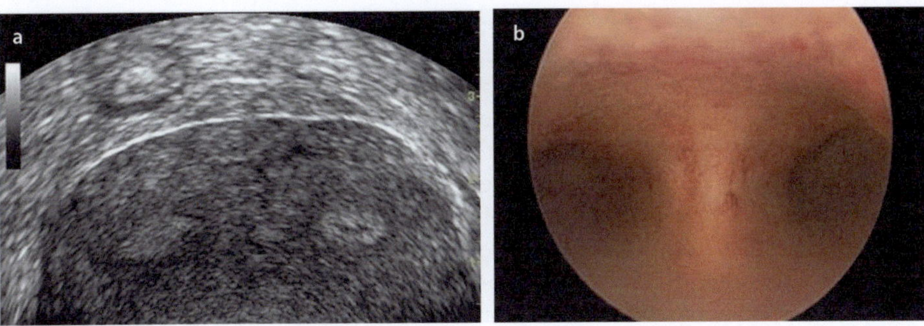

■ **Fig. 6.1**   Uterus subseptus. **a**: sonographic finding, cross-section, "cat's eye phenomenon", **b**: hysteroscopic finding with broad septum dividing the uterine cavity into two halves. (After Schill T [Specialization in Reproductive Medicine])

malformation is referred to as **uterus bicornis bicollis**, but also as uterus didelphys or uterus duplex. In addition, there are numerous variants such as absence of a uterine horn or incompletely (rudimentary) developed uterine horns.

Operative Therapy for Uterine Malformations

In cases of infertility, septum resection can be performed hysteroscopically in women with a uterus septus or subseptus, after individual assessment, in the presence of symptoms, and depending on the extent of the septum (■ Fig. 6.1). Symptoms include implantation failure, recurrent miscarriages, or preterm births. It is discussed that blood supply and placental development may not be sufficient for successful embryo implantation over a septum (Müller and Hohl 2020). Reduced uterine capacity, i.e., a uterine cavity too small for pregnancy, is also debated as a risk factor for pregnancy. In cases of double uterine malformations such as uterus bicornis bicollis, so-called metroplasty (reconstruction of the uterus) can be performed after careful consideration in cases of recurrent miscarriages and preterm births (AWMF guideline 2020). There is evidence that the birth rate increases after metroplasty and that fewer miscarriages and preterm births occur. In summary, there are no clear indications for the surgical correction of uterine malformations.

Myomas

Myomas are only operated on in cases of infertility in special circumstances (see ▶ Chap. 4). A quarter of women over 30 have myomas, but only 25% of affected women report symptoms. The decision for myomectomy should be individualized and made together with the patient, depending on the symptoms and the size of the myomas. Myomas larger than 3 to 5 cm are usually symptomatic (pressure sensation, bleeding disorders with anemia). Surgical therapy can generally be performed hysteroscopically or laparoscopically. Submucosal myomas are resected hysteroscopically. Intramural or subserosal myomas can usually be enucleated laparoscopically. The uterine cavity should, if possible, not be opened to avoid rupture in a subsequent pregnancy. Surgery on the uterus should always be performed as gently as possible to minimize risks such as Asherman syndrome (see ▶ Chap. 4).

An alternative treatment method to myomectomy is magnetic resonance-guided focused ultrasound (MRgFUS). This treatment is performed in specialized centers.

Some systems are now approved throughout Europe for women wishing to conceive, e.g., the ExAblate ONE system (Insightec/GE). However, this method is not suitable for every patient with myomas. Selection criteria for MRgFUS in myomas include vascularity, location, size, and number of myomas. Conservative options include medical therapies with GnRH agonists, antagonists, a selective progesterone receptor modulator (SPRM), or progestins.

Asherman Syndrome

Asherman syndrome results from injury and destruction of the lower layer of the endometrium, the basalis. In about 90% of cases, this is caused by curettage during pregnancy, but in about 10% by intrauterine surgery such as myomectomy or septum resection. Surgical therapy is performed hysteroscopically with special instruments (e.g., micro scissors), which usually allows reconstruction of a functional uterine cavity. The few centers equipped for this perform up to 700 Asherman syndrome cases per year. To prevent postoperative adhesions, catheters or intrauterine devices are often prophylactically inserted into the cavity, and postoperative antibiotic treatment for several weeks is given to treat possible inflammation (endometritis). In addition, high-dose estrogens are often administered to support the healing process and stimulate the endometrium. Depending on the extent of adhesions, clinical classification is into mild, moderate, and severe. Clinical pregnancy rates, depending on severity, range from 70% to 40%.

Endometriosis

Endometriosis is a chronic disease. The goal of surgical therapy is to remove the endometriotic tissue as completely as possible to achieve **symptom relief**. Depending on the extent and location of the lesions, **surgical management** may be necessary via laparoscopy, laparotomy, or vaginally (see ▶ Chap. 4). Frequently, hormonal follow-up treatment with GnRH agonists or progestins is given. Endometriosis surgeries are often performed in **endometriosis centers** that collaborate with fertility centers, as even after surgical endometriosis treatment, **IVF treatment** is usually necessary for women wishing to conceive.

Principles of Ovarian Stimulation Therapy

In ovarian stimulation therapy, follicles are stimulated to grow so that one or more mature eggs develop. This treatment is also referred to as **ovulation induction** (OI). Stimulation therapy is used in both patients without ovulation and those with ovulation. The natural hormones LH and FSH are called gonadotropins because they stimulate the gonads. Ovarian stimulation treatment with gonadotropins was first successfully performed in women without ovulation in the early 1960s. Ovulation was triggered with the gonadotropin hCG. Anovulatory women usually have primary or secondary amenorrhea. The causes for this are varied (see ▶ Chap. 4).

The goal of stimulation treatment is a **singleton pregnancy** resulting in the birth of a healthy child. Achieving a "perfect outcome" with the development of only one follicle is not always possible, as the individual ovarian response to hormone therapy cannot be reliably predicted. If more than one follicle matures, there is a risk of a **multiple pregnancy**. Therefore, hormone treatment is monitored by ultrasound and usually also by hormone measurements. If more than two to three follicles mature, the cycle should be canceled. Alternatively, excess follicles can be aspirated before ovulation through a **selective follicle reduction** on an individual basis.

Ovarian stimulation therapy is also generally performed in infertile women with a normal cycle. During stimulation treatment, hormone levels for estradiol and progesterone rise into the therapeutic range. This is intended to improve the conditions for successful fertilization and implantation. A cycle in which only one follicle matures is called **monofollicular**, while a cycle with the development of several follicles is referred to as **poly-** or **multifollicular**.

The **stimulation medications** used for ovulation induction include clomiphene, letrozole, the gonadotropins LH and FSH, and GnRH. Their use and the treatment protocols with adjunct medications in assisted reproduction are shown in Fig. 6.2. There is a manageable number of hormone preparations approved for hormone stimulation (Table 6.2). Ovarian stimulation treatment with the hormone GnRH is only performed in exceptional cases. This treatment is very effective when hypothalamic GnRH release is absent, as in isolated hypothalamic hypogonadism (IHH) or Kallmann syndrome. If stimulation medications are used off-label for fertility treatment, the specifics of **off-label use** must be considered. Documented patient counseling is recommended (sample consent form in Appendix 6.1).

Pulsatile GnRH Stimulation

In women with **hypothalamic amenorrhea**, ovulation induction can be performed with **pulsatile GnRH** (Fig. 4.5). The pituitary gland must be functional. Hormone treatment is administered subcutaneously using a mini-infusion pump that delivers about 20 μg GnRH subcutaneously every 90 minutes (LutrePulse®). In this way, the natural hypothalamic GnRH stimulation of the pituitary is mimicked. Once a preovulatory follicle has matured, a natural LH surge and ovulation occur under GnRH therapy. Pulsatile GnRH stimulation is very effective

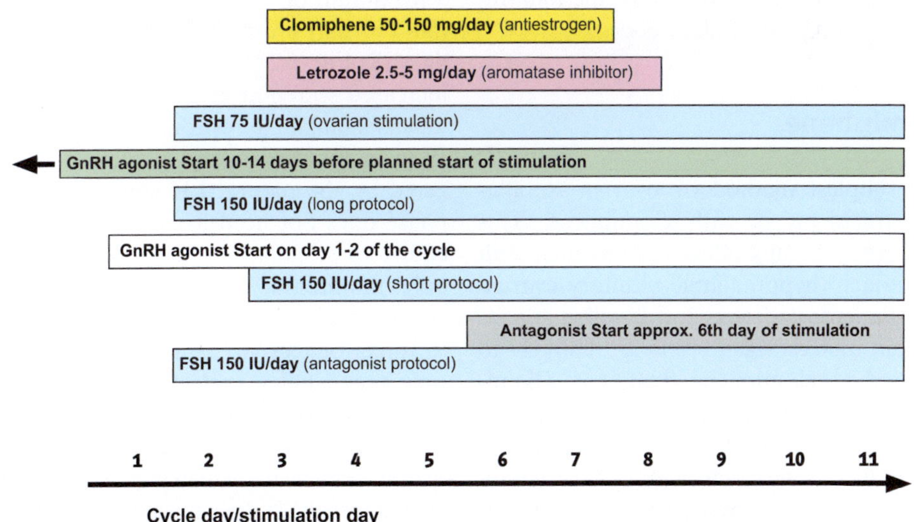

Fig. 6.2 Stimulation protocols for ovulation induction (OI) and for controlled ovarian stimulation (COS) in the context of assisted reproduction, "I.U." = "International Unit", "die" = "day"

▫ Table 6.2   Medications for ovarian stimulation (OI) and controlled ovarian stimulation (COS)

Medications	Active ingredient	Medication[R]	Production	Stimulation
hMG	Menotropin (LH and FSH)	Menogon HP, Meriofert	urinary	OI, COS
U- FSH	FSH	(not available)	urinary	OI, COS
R-FSH	Follitropin α, β and δ, Corifollitropin α	Gonal-f, Bemfola*, Ovaleap*, Puregon, Rekovelle, Elonva	recombinant	OI, COS
R-FSH/LH	Follitropin α/Lutropin α	Pergoveris	recombinant	OI, COS
U-hCG	Chorionic gonadotropin	Brevactid 5,000 I.U.	urinary	OI, COS
R-hCG	Chorionic gonadotropin α	Ovitrelle 250 μg/0.5 ml	recombinant	OI, COS
R-LH	Lutropin α	Luveris	recombinant	OI, COS
GnRH agonist	Triptorelin, Nafarelin	e.g., Decapeptyl Gyn 3.75 mg, Decapeptyl IVF 0.1 mg/1 ml, Synarela nasal spray	chemical	COS
GnRH antagonist	Ganirelix, Cetrorelix	e.g., Orgalutran, Cetrotide	chemical	COS

hMG: human menopausal gonadotropin; *: biosimilar

when physiological hypothalamic GnRH secretion is absent, with ovulation rates of 80 to 100%. Trained support staff should be available for programming the handheld computer (LutrePulse® Manager) and instructing patients in the use of the mini-infusion pump (LutrePulse® Pod).

Clomiphene

The simplest method of ovarian stimulation treatment is with clomiphene. This medication is only effective in women with an intact hypothalamic-pituitary-ovarian axis. Patients with very low baseline gonadotropin and estrogen levels are unlikely to respond to clomiphene treatment. Clomiphene is an **antiestrogen** (estrogen receptor modulator) and is structurally very similar to the drug tamoxifen. Clomiphene stimulation has been practiced since the 1960s. The medication is approved for ovulation induction in women seeking pregnancy who do not ovulate. This mainly includes women with polycystic ovary syndrome (PCOS). In four out of five women with PCOS, ovulation can be induced in this way. At the beginning of the cycle, one to a maximum of three tablets of clomiphene (50–150 mg) are taken on five consecutive days (▫ Fig. 6.2). The body responds with increased secretion of LH and FSH, as the tablets simulate an estrogen deficiency. The cycle is monitored and ovulation is triggered by the natural LH surge. The luteal phase does not need to be supported. The course of stimulation cannot be influenced, only monitored. There are polyfollicular courses with the growth of more than two to three follicles. To avoid the risk of multiple pregnancies, cycle monitoring is necessary and, if needed, the cycle should be canceled. Clomiphene treatment is ineffective in women with unexplained infertility, as this treatment does not result in a higher pregnancy rate than expectant management (Bhattacharya et al. 2008).

Letrozole

Hormone stimulation with the medication letrozole is increasingly being practiced. Letrozole is an **aromatase inhibitor**. Aromatase is required for estrogen biosynthesis in tissue, as it converts androgens into estrone and estradiol. In premenopausal women, the estrogen level drops and there is increased secretion of LH and FSH, stimulating the ovaries. Administration is similar to clomiphene, with, for example, 2.5 mg letrozole taken daily for five consecutive days starting on cycle day 3 to 5 (◘ Fig. 6.2). Pregnancy rates after letrozole appear to be higher than after clomiphene (Franik et al. 2022). Letrozole is not approved for fertility treatment, but only for breast cancer in menopause. Use for fertility treatment is therefore off-label.

Gonadotropin Stimulation

Human **menopausal gonadotropin (hMG)** contains the gonadotropins **LH** and **FSH**. It is isolated from the urine of postmenopausal women. Another gonadotropin is human **chorionic gonadotropin (hCG)** from the placenta. hCG has a very similar structure to LH. Like LH, it binds to the theca cells in the follicle, so it can be used in ovarian stimulation treatment to trigger ovulation. Lunenfeld was the first to successfully perform ovulation induction with hMG in humans in 1962 (Lunenfeld 1963). He is considered a pioneer in gynecological endocrinology. He treated a hypogonadotropic patient with primary amenorrhea. This therapy resulted in the birth of a healthy child. This first successful hMG stimulation attracted great attention.

The goal of gonadotropin stimulation is **monofollicular oocyte maturation**. In gonadotropin stimulation, **ovulation triggering** must always be performed. The standard trigger medication is hCG, as LH is not available in the required trigger dose (see below). Starting on cycle day 2 or 3, gonadotropins are self-injected subcutaneously daily until ovulation is triggered (◘ Fig. 6.2). To avoid complications, cycle monitoring with vaginal ultrasound and hormone measurements is important. If follicle growth is insufficient, the gonadotropin dose can be increased. If there are risks for severe ovarian hyperstimulation syndrome (OHSS), the gonadotropin dose should first be reduced and, if unsuccessful, the stimulation cycle should be canceled.

If at least one follicle is 15 mm or larger, ovulation can be triggered with 5,000–10,000 I.U. hCG or 250 µg recombinant hCG, as this gonadotropin acts like LH on the maturing follicle (see above). LH itself is not used for ovulation triggering due to the very high dose required, about 25,000 I.U. (Beckers et al. 2003). If more than two to three follicles have matured, each $\geq$ 15 mm in diameter, to avoid higher-order multiple pregnancies, cycle cancellation and protected intercourse should be discussed. Alternatively, selective follicle reduction can be offered at a fertility center, as follicle punctures are usually routine procedures. After gonadotropin stimulation, the luteal phase must always be hormonally supported. Luteal phase support is possible with hCG and/or progestogens, which can be combined with estrogens if necessary. Without luteal phase support, breakthrough bleeding often occurs just a few days after ovulation (Beckers et al. 2003). The chances of successful implantation and ongoing pregnancy are then generally lost.

The **risks** of gonadotropin therapy are severe **ovarian hyperstimulation syndrome (OHSS)** and **multiple pregnancies**. Ovarian hyperstimulation syndrome only develops after ovulation has been triggered with hCG. If there are risks for OHSS, the gonadotropin dose should first be reduced and, if unsuccessful, the stimulation cycle should be canceled and repeated with an adjusted dose. Individual **dose finding** can be complicated, and the "therapeutic window" of gonadotropins is narrow. Therefore, as required in assisted reproduction, physicians should also have obtained qualification in gynecological endocrinology and reproductive medicine for gonadotropin stimulation alone.

Natural Cycle

In women with regular ovulation, fertility treatment can also be performed in a natural cycle (spontaneous cycle). It is necessary to determine the optimal timing for fertilization using ultrasound and hormone measurements. An egg is fertilizable for about 10 to 12 hours, whereas sperm survive for several days in the uterus and fallopian tube. The chances for spontaneous conception (natural fertilization) are therefore best if intercourse occurs 1 to 2 days before or around the time of ovulation. The German IVF Registry uses the term **"intercourse at the optimal time" (timed intercourse)**, abbreviated as **"VZO" (TI)**, for this.

Intrauterine Insemination (IUI)

In reproductive medicine, insemination refers to the transfer of semen into the female genital tract to fertilize an egg. This is the simplest method of artificial fertilization. In practice, insemination is performed into the uterine cavity. This method is called **intrauterine insemination (IUI)**. Sperm in high concentration and the egg are brought together as close as possible in the woman's body to facilitate fertilization. The passage through the cervix is bypassed with a catheter. The semen transfer is performed at the time of ovulation. For this, the time of ovulation must be determined by cycle monitoring. This treatment method can overcome **fertility barriers**. These include organic male or female disorders such as hypospadias (◘ Table 5.2) or vaginismus. An abnormal semen analysis is also a factor for infertility that can be treated with IUI. However, sperm concentration and motility must still be sufficient for successful fertilization. Treatment with the partner's semen is called **homologous IUI**. Another indication for IUI is in same-sex couples who wish to be treated with donor sperm (**donor** or **heterologous insemination**). Success rates are disappointing if there are no identifiable fertility barriers that can be overcome with IUI. This is the case in couples with idiopathic infertility.

The goal of fertility treatment with IUI is to achieve an ongoing pregnancy and the birth of a child as quickly as possible. Therefore, IUI is often combined with **medications** for ovarian stimulation. The pregnancy rate of a combined clomiphene stimulation with IUI is age-dependent and, in women under 35, is at most 10% per cycle. Thus, this combined treatment of IUI with clomiphene stimulation, like sperm transfer alone or expectant management, is ineffective (Bhattacharya et al. 2008). Only switching to hormone stimulation with gonadotropins leads to an improved live birth rate (Wessel et al. 2022). The **German Register for Insemination (DERI)** has evaluated IUI cycles for the second year in a row (Hammel et al. 2024). This register is an initiative of the Working Group Donor Insemination (AK DI). About one in four IVF centers is already a DERI center. Pregnancy and birth rates are calculated separately for homologous inseminations in couples (**IUI-H**), for donor (heterologous) insemination in couples (**IUI-D**), and for donor insemination in same-sex partnerships and single women. Treatment with donor sperm is also referred to as "**artificial insemination with donor sperm**" (**AID**). In recent years, AID in lesbian couples and single women has grown significantly to two-thirds of all AID cycles.

Pregnancy and birth rates in heterosexual couples (**IUI-H**) are disappointingly low. The pregnancy rate per insemination was 10% and the birth rate was 6%. The treatment results were somewhat better for donor sperm treatment (**IUI-D**), with a maximum pregnancy rate of 16.1% and a birth rate of 12.4%. These sobering figures are an important **basis for counseling** affected women, who often wish to become pregnant with AID in a natural cycle and do not want hormone stimulation if they have a regular cycle. A separate register analysis of IUI cycles by stimulation medication has not yet been published. It can be assumed that many IUIs are performed in the natural cycle or after stimulation with clomiphene. The results of IUI treatment would probably be within an acceptable range if IUI were combined with low-dose gonadotropin stimulation (daily dose 37.5 to 75 I.U.).

Performing an IUI

Like IVF, IUI falls under the Tissue Act, so the necessary spatial, personnel, and equipment requirements must be met (see ▶ Chap. 1). Once the indication for IUI has been established and the diagnostic preparations, including infection diagnostics in the man, are complete, the treatment cycle can begin promptly. If AID treatment is planned, organizational preparations such as ordering and delivery of samples to the fertility center must be completed before treatment begins. **Monitoring** is performed in the natural cycle or in a stimulated cycle. If the endometrium is at least 6–8 mm thick and a preovulatory follicle of at least 15–17 mm has developed, ovulation can be triggered by an hCG injection. Alternatively, the LH surge can be awaited. This is determined by LH measurement in a blood sample or by semi-quantitative measurement with ovulation self-tests. Insemination

is performed either one day after the LH surge or about 36 to 40 hours after pharmacological **ovulation triggering**. For organizational reasons, ovulation induction with hCG is usually preferred for scheduling the insemination, as IUIs can be better planned for weekdays in fertility centers.

The **identity check** of both partners must be strictly observed at each step of the process in the semen collection room, laboratory, and procedure room, and documented on the sample accompanying forms with the signatures of staff and patients. On the day of treatment, the partner must provide a semen sample according to WHO guidelines (see ▶ Chap. 5). This must be prepared for intrauterine insemination so that the best sperm can be selected and concentrated for treatment. The selected sperm are suspended in culture medium and warmed in the incubator until IUI. Depending on the **preparation method**, sample preparation takes about 1–2 hours. After the identity check, the **intrauterine transfer** of the prepared sperm cells is performed in a small volume (about 0.2–0.5 ml) using a catheter. The procedure must be performed under sterile conditions. Under ultrasound guidance, the position of the insemination catheter in the uterine cavity and the transfer of fluid can be visually monitored by turbulence at the catheter tip.

After gonadotropin stimulation, the luteal phase must be supported with medication using hCG or progesterone (possibly in combination with estrogen). **Luteal phase support** is also possible in the natural cycle or after clomiphene stimulation, but is generally not necessary, as neither pregnancy rates nor miscarriage rates can be demonstrably improved (Casarramona et al. 2022). The **pregnancy test** should be performed no earlier than 14 days after IUI in a blood sample. If hCG was used for luteal phase support, at least seven days must have passed between the last hCG administration and the pregnancy test. Otherwise, the pregnancy test could be falsely positive, as residual injected hCG in the blood would still be measured.

In Vitro Fertilization (IVF) and Intracytoplasmic Sperm Injection (ICSI)

The first child conceived through in vitro fertilization was born in 1978. IVF treatment is the most effective, but also the most complex, method of assisted reproduction. A successful pregnancy is not guaranteed, as the natural factor cannot be reliably calculated. Many couples are initially disappointed by the pregnancy prognosis of 30 to 40% per cycle, which, after several years of unfulfilled desire for children without treatment, would be less than five percent. IVF treatment makes it possible to examine **oocytes** and their fertilization potential directly under the microscope. The fertilization process, including the **sperm-oocyte interaction** and the development of the fertilized oocyte into an **embryo**, can also be visually monitored. IVF treatment is the method of choice for women who have no fallopian tubes or whose tubes are nonfunctional. This also includes women with endometriosis. Nowadays, the treatment is also performed in couples without a tubal factor who, for example, have not become pregnant with hormone stimulation and insemination treatment. Women of **advanced reproductive age** often choose IVF treatment as a primary option to increase their remaining chance of pregnancy, since ovarian stimulation can significantly increase the number of oocytes available for fertilization in a single IVF cycle. In one year, not just 12 oocytes, but a multiple of that number can be fertilized through repeated IVF cycles. This allows for the development of more viable embryos, which increases the chances of an ongoing pregnancy at the end of the reproductive phase.

For many couples, the actual **cause of infertility** only becomes apparent during an IVF cycle. This is especially true for couples with so-called "idiopathic infertility." Some women, for example, surprisingly have many empty follicles ("empty follicle syndrome") or a high proportion of immature oocytes. In some couples, fertilization does not occur, or the fertilized oocytes arrest at various stages of development up to the blastocyst stage (embryo arrest). In such cases, the preliminary diagnostics should be reviewed before further treatment, and, if necessary, a chromosomal analysis should be performed. Poor oocyte quality as a cause is indeed treatable if a woman is not sufficiently **healthy for pregnancy**. This applies, for example, to women with impaired glucose tolerance (**prediabetes**). Preconceptional impaired glucose tolerance and exceeding the thresholds for gestational diabetes in the glucose tolerance test are not currently indications for treatment in diabetology prior to pregnancy (Bals-Pratsch and Fill Malfertheiner 2017). The necessary medications and test strips for self-monitoring of blood glucose must be paid for out of pocket by women with statutory health insurance who wish to conceive. It should be noted that, due to the long oocyte maturation period of about one year (see ▶ Chap. 2), oocyte quality often only improves 6 to 12 months after the start of metabolic optimization. Glucose levels should therefore be within the target range for pregnancy for this length of time before further treatment is considered. In cases of failed fertilization or a low fertilization rate, intracytoplasmic sperm injection (ICSI) should be performed in a subsequent cycle as an extension of IVF treatment.

The **ICSI method** represents another milestone in the rapid development of assisted reproduction (◘ Fig. 6.3). Previously, IVF treatment was usually unsuccessful in cases of poor semen quality. Researchers

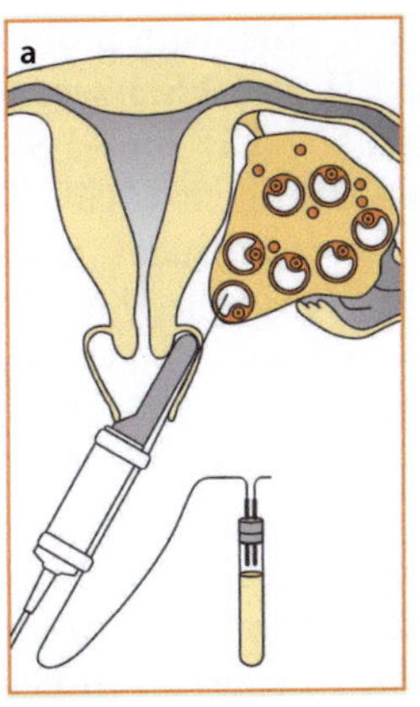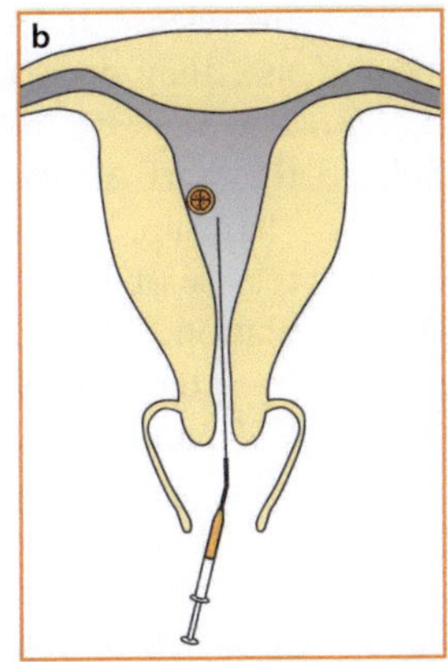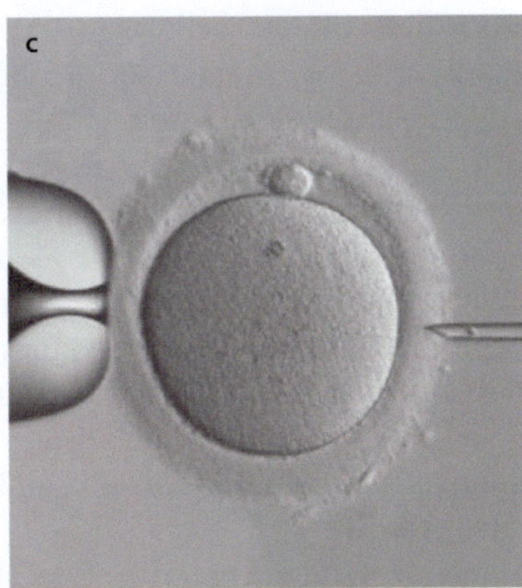

◘ Fig. 6.3 Oocyte retrieval, embryo transfer, and ICSI technique. **a**: Ultrasound-guided follicular puncture **b**: Embryo transfer **c**: ICSI method MII oocyte (polar body at the top). On the right, injection capillary with a sperm cell at the tip of the needle; on the left, holding pipette

therefore attempted to use a micromanipulator to introduce individual sperm cells into the space between the zona pellucida and the oocyte membrane. Accidentally, sperm cells were injected directly into the oocyte. Surprisingly, these oocytes were fertilized the next day. This groundbreaking discovery in 1992 opened up the possibility for men with severely impaired semen quality to father their own children using ICSI. Injection of surgically retrieved sperm from the epididymis or testes also resulted in fertilization of oocytes.

Modern IVF treatment also includes **cryopreservation**. Cryopreservation of sperm cells has been established for decades. Today, with the new method of vitrification, both unfertilized and fertilized oocytes at all stages of development can be safely frozen.

Controlled Ovarian Stimulation (COS)

IVF treatment is usually performed in combination with ovarian stimulation. The goal is for several (about six to eight) follicles to mature. This requires a higher hormone dose than for monofollicular oocyte maturation as in IUI. For safe and effective therapy, the optimal treatment protocol and appropriate stimulation medications should be selected. PCOS patients should preferably be stimulated with FSH instead of hMG due to the increased risk of OHSS. Today, various urinary and recombinant FSH medications are available. Follitropin α, β, and corifollitropin α are produced by genetic engineering on ovary cell lines of the Chinese hamster (◘ Table 6.2). In addition, there is another gonadotropin (follitropin δ) produced on a human fetal retina cell line. Corifollitropin α is the only depot preparation and is administered as a single dose. All other gonadotropins must be self-injected daily. Ovulation induction is performed with 5,000 to a maximum of 10,000 IU hCG or 250 μg choriogonadotropin α (equivalent to about 6,500 IU hCG).

In special cases, such as when there is a risk of OHSS and ovulation should be triggered with the GnRH agonist triptorelin for safety, usually 2 prefilled syringes of Decapeptyl IVF 0.1 mg® or Triptofem 0.1 mg® can be injected (off-label use). However, due to the subsequent, inadequately treatable corpus luteum insufficiency, cryopreservation of the cells is usually necessary, so embryo transfer should be postponed to a subsequent cycle.

Hormonal preparation for IVF is called controlled ovarian stimulation, abbreviated COS. Sometimes the term controlled ovarian hyperstimulation (COH) is also used. According to general understanding, a **COS treatment** must fulfill three criteria:

1. **Gonadotropin stimulation for multifollicular growth**
2. **Adjunctive treatment with GnRH agonists or GnRH antagonists (pituitary suppression to prevent premature LH surge)**
3. **Ovulation induction 32 to 40 hours before oocyte retrieval**

Gonadotropin stimulation can be well controlled by dosage. A higher hormone dose leads to multifollicular oocyte maturation. Stimulation must be performed with adjunctive medications to prevent premature ovulation (so-called GnRH agonists and antagonists) according to one of the established standard protocols. Otherwise, about 30% of IVF cycles result in premature ovulation. In addition, ovulation must be induced pharmacologically. This is necessary because the adjunctive medications suppress the natural LH surge. Oocyte retrieval should be performed about 36 +/− 2 hours after ovulation induction, so that the follicles have not yet ruptured and the oocytes are fertilizable. Administration of hCG activates oocyte maturation, so that the oocytes continue meiosis I and the first polar body is extruded. At the time of follicular puncture, the oocytes are in metaphase II (MII oocytes), i.e., meiosis II has begun.

Adjunctive treatment with GnRH agonists or antagonists effectively suppresses a premature natural LH surge, allowing the follicles to mature to a diameter of 15 to 20 mm. **GnRH agonists** stimulate gonadotropin synthesis in the pituitary and increase the release of LH and FSH; with prolonged use, they decrease LH and FSH secretion. The massive release of LH and FSH at the start of agonist treatment is called the "flare-up," while the subsequent minimal release of LH and FSH is called "downregulation." The flare-up effect is characterized by a temporary sharp increase in LH and FSH and typically begins about two days after starting agonist treatment. As a sign of the onset of downregulation, LH and FSH levels drop to subnormal levels after about 10 to 14 days. In contrast to GnRH agonists, the effect of **GnRH antagonists** is immediate. They block the release of gonadotropins from the pituitary gland. After discontinuation of antagonist treatment, natural stimulation of the pituitary by hypothalamic GnRH and the release of LH and FSH resume immediately.

Stimulation Protocols

GnRH agonists and antagonists are used in **three different protocols** for COS in the context of IVF treatment. For ovarian stimulation, in addition to hMG, the newer recombinant gonadotropins are available as original preparations or as biosimilars (◘ Table 6.2). The treatment cycle can be scheduled for the desired time with a preceding pill cycle.

One protocol for COS is the so-called **long protocol** (◘ Fig. 6.2). Adjunctive treatment is performed with a **GnRH agonist**. This is available as an injection or nasal spray for daily administration and as a depot for single administration. The GnRH agonist is started 10 to 14 days before the start of stimulation, i.e., in the preceding cycle. Daily agonist administration is continued until ovulation induction, about three to four weeks later. To avoid ovarian cysts triggered by the "flare-up effect," treatment with a GnRH agonist should begin in the luteal phase or while taking the pill. After the onset of withdrawal bleeding, which occurs about ten days after starting the agonist, gonadotropin stimulation should only begin after hormone and ultrasound monitoring to confirm downregulation and exclude cysts. Pregnancy must be ruled out before starting stimulation, as spontaneous pregnancies have repeatedly been observed after starting GnRH agonists before stimulation. The long protocol can only be performed in women with good ovarian reserve. Ovulation induction can only be performed with hCG preparations due to pituitary downregulation. If there is a risk of ovarian hyperstimulation syndrome, discontinuation of treatment before hCG administration should be considered, as excessive follicular growth combined with hCG administration carries a high risk of hyperstimulation syndrome.

In the so-called **short protocol** (◘ Fig. 6.2), the **GnRH agonist** is started daily at the onset of bleeding, around cycle day 1 to 3. Usually, hormone and ultrasound checks are performed to exclude cysts. Gonadotropin stimulation then starts around cycle day 2 to 4. The "flare-up effect" at the beginning of the cycle, with a sharp release of LH and FSH, strongly supports gonadotropin stimulation. GnRH agonist treatment is continued until ovulation is triggered. Stimulation with the short protocol is an option for women with low ovarian reserve. Due to downregulation, ovulation induction, as in the long protocol, can only be performed with hCG preparations.

In the **antagonist protocol**, gonadotropin stimulation is started on the second or third day of the cycle, usually after cyst exclusion and hormone monitoring (◘ Fig. 6.2). Depending on the progress of stimulation, daily administration of **GnRH antagonists** is started around the sixth day of stimulation and continued until the day of ovulation induction. Downregulation with the risk of hormone deficiency symptoms, as in the long protocol, does not occur, and the duration of hormone therapy is limited to the period of gonadotropin stimula-

tion. The antagonist protocol can be used in any woman. Today, this protocol is the most commonly used in fertility centers. In women with a high **risk of hyperstimulation**, this protocol is used because ovulation can be triggered not only with hCG but also with a single dose of a GnRH agonist. A high risk of OHSS is avoided, as agonist administration triggers natural ovulation via the body's own LH through the "flare-up effect."

Individualized Therapy Options

When planning an IVF cycle, individual prognostic factors, the patient's fears and wishes, and the course of previous treatment cycles must be taken into account. Women often have concerns about hormone treatment and, despite limited chances of success, wish to undergo IVF in a natural cycle. In a spontaneous cycle, however, ovulation induction with hCG cannot be omitted in IVF treatment, as oocyte retrieval should be performed about 36 +/− 2 hours after ovulation is triggered. Otherwise, there is a high risk that no fertilizable MII oocytes can be obtained during retrieval (see above). If a woman has previously experienced severe ovarian hyperstimulation syndrome during IVF treatment, recurrence of this serious complication can be ruled out in a natural cycle. Alternatively, controlled ovarian stimulation can also be proposed using the GnRH antagonist protocol. The risk of OHSS is minimal in this protocol if ovulation is triggered by a single dose of a GnRH agonist, since, unlike ovulation induction with hCG, a bolus of a GnRH agonist triggers ovulation via the natural LH surge (Itskovitz-Eldor et al. 2000). Many women with PCOS also benefit from stimulation in the GnRH antagonist protocol, as they are prone to hyperstimulation syndrome. However, embryo transfer after ovulation induction with a GnRH agonist should generally be postponed to a later thaw cycle.

Procedure for IVF and ICSI

An IVF cycle is complex and expensive. Therefore, such treatment should be well planned in terms of timing, so that it is feasible for both the couples and the fertility center (◘ Fig. 6.4). In addition, the number of embryos to be transferred should be actively discussed during planning. To achieve the goal of a singleton pregnancy, transfer of a single embryo is usually recommended, depending on prognostic factors such as age. An IVF cycle can be divided into five phases: pre-cycle (1), stimulation (2), follicular puncture (3), embryo transfer (4), and pregnancy test (5).

In the **pre-cycle**, the stimulation protocol and the start of stimulation are determined. In the short protocol and the antagonist protocol, the start of stimulation depends on the expected menstrual period. However, the start of the cycle can also be modified by using an oral contraceptive (e.g., cycle extension with the pill). In the long protocol, the onset of bleeding can be delayed by about a week if the GnRH agonist is started in the luteal phase and not while on the pill, because the "flare-up effect" temporarily stimulates the corpus luteum and can prolong the luteal phase.

Ovarian **stimulation** is usually performed after cyst exclusion and hormone monitoring for about 10 to 12 days. The subcutaneous self-injections are usually administered in the evening (◘ Fig. 6.4). The goal is for several (about six to eight) follicles to mature. Two to three **monitoring appointments** should be scheduled to monitor follicle maturation. These are useful for checking the hormone dose, as an insufficient dose may result in only a few follicles growing. If only two to three follicles mature, the IVF cycle is often canceled due to the lower chances of success. An excessively high hormone dose can also lead to cycle cancellation, as this increases the risk of OHSS. Ovulation is usually triggered with hCG. In the case of impending ovarian hyperstimulation syndrome, ovulation can alternatively be triggered with an agonist only in the an-

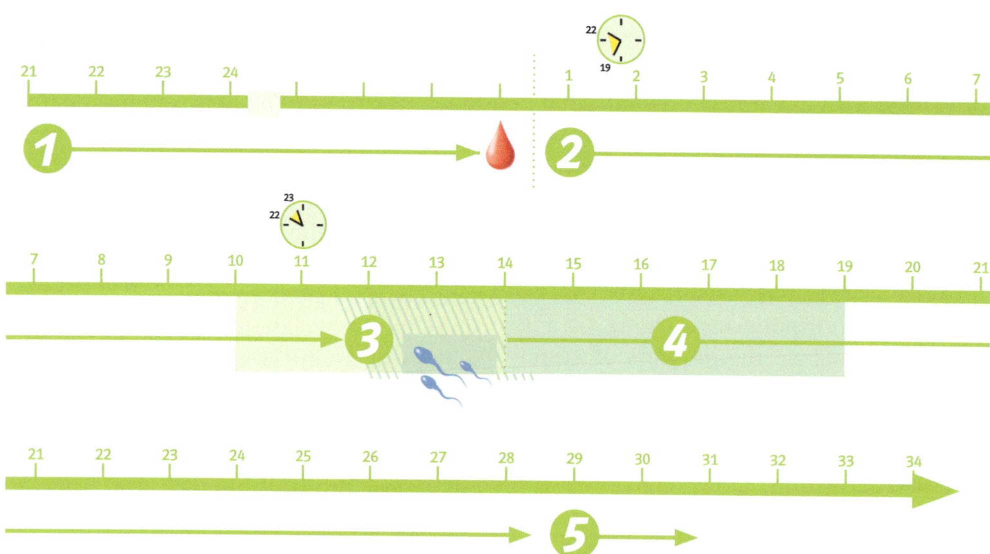

◘ **Fig. 6.4** Timeline of the IVF treatment. 1: Pre-cycle, 2: Stimulation treatment, 3: Follicular puncture, 4: Embryo transfer, 5: Pregnancy test

tagonist protocol (see above). After about 10 to 12 days of stimulation, the so-called "**trigger ultrasound**" is performed to check whether enough follicles with a diameter of at least 15 mm have developed. If this goal is achieved, follicle aspiration and sperm collection for IVF treatment can be scheduled together with the ART laboratory.

The exact timing of **follicle aspiration** is determined by the "**trigger injection**." The trigger medication must be injected in the evening exactly 36 hours before the planned oocyte retrieval. For example, if follicle aspiration is scheduled for 10 a.m. two days later, the trigger medication must be administered at 10 p.m. the evening before (◘ Fig. 6.4). If the medication is injected a few hours early, the follicles may have already ruptured before aspiration. If the medication is injected late, the oocytes may not yet be in metaphase II and thus not fertilizable. It may also not be possible to retrieve the oocytes during follicle aspiration, as they may not yet have detached from the follicle wall. Follicular puncture takes about five to ten minutes and is performed on an outpatient basis, usually under short anesthesia (◘ Fig. 6.3). First, the sperm sample is collected at the center, followed by oocyte retrieval. The aspiration is performed transvaginally under ultrasound guidance. Oocytes, as the largest cells in the human body, are very sensitive. Therefore, they must be immediately transferred to prepared culture dishes in the laboratory, warmed in the incubator, and then prepared for subsequent IVF or ICSI treatment. The patient is discharged about two hours after aspiration. During the **post-procedure consultation**, the hormones for luteal phase support are finally determined. For organizational reasons, the date for the pregnancy test is often scheduled about 15 days after oocyte retrieval. The date for embryo transfer is set if fertilization has occurred as expected.

The **fertilization check of the oocytes** is performed one day after aspiration and oocyte treatment with IVF or ICSI (◘ Fig. 1.2). In this so-called "**PN check**", it is checked whether the oocytes are fertilized. As evidence of fertilization, the two pronuclei must be clearly visible and the second polar body must be extruded. Patients are usually informed of the PN check results by phone. At this point, the couple's decision is confirmed as to whether one embryo, and in exceptional cases two (maximum three) embryos, should be transferred. The timing of the **embryo transfer** is also determined according to the desired culture duration. According to the couple's decision and prognostic criteria, as many PN cells are cultured as needed so that one embryo or two (maximum three) embryos are available at transfer (see ▶ Chap. 1). Embryo transfer is performed under sterile conditions, e.g., in a procedure room. First, under ultrasound guidance, the transfer sheath is advanced through the cervical canal (◘ Fig. 6.3). Then, one or more embryos are loaded into the catheter. This is immediately advanced through the transfer sheath into the upper third of the uterine cavity. Embryos are transferred in a small drop of culture medium. The position of the transferred embryos can be visualized indirectly on ultrasound, as air bubbles are also transferred during the procedure. These should appear as bright echoes in the upper third of the uterine cavity immediately after transfer. As a precaution, the ART laboratory flushes the embryo transfer catheter after the procedure to ensure that no embryo has remained in the catheter. If this is the case, the embryo transfer is repeated.

The **pregnancy test** is usually performed 15 to 17 days after follicular puncture using a blood sample. HCG values > 5 U/L are considered evidence of a **biochemical pregnancy**. If the measured hCG value is in the low range below 25 to 50 U/L, a repeat test is recommended within 2 to 10 days. If hCG levels fall, luteal phase support is discontinued. The resulting hormone drop leads to withdrawal bleeding. Sonographic evidence of a **clinical pregnancy** with visualization of a **chorionic cavity** (gestational sac) is usually possible two to three weeks after the pregnancy test.

Frozen Embryo Transfer (FET) Cycles

In a frozen embryo transfer (FET) cycle, embryos are transferred that have developed from fertilized eggs after a thawing procedure. These were obtained in a previous IVF cycle and cryopreserved.

Cryopreservation and Freezing Methods

Cryopreservation is nowadays an essential component of **fertility treatment** for both women and men. This laboratory method is a prerequisite for establishing a depot of oocytes and sperm for **fertility preservation** and for **social freezing**. Oocytes and developed fertilized oocytes from the pronuclear stage to the blastocyst are now predominantly cryopreserved using the so-called **vitrification (glassification)** method. With this technique of ultra-rapid freezing, the cells are frozen within fractions of a second, preventing the

formation of cell-damaging ice crystals. Oocytes, being the largest cells in the body, are more sensitive than sperm, which are still mainly cryopreserved using the so-called **"slow freezing"** method, which achieves good "revival rates." In this technique, the cells are gradually cooled over about two hours down to minus 196 degrees. Cryopreserved oocytes and sperm are stored in liquid nitrogen tanks at minus 196 degrees. In some cases, **storage** also takes place in the vapor phase of liquid nitrogen at minus 150 degrees.

Indications for Cryopreservation

Cryopreservation of unfertilized and fertilized oocytes is important for the **health protection** of **women** undergoing fertility treatment. This method allows the **fertilization** of oocytes to be **postponed** or enables cells to be cryopreserved for an **additional embryo transfer**. This can help avoid repeated stimulations with an OHSS risk and follicle punctures with the general risks of surgery and anesthesia. Oocytes can also be preserved for later fertilization in stimulation and puncture cycles if they are retrieved but unexpectedly cannot be fertilized (◘ Table 6.3). If, in

◘ **Table 6.3**   Cryopreservation of oocytes and embryos as (additional) treatment in ART ("FoPu" = follicular puncture, "d" = day or days)

Time point	matureoocytes, fertilized oocytes, "unplanned" embryos
FoPu	mature oocytes, if no sperm available for egg cell treatment
FoPu	mature oocytes, if no motile sperm available for egg cell treatment
FoPu	mature oocytes for fertility preservation
FoPu	mature oocytes for social freezing
FoPu +1 d	2-PN cells (fertilized egg cells) for fertility preservation
FoPu +1 d	2-PN cells (fertilized egg cells) if surplus
FoPu +1 d	2-PN cells (fertilized egg cells) according to the motto "one and done"
FoPu +1–5 d	2-PN cells or embryos in case of ovarian hyperstimulation (OHSS) risk
FoPu +2–5 d	"Unplanned" embryos in blastocyst culture (to avoid multiples)
+5 d	Preimplantation genetic diagnosis (trophectoderm biopsy TED)

a puncture cycle, there are more fertilized and developmentally competent surplus cells, these can also be used for a later additional embryo transfer. However, less than 50% of couples currently take advantage of cryopreservation, as it is **expensive** and cells are not always available for cryopreservation.

An embryo transfer in a fresh cycle should not be postponed without a medical reason such as impending OHSS. Currently, in about 11% of puncture cycles with egg cell treatment, all fertilized egg cells are frozen instead of performing an embryo transfer in the fresh cycle (D·I·R Annual Report 2024). This now high proportion of **"Freeze All"** raises the suspicion that stimulation treatment is no longer sufficiently individualized and that postponing embryo transfer in the fresh cycle is necessary to reduce the OHSS risk. However, couples generally wish to become pregnant as quickly as possible and to avoid unnecessary costs for cryopreservation and a FET-cycle.

Significance of FET Cycles in Fertility Therapy

The proportion of FET cycles is now high among treatment cycles involving assisted reproduction. About **34%** of the **treatment cycles** documented in the DIR are **FET cycles** with pronuclear stages or embryos (D·I·R Annual Report 2023). The number of cycles with **"fertilization after egg cell thawing"** is still low but increasing. Of these approximately 500 cycles per year, 25% are now performed after prior egg cryopreservation for social freezing or fertility preservation (D·I·R Annual Report 2023). However, unfertilized egg cells are not only cryopreserved as planned for an egg cell depot, but also unexpectedly in puncture cycles when, for unforeseen reasons, no sperm are available for fertilization (see above). Such unexpected situations arise when the

man is unable to provide an ejaculate at the time of follicle puncture, or when no or no suitable sperm can be found in the semen or in surgically retrieved testicular tissue (◘ Table 6.3). Advances in freezing and thawing methods have also improved the **success rate** in the **FET cycle**. Pregnancy rates are now comparable at about 30% per embryo transfer in both FET cycle and the so-called fresh cycle. If the cumulative pregnancy rate is calculated from several embryo transfers from a single follicle puncture, 50% of couples can expect the birth of a child after a fresh transfer and at least two subsequent embryo transfers (D·I·R Annual Reports 2023).

Basic Principle of the FET Cycle

In theFET cycle, the age of the thawed fertilized **egg cells** must be **synchronized with the developmental age of the endometrium**, calculated from the time of ovulation. Cryopreserved pronuclear stages are thawed one day after ovulation and cultured for one to four days until the four-cell stage or blastocyst. A four-cell embryo is transferred two days after ovulation, and a blastocyst five days after ovulation into the uterine cavity (◘ Fig. 6.5). At these times, the endometrium is receptive for implantation, as it has already matured or transformed for two or five days after ovulation due to rising progesterone levels. To determine the correct time for thawing, a FET cycle must be planned with cycle monitoring.

Transfer after a thaw treatment can be performed not only in an artificial cycle (**hormonal endometrial preparation**) but also in a **stimulated cycle** or in a natural cycle (**spontaneous cycle**). In the modified spontaneous cycle, the natural LH surge is not awaited; instead, ovulation is triggered with hCG. In principle, **pregnancy rates** do not differ between the three options for prepar-

6

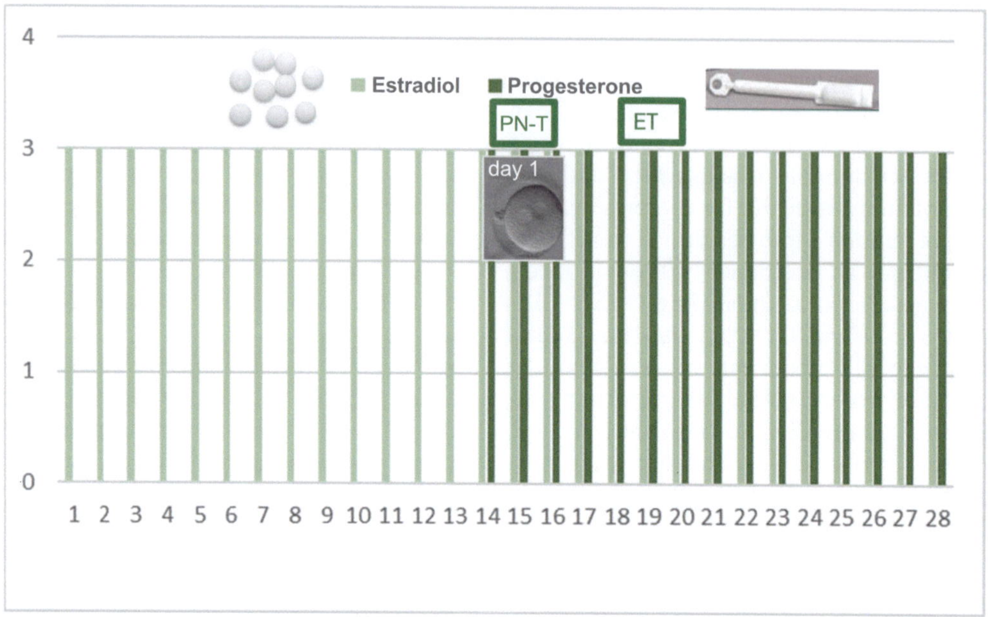

◘ Fig. 6.5 Standard protocol for hormonal endometrial preparation: thawing of pronuclear stages. PN-T (PN thawing), ET (embryo transfer)

ing a thaw treatment. However, with **hormonal endometrial preparation**, the **miscarriage rate** and the **cesarean section rate** are eight to nine percent higher than in the natural or stimulated cycle (D·I·R Annual Report 2022). There are, however, indications for hormonal endometrial preparation where no alternative preparation for embryo transfer after thawing is possible (◘ Table 6.4). This indication applies to women with congenital or acquired loss of ovarian function, such as after chemotherapy or after oophorectomy.

The absence of the corpus luteum after hormonal endometrial preparation may pose a **health risk** for **mothers** and **children**. An increased rate of preeclampsia (gestosis) has been reported. For this reason as well, **thaw treatment** is currently preferably **recommended in the spontaneous cycle** or in the **stimulated cycle** (Epelboin et al. 2023). As shown by the special analysis of the D·I·R, the proportion of natural cycles almost doubled in the short interval from 2020 to 2022 (D·I·R Annual Report 2023). At the same time, the proportion of cycles

◘ Table 6.4   Indications for hormonal endometrial preparation for FET cycles

Indication	Reasons
Ovaries absent	after surgical treatment for malignant and benign ovarian tumors
naturally ceased ovarian function	due to age, chromosomal disorders such as Ullrich-Turner syndrome, developmental disorders, etc.
ceased ovarian function after medical treatments	tumor therapy (radiation therapy, chemotherapy), treatments with cytotoxic drugs, e.g., for rheumatism
absent ovulation	as a cost-effective alternative to hormonal stimulation

with hormonal endometrial preparation has slightly decreased. In the D·I·R analyses, the methods of endometrial preparation are usually not differentiated in thaw treatments.

Hormonal Endometrial Preparation

In hormonal endometrial preparation, also called artificial (artificial) cycle, the **hormone profile** for **estrogen** and **progesterone** in the natural cycle is **mimicked** by sequential hormone therapy. This means that from the beginning of the cycle, an estrogen preparation is given for 28 days to build up the endometrium, and from day 15, a **progesterone preparation** is additionally administered. This causes the **endometrium** to undergo secretory transformation and become **receptive** for embryo implantation. This means that pronuclear stages are thawed on the second day of additional progesterone treatment and, after one to four days of embryo culture, are transferred as four-cell embryos or already as blastocysts (◘ Fig. 6.5). The **pregnancy test** is performed on day 28. A prerequisite for thawing is that the endometrium is sufficiently built up. If the endometrium is less than 6 mm thick on ultrasound, estrogen treatment alone can be extended by about seven days. If the endometrium does not continue to build up, the cycle must be canceled. Usually, a pill preparation is given for 10 to 14 days to induce bleeding. A new FET cycle can be started from the onset of bleeding. Estrogen can be administered as a tablet, gel, or hormone patch. Progesterone is usually applied vaginally as a capsule, tablet, or gel, but can also be given as an injection.

Advantages of hormonal endometrial preparation include good **planning ability** for both the patient and the center, as weekends, holidays, and vacations can be accommodated by extending the estrogen phase and thus delaying the start of additional progesterone administration. In addition, the effort required from the patient is low and **cost-effective**, as monitoring is usually limited to a single ultrasound to determine endometrial thickness. However, there are also **disadvantages**: **Estrogen-progesterone therapy** must be continued until the **12th week of pregnancy**, as ovulation usually does not occur due to the hormone therapy. Thus, the corpus luteum is absent for endogenous progesterone and estrogen production in the ovary. If substitution therapy with estrogen and progesterone is discontinued prematurely, bleeding occurs and the pregnancy is usually lost. In addition, despite estrogen therapy from the onset of bleeding and the associated suppression of follicle maturation, **ovulation** can still occur. In this case, a corpus luteum can usually be visualized on ultrasound and a rise in progesterone can be measured in the blood sample. If this goes unnoticed, the synchronization of endometrial maturity with embryo age is lost. Pregnancy then does not occur.

Thaw Treatment in the Spontaneous or Stimulated Cycle

In thaw treatment in the spontaneous or stimulated cycle, there is a risk of **additional "in vivo pregnancies."** Therefore, protected intercourse is generally recommended during this preparation. Thaw treatment in the spontaneous cycle means that the **day of ovulation** must be determined precisely so that the timing of thawing can be synchronized with endometrial maturity. This requires **extended cycle monitoring** with increased effort for the patient. Usually, repeated ultrasound examinations and measurements of estradiol and LH levels are necessary until the LH surge, so that thawing can be performed in the appropriate cycle phase. When the LH surge occurs, ovulation is the following day. Accordingly, pronuclear stages must be thawed two days after the LH surge. In practice, the **modified**

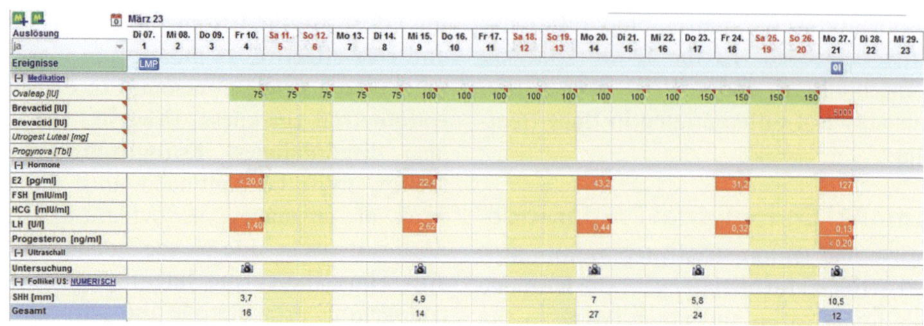

März 23

Auslösung / ja	Di 07. / 1	Mi 08. / 2	Do 09. / 3	Fr 10. / 4	Sa 11. / 5	So 12. / 6	Mo 13. / 7	Di 14. / 8	Mi 15. / 9	Do 16. / 10	Fr 17. / 11	Sa 18. / 12	So 19. / 13	Mo 20. / 14	Di 21. / 15	Mi 22. / 16	Do 23. / 17	Fr 24. / 18	Sa 25. / 19	So 26. / 20	Mo 27. / 21	Di 28. / 22	Mi 29. / 23
Ereignisse	LMP																				OI		
[–] Medikation																							
Ovaleap [IU]				75	75	75	75	75	100	100	100	100	100	100	100	100	100	150	150	150	150		
Brevactid [IU]																					5000		
Brevactid [IU]																							
Utrogest Luteal [mg]																							
Progynova [Tbl]																							
[–] Hormone																							
E2 [pg/ml]				< 20,0					22,4					43,2					31,2		127		
FSH [mIU/ml]																							
HCG [mIU/ml]																							
LH [U/l]				1,40					2,62					0,44					0,32		0,13		
Progesteron [ng/ml]																					< 0,20		
[–] Ultraschall																							
Untersuchung				🔍					🔍					🔍			🔍				🔍		
[–] Follikel US: NUMERISCH																							
SHH [mm]				3,7					4,9					7			5,8				10,5		
Gesamt				16					14					27			24				12		

Fig. 6.6 Stimulated FET cycle in a PCOS patient (hCG on cycle day 21 with 19 mm follicle, ovulation on cycle day 23, thawing of PN cells on cycle day 24). LMP (last menstrual period), OI (ovulation induction)

6

spontaneous cycle is usually performed, often requiring only one monitoring appointment. This takes place about one to two days before the expected ovulation. If a pre-ovulatory follicle of at least 15 mm in diameter and an endometrial thickness of at least 6 mm are measured, ovulation can be triggered in the evening with hCG (◘ Table 6.2). **Ovulation induction**, for example on cycle day 13, means that ovulation occurs on day 15 and pronuclear stages are thawed on day 16. Embryo transfer would then take place according to the culture duration on day 17 for a four-cell embryo or on day 20 for a blastocyst. The **pregnancy test** can be reliably performed no earlier than 14 days after ovulation.

Thaw treatment is also possible in the **stimulated cycle**. The goal is monofollicular growth. If multiple follicles develop, no interventions are necessary in the absence of OHSS risk, as protected intercourse is strictly recommended anyway to avoid additional "in vivo pregnancies." At the start of stimulation, a low-dose hormone therapy with 37.5 to 75 IU hMG or FSH should be individually selected. Monitoring is performed as in ovarian stimulation. The duration of stimulation may also be prolonged, e.g., in PCOS patients, as the ovaries often only respond to hormone ther-

apy after reaching the individual threshold dose, and ovulation may, for example, only be triggered on cycle day 21 (◘ Fig. 6.6). In a stimulated cycle, the endometrium may build up better due to higher estrogen and progesterone levels. This could improve the conditions for successful implantation. Future registry analyses will show whether a stimulated cycle leads to higher pregnancy and birth rates.

Andrological Therapy Prior to ART Methods

The basic principle in reproductive medicine is: If the man is infertile, the woman is treated, since in ART the hormonal treatments and surgical interventions are performed on the woman. However, **fertilizable sperm cells** must be available for these treatments. There are only a few **exceptions** in which the male fertility disorder can be **causally treated** (◘ Table 6.5). If the man has not already been referred by a physician with additional training in andrology, it is the responsibility of the reproductive medicine specialist to identify these exceptional situations through basic andrological diagnostics (hormone levels and semen analysis with culture). If abnormalities are found,

◻ Table 6.5 Male fertility disorders with therapeutic options

Disorder	Impact on fertility, therapeutic approaches
Infections	Treatment of sexually transmitted pathogens (e.g., chlamydia, Gardnerella vaginalis)
Ejaculation disorders	Specialist co-management, e.g., in aspermia due to spinal cord injury, retrograde ejaculation, psychological causes
Substance abuse, medications	Cessation or discontinuation, e.g., nicotine and alcohol, anabolic steroids and antiandrogens
Metabolic disorders, obesity	e.g., management of diabetes mellitus, weight reduction
Varicocele	Specialist co-management, impairment of fertility due to increased temperature and fragmentation of genetic material (DNA)
Obstruction of the seminal tract	Surgical therapy, e.g., after infections, in cases of malformations, after vasectomy
Hormone deficiency	Stimulation with FSH and hCG in the presence of functional testicular tissue

further diagnostics and therapy should be carried out by an andrologist.

Antibiotics for Sexually Transmitted Infections (STI)

The **microbiological ejaculate diagnostics** for chlamydia and Gardnerella vaginalis as sexually transmitted pathogens is also useful in parallel with the microbiological diagnostics in the woman, since infections are not only an infection risk during vaginal follicle puncture, but especially in in vitro fertilization also pose a risk of contamination of the **oocyte culture**. An infection can also disrupt implantation after embryo transfer. In addition, infections are known causes of miscarriage. Gardnerella vaginalis can also **reduce sperm motility** and **sperm morphology** and trigger **apoptosis** (cell death) (Damke et al. 2018). Sperm concentration and motility can significantly improve after antibiotic treatment (Goulart et al. 2020). For these reasons, if chlamydia or Gardnerella are detected, **antibiotic therapy** as a **couple's treatment** should be recommended, even in the absence of symptoms.

Treatment of Ejaculation Disorders

Ejaculation disorders can have either an organic or psychological cause. In **aspermia** (see ◻ Tables 5.1 and 5.6), there is no ejaculation. This disorder is known to occur in spinal cord injury, but also in chronic neurological diseases such as multiple sclerosis and diabetes mellitus. Often, **penile vibratory stimulation** can be used to stimulate the nerve fibers. The ejaculate that drips from the urethra can be collected and used for insemination. If this method fails, **transrectal electroejaculation** is recommended in cases of spinal cord injury. Anesthesia is usually not necessary due to the spinal cord injury. Only a few medical facilities, such as trauma clinics, have experience with this treatment method. In **retrograde ejaculation**, ejaculation occurs into the bladder. This ejaculation disorder is a typical complication after radical prostate surgery, which impairs the bladder musculature. Two out of three prostate patients are affected. Medication can be used in an attempt to ensure that the bladder neck closes sufficiently for sperm emission. If unsuccessful, urine can be alkalinized with medication and sperm retrieved from the urine after masturbation. The quality of the sperm obtained is rarely sufficient. In these cases, sperm obtained after **sperm preparation from urine** can be used for insemination or for IVF with ICSI. Conservative treatment options for aspermia or retrograde ejaculation are often unsuccessful, or transrectal electroejaculation is not available. In these cases, sperm can be surgically retrieved from the testis (see below).

In cases of **psychogenic ejaculation disorder**, co-management by a sexual medicine specialist is recommended. The request for sperm collection at the time of ovulation or follicle puncture often leads to failure to ejaculate during masturbation attempts in sensitive patients. To reduce stress from the treatment situation during IUI or in vitro fertilization, **relaxation techniques** can be helpful. If no sperm can be obtained at the time of IVF, the retrieved oocytes can be frozen for a postponed oocyte treatment. Sperm can also be cryopreserved in advance of a treatment procedure. This can relieve patients, as **cryosperm** samples can be thawed and used at the time of IUI or IVF and ICSI, ensuring that oocyte treatment can proceed.

Lifestyle Interventions and Cessation of Medication Abuse

Fertility can also be impaired by an unhealthy **lifestyle** and **lifestyle medications**. Smoking reduces fertility, even if ejaculate parameters such as concentration, motility, and morphology are not directly reduced and may still be within the normal range. It is believed that nicotine abuse damages the genetic material in sperm cells and impairs embryo development and the developmental potential of embryos. This explains why nicotine abuse, especially in IVF treatment, halves the pregnancy rate by more than 50% (Zitzmann and Nieschlag 2004). **Nicotine abstinence** improves fertility in the long term. Medications can also impair sperm quality. Self-medication with **anabolic steroids** among bodybuilders even more frequently leads to azoospermia. Anabolic steroids suppress LH and FSH secretion, resulting in a lack of stimulation of spermatogenesis. Finasteride is a medication associated with decreased sperm quality and increased genetic damage in the form of DNA fragmentation. It is an inhibitor of the potent testosterone derivative dihydrotestosterone (DHT) and is used against hair loss. Only a thorough medical history with targeted review of medication use can reliably identify a medication-induced cause of fertility disorder, which can be resolved by **discontinuing** the **harmful medication**. Unhealthy diet and lack of exercise are the main causes of overweight and obesity. According to regular studies by the Robert Koch Institute (RKI) and the Federal Statistical Office (Destatis), over 60% of men in Germany are overweight. More than 20% of young men up to 39 years old are already obese. Obesity is a risk factor for prediabetes and type 2 diabetes mellitus. Elevated blood glucose levels (hyperglycemia) are toxic to cells. Oocytes, as the largest cells in the human body, are particularly sensitive, but sperm cells and the germinal epithelium in the seminiferous tubules are also sensitive to cell-damaging influences. Overweight and obese men should therefore be advised on **dietary changes** and **physical training**, possibly with **medication support**. Affected patients should seek professional advice about the "weight loss injection" such as Wegovy® or Ozempic®. Type 2 diabetes mellitus should be identified as part of obesity counseling by cooperating physicians or general practitioners and should be optimally managed in cases of fertility desire to allow recovery of spermatogenesis. The same applies to patients with already diagnosed type 2 diabetes. Blood glucose control can be easily checked in the fertility center by determining HbA1c (blood sugar memory) in a blood sample.

Varicocele Treatment

If a **varicocele** is diagnosed during specialist clinical-andrological examination, it should be treated surgically if symptoms (pain, pressure sensation) are present. If the varicocele is asymptomatic, there is an unfulfilled desire for children, and a semen analysis is abnormal, andrologists, urologists, radiologists, and reproductive medicine specialists should decide interdisciplinarily whether varicocele treatment should be offered to the patient. Relative indications for such a surgical intervention are mainly an abnormal semen analysis, previous unsuccessful artificial inseminations, or increased DNA fragmentation. However, an increase in pregnancy success after varicocele therapy has not been proven. Surgical treatment of a varicocele is performed through a small incision in the groin, by injecting a liquid into the dilated vessel (obliteration or sclerotherapy), by inserting small metal coils ("coils"), or by using a tissue adhesive (embolization).

Hormone Therapy in Failure of Hypothalamus and Pituitary

A **hormone deficiency** with **functional testicular tissue** is rare. Affected patients present with azoospermia and low ejaculate volume. Hormone analysis shows low levels of the regulatory hormones LH and FSH and a reduced testosterone level. These patients can usually be successfully treated with testicular stimulation therapy alone and can have their own child. The indications for gonadotropin stimulation in central hypogonadism are the same as in women (◙ Table 6.6). In **isolated hypogonadotropic hypogonadism (IHH)** and in **Kallmann syndrome**, the hormone deficiency is due to the absence of GnRH signals from the hypothalamus. As a result, the pituitary is no longer stimulated, and the release of the regulatory hormones LH and FSH from the pituitary ceases. Testosterone production and sperm maturation in the testicular tissue stop, and testicular volume decreases. In contrast to IHH, Kallmann syndrome is a genetic disorder associated with olfactory disturbance and loss of hypothalamic GnRH secretion. It usually affects men (1:10,000) and less frequently women (1:50,000). A prolactin-producing pituitary tumor (**prolactinoma**) can also lead to loss of LH and FSH and thus to infertility. The tumor is rare in men, is generally benign, but grows expansively. Depending on tu-

◙ **Table 6.6**   Indication for gonadotropin stimulation in women and men

Diagnosis	Level of brain structure failure
isolated hypogonadotropic hypogonadism (IHH)	Hypothalamus (idiopathic)
Kallmann syndrome (with additional olfactory disturbance)	Hypothalamus (genetic)
Pituitary adenoma (hormone-active or -inactive)	Pituitary
Prolactinoma (microprolactinoma <1 cm)	Pituitary (special form of pituitary adenoma)
Hypopituitarism	Pituitary (e.g., postoperative, trauma, radiation)

▣ Table 6.7 Differences in gonadotropin stimulation in men and women

Woman	Man
Ovulation induction (OI) and triggering, for IVF or ICSI treatment controlled ovarian stimulation (COS), stimulation goal approx. 6–8 mature follicles	Stimulate sperm maturation
Stimulation duration approx. 10–12 days (maturation of antral follicles)	Stimulation duration at least 6 months to >1 year
FSH sufficient for stimulation, LH added in case of gonadotropin deficiency (rare)	FSH and hCG (as a substitute for LH) necessary
Prescription according to the guidelines of the Federal Joint Committee	Prescription by urologists, andrologists
Repeated monitoring of ovarian stimulation with ultrasound and hormone measurement	Monitoring every 3 months: clinical, hormone measurement, semen analysis

mor size, this leads to loss of pituitary gonadotropin secretion with testicular inactivity. Depending on the clinical situation, gonadotropin stimulation may be considered in cases of fertility desire. However, drug therapy of the tumor is carried out as in women with a dopamine agonist (see ▶ Chap. 4). Pituitary surgery is considered in cases of compression of the optic chiasm with visual field defects and in case of failure or intolerance of drug therapy. There are surgical centers for pituitary surgery. The operation is performed through the nose. After pituitary surgery, radiation therapy, or trauma (e.g., pituitary stalk transection), complete loss of pituitary function can occur. This complete loss of pituitary function is also referred to as **panhypopituitarism**. In this case, not only male hormones but also the vital hormones of the thyroid and adrenal glands must be replaced. In cases of failure of the hypothalamus and/or pituitary, interdisciplinary management and therapy should always be carried out together with specialists in internal medicine and endocrinology.

Testicular Gonadotropin Stimulation

In cases of fertility desire, **gonadotropin stimulation** is performed with the same medications as in women, but there are differences (▣ Table 6.7). In men, FSH preparations are administered three times per week at a dose of 150 IU (e.g., Mondays, Wednesdays, and Fridays) and hCG twice per week at a dose of 1,500 to 2,500 IU (e.g., Mondays and Fridays). FSH is necessary for stimulation of spermatogenesis, and hCG serves as a substitute for LH for testosterone production. The treatment is always a long-term therapy lasting at least 6 to 12 months. For therapy monitoring, serial **semen analyses** and **hormone measurements** should be performed at three-month intervals, corresponding to the duration of spermatogenesis. In 90% of cases, spermatogenesis can be successfully initiated. Spontaneous conception occurs in half of the couples. At the time of conception, semen parameters are usually still below the normal range. Testicular stimulation therapy should be discontinued when the partner is continuously pregnant in the 12th week of gestation. Before switching stimulation therapy to **testosterone replacement**, the patient can be offered cryopreservation of the ejaculate. Thus, in the future, if there is a renewed desire for children, **cryopreserved sperm** could be used for fertility treatment without the need to repeat the lengthy and

⬛ Table 6.8	Indications for Surgical Sperm Retrieval
Indication	**Causes of Disorder**
Non-obstructive azoospermia (NOA)	idiopathic, germ cell-damaging tumor therapy, genetic (azoospermia factor, Klinefelter syndrome), testicular malposition, unsuccessful GnRH or gonadotropin stimulation (>12 months) in IHH or pituitary lesions
Obstructive azoospermia (OA)	vasectomy, post-inflammatory (e.g., after STI), malformations of vas deferens and epididymis (e.g., in cystic fibrosis), malformation of the urogenital tract (e.g., after correction of bladder exstrophy)
Aspermia	neurogenic, e.g., spinal cord injury, multiple sclerosis (MS), diabetes mellitus
Retrograde ejaculation	after exhaustion of conservative therapeutic approaches
Relative indication (including necrozoospermia)	e.g., high DNA fragmentation index (DFI), necrozoospermia, psychogenic ejaculatory disorder (after diagnosis and counseling)

expensive stimulation with FSH and hCG. However, ICSI treatment would be preferred, as motility after thawing is usually insufficient for insemination.

Pulsatile GnRH Stimulation

Spermatogenesis in patients with hypothalamic hypogonadism can also be stimulated with GnRH (LutrePulse®). The treatment is similar to that in women, using a mini-infusion pump (pod) controlled by a handheld computer (manager) (see above). The treatment duration, as with gonadotropin stimulation, is at least 6 to 12 months. 5–20 μg **GnRH pulsatile** is administered every 120 minutes. Pulsatile GnRH stimulation mimics natural GnRH secretion. Continuous infusion of GnRH would be unsuccessful, as the GnRH receptors in the pituitary gland would then be "downregulated," making the stimulation therapy ineffective.

Surgical Procedures in Men

The incidence of azoospermia is about one percent. If no conservative treatment options are available, a testicular biopsy may be considered for the surgical retrieval of sperm cells in cases of azoospermia. In 1993, the birth of a child conceived with surgically retrieved sperm from testicular tissue was reported for the first time (Schoysman et al. 1993). The indications for surgical sperm retrieval are summarized in ⬛ Table 6.8.

Congenital and Acquired Causes of Azoospermia

If the testicular tissue is impaired or non-functional, this is referred to as **non-obstructive azoospermia (NOA)**. Spermatogenesis mainly halts at a meiotic stage, for example at the level of spermatocytes (⬛ Figs. 2.2 and 2.5). In most cases, NOA is idiopathic, meaning the cause of the spermatogenesis disorder is unknown. More commonly, a history of undescended testes or chromosomal abnormalities is present. If gene segments are missing in the azoospermia factor region on the Y chromosome (see ▶ Chap. 5), the degree of spermatogenesis impairment depends on the affected gene segments. In some of these cases, the germinal epithelium is completely absent (Sertoli cell-only syndrome, ⬛ Fig. 5.2). If there is a transport disorder with intact testicular tissue, this is referred to as **obstructive azoospermia (OA)**. The causes may be genetic, such as absence of the vas deferens, or acquired, such as obstruction of the vas deferens after vasectomy. After vasectomy, surgical sperm retrieval is indicated if the patient opts against or has had an unsuccessful reversal. In general, the prognosis for successful surgical sperm retrieval is poor in non-obstructive azoospermia and good in obstructive azoospermia. The diagnostic workup prior to surgical sperm retrieval is complex and should be performed in cooperation with an andrologist. In addition to clinical-andrological examination and laboratory diagnostics, **human genetic diagnostics** (chromosome analysis and, if necessary, molecular genetics) are usually recommended (◘ Table 6.9). If abnormalities are found, additional human genetic counseling is recommended. For example, if the man has cystic fibrosis or is a carrier, the couple should receive genetic counseling and the woman should be tested for cystic fibrosis. The aim is to clarify the risk of cystic fibrosis for a child, which should be known to the couple before starting ICSI-TESE treatment. Couples with abnormalities in the azoospermia factor region should also be counseled, as this genetically determined spermatogenesis disorder would be passed on to all sons.

Testicular Sperm Extraction (TESE)

The retrieval of sperm cells from testicular tissue is referred to as testicular sperm extraction (TESE). With the subsequent ICSI method, it is now possible to successfully fertilize oocytes with the still immotile sperm cells from testicular tissue. With the combined **TESE-ICSI treatment**, most affected couples can still have their own child. Unfavorable prognostic factors for TESE are elevated LH and FSH levels, indicating a severe spermatogenesis disorder. The probability of a successful biopsy in such cases is only about 50% (Aljubran et al. 2022). Typically, a testicular biopsy is performed before starting an ICSI cycle. This ensures that sperm cells are available for fertilization at the time of follicular puncture. The tissue should be examined for sperm cells intraoperatively as a **diagnostic-TESE** or fresh TESE. After the testicular biopsy, the tissue samples (biopsies) are preserved for ICSI in the treatment cycle for later "**cryo-TESE**." However, the clinical significance of TESE-ICSI cycles is low. The proportion of these cycles is well below five percent (D·I·R Annual Report 2023). Fertilization, transfer, clinical pregnancy, and birth rates are lower with testicular sperm compared to fresh ejaculate sperm.

◘ **Table 6.9**   Pre-diagnostic Workup before Surgical Sperm Retrieval

Diagnostics	Obstructive Azoospermia (OA)	Non-obstructive Azoospermia (NOA)
Medical history	Surgeries, infections	Undescended testes, tumor therapy
Examination	Vas deferens not palpable	Firm consistency of testes
Ultrasound	Epididymis dilated	Small testicular volume
Ejaculate	Azoospermia, low volume	Azoospermia
Blood	LH, FSH, testosterone normal	LH, FSH elevated, testosterone deficiency
Chromosomes	unremarkable	abnormal, e.g., 47,XXY
Azoospermia factor	unremarkable	abnormal (AZF a-c)
CFTR gene	mutation in cystic fibrosis	unremarkable

Performing a Testicular Biopsy

Testicular biopsies for subsequent ICSI-TESE treatment should preferably be performed by an experienced team of andrologists or urologists and embryologists, ideally in cooperation with a fertility center. The testicular biopsy can be performed as an "open biopsy," allowing for inspection of the testis and epididymis after opening the tunica and exposing the area (Fig. 6.7). Typically, pea-sized tissue samples are taken from the upper and lower poles of each testis. A small portion of the testicular tissue is usually examined intraoperatively for sperm cells (**diagnostic-TESE**). The larger portion of the testicular tissue is divided and cryopreserved for later ICSI treatment. A small tissue sample from each testis should also be examined histologically, preferably using the special semithin section technique (see below).

In cases of non-obstructive azoospermia, the testicular biopsy can be performed under an **operating microscope** to increase the chances of successfully retrieving sperm cells for ICSI-TESE. The testis is exposed, incised circumferentially, and the tissue is examined for dilated seminiferous tubules. In this so-called **micro-TESE**, tubules that appear dilated under the microscope are selectively biopsied, as these are likely to still have active spermatogenesis. Narrow tubules may lack germinal epithelium and should therefore not be biopsied. If suitable sperm cells are found during a testicular biopsy, a promising ICSI-TESE treatment is possible. Morphologically mature sperm cells (spermatozoa) consist of a head, midpiece, and tail. The so-called **round** or **elongated spermatids** as precursors of sperm cells are not yet suitable for ICSI, as they are not sufficiently mature and cannot fertilize oocytes regularly, even with ICSI (Fig. 2.5).

Special Considerations in Testicular Biopsy and Testicular Sperm Extraction (TESE)

Sperm maturation is often unevenly impaired in testicular tissue. In addition to islands of intact spermatogenesis, areas without spermatogenesis can be found. These disturbances can also occur in adjacent

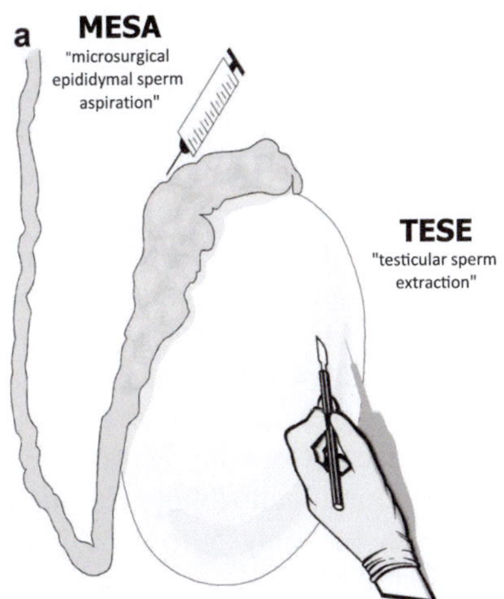

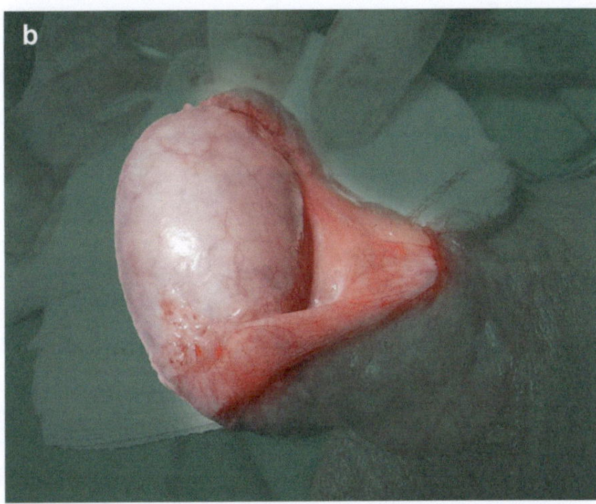

Fig. 6.7 Testicular biopsy for testicular sperm extraction (TESE) and aspiration of sperm from the epididymis (MESA). **a** schematic representation of a testicular biopsy for TESE and MESA; **b** open testicular biopsy

seminiferous tubules, a phenomenon referred to as **"patchy atrophy of spermatogenesis."** For this reason, in non-obstructive azoospermia, biopsies should be taken from two sites in each testis whenever possible. In micro-TESE, the chances for successful TESE in cases of patchy atrophy are maximized.

In obstructive azoospermia, microsurgical epididymal sperm aspiration (**MESA**) can generally be performed. Under the operating microscope, sperm cells are aspirated from the epididymis. This procedure is suitable, for example, after vasectomy. However, it has not become the standard procedure, as MESA should be performed in conjunction with a testicular biopsy and histology, since **testicular tumors** peak in incidence between ages 25 and 45 and can only be reliably detected by tissue examination. This should be performed using semithin section histology, a special method for examining testicular tissue. With this technique, not only malignancies (e.g., seminomas) and their precursors (**intratubular neoplasia**, abbreviated **TIN**) can be reliably diagnosed, but also the exact nature of the spermatogenesis disorder can be determined.

Donor Sperm

Donor (heterologous) inseminations are performed with donor sperm, homologous inseminations with the partner's sperm (see above). Before ICSI or TESE-ICSI treatments became possible, couples with severely impaired semen quality or azoospermia often underwent donor treatment. Prior to the legal revision of preimplantation genetic diagnosis (PGD), couples also more frequently opted for heterologous treatments with donor sperm if the partner was a carrier of a serious hereditary disease and there was a high risk of having a child with the condition. Since the entry into force of the Sperm Donor Registry Act (SaRegG), not only heterosexual couples are treated, but especially **lesbian couples** and increasingly also **single women**. Women in lesbian partnerships or women without a partner can only become pregnant in medical facilities with a donor.

Legal Regulation of Donor Sperm Treatment

In addition to social change and the acceptance of heterologous treatments for lesbian couples and single women, legal certainty has certainly contributed to the increase in treatments. Not only has the Sperm Donor Registry Act (**SaRegG**) been enacted, but an amendment to the Civil Code (**BGB**) has also been made (§ 1600 para. 4). Thus, the legal paternity of a donor is excluded, ending discussions about, for example, maintenance obligations or inheritance claims of a donor child. Previously, there was great concern among all parties about the determination of the donor's legal paternity. It is understandable that physicians previously wanted to protect the identity of their donors.

The essential content of the law for donor children is the regulation of the **right of personality**, as every person has the right to know their origins. This fundamental right is enshrined in Articles 1 and 2 of the Basic Law. Prior to the legislation, donor children repeatedly sued the treating physicians of their mothers and demanded the release of donor records. These were usually no longer available. Many donor children have therefore searched DNA databases for their genetic father or half-siblings, often successfully. Estimates suggest that about 100,000 donor children live in Germany. Most donor children have found half-siblings through DNA databases, but only 5 to 10% have been able to identify their genetic father.

According to the SaRegG, sperm banks are **retrieval facilities (EE)** and sperm cells are considered tissue under the Tissue Act. Donor sperm is collected, cryopreserved, and stored in EEs, and above all, clearly labeled with the **"Single European Code" (SEC)**. Fertility centers are **medical care facilities (EMV)** where patient care takes place. These must enter into a contract with the cooperating sperm bank to delineate responsibilities. Documentation of treatment with donations is carried out at the **German Institute for Medical Documentation and Information (DIMDI)**. The institute is an agency of the Ministry of Health based in Cologne.

According to SaRegG § 3, sperm banks may only supply sperm samples to reproductive medicine centers that are under continuous medical supervision and where medical services are provided by physicians. This regulation is in line with the Transplantation Act § 1a sentence 9 and the Embryo Protection Act § 9 (requirement for physician involvement). Distribution to non-physicians or private individuals is not permitted.

SaRegG § 4 sets out the **information and documentation obligations** for the fertility center (◻ Table 6.10). The law also applies if the sperm samples come from a foreign sperm bank. Contractual agreements between the fertility center as EMV and the foreign sperm bank as EE must ensure that the necessary donor data are provided to DIMDI. The recipient must be informed that she must report the date of birth and the number of children born to the fertility center within three months of delivery. The recipient's counseling prior to sperm donation and her consent to the notifications to DIMDI should be documented in writing (template in Appendix 6.2).

The transmission of stored data according to SaRegG § 5 (◻ Table 6.11) to DIMDI takes place as soon as the recipient has informed the fertility center about the birth and the number of children born. The stored data must also be transmitted if, despite inquiries, the fertility center has not received information about the birth four months after the expected due date (EDD). DIMDI stores the data for 110 years. In the case of unsuccessful AID treatments or six months after data transmission to DIMDI, the fertility center must delete the stored data.

A **right to information** under SaRegG § 10 about the donor is granted only to the person conceived by sperm donation. Sperm donors have no right to information.

◻ **Table 6.10** Information for the Recipient about Sperm Donation according to SaRegG § 4 by the Medical Care Facility (EMV)

Obligations of the EMV	Counseling Content
Counseling	Child's right to information, non-medical counseling on the consequences of sperm donor treatment
Documentation obligation	Family name, maiden name, place of birth, and address of the patient, storage for 10 years
Obligation to transmit	Transmission of data to DIMDI, storage there for 110 years
Provision of information	Obligation of DIMDI to provide information to authorized persons
Donor	Exclusion of the donor's legal paternity (§1600 BGB)
Counseling on information	Procedure for providing information
Patient's obligation	Within 3 months after the birth of the child(ren) with date of birth
Patient's consent	Written confirmation by the patient that everything is understood

□ Table 6.11   Data Collection, Storage for Transmission to DIMDI by the Medical Care Facility (EMV) before and after Donor Sperm Treatment according to SaRegG § 5

Data Collection and Storage	Explanation
Recipient's data	Family name, maiden name, place of birth, and address
EE documentation	Name and address of the retrieval facility (EE) from Germany or abroad
Donations	SEC code of the sperm samples
Treatment data	Time of use IUI/IVF/ICSI, confirmation of pregnancy and expected due date (EDD)
Birth	Date of birth, number of children, if applicable, miscarriage
No notification from recipient	Follow-up with recipient if no information is received, at the latest 4 months after EDD
Deletion of treatment data	6 months after transmission to DIMDI or in case of unsuccessful treatments

However, parents and other legal representatives may assert a right to information before the child turns 16, provided they present the child's birth certificate and copies of their identity cards and, if applicable, proof of legal representation. From the age of 16, a donor child can obtain information about the personal details of their donor by presenting their identity card and birth certificate. When providing information, DIMDI informs donor children or their parents or representatives about the possibility of specific counseling and existing counseling services to prepare for contact. Donors are notified four weeks before a contact attempt by the donor child. If no current address for the donor is available, the donor is not notified. DIMDI stores only data on sperm donations, not on **embryo donations**, which can be legally performed. By analogy with DIMDI, donor data (woman and man) are stored for 110 years by the German Network for Embryo Donation Germany e. V.   (▶ https://www.netzwerk-embryo-nenspende.de) in a cooperating notary's office. The network is a non-profit association and arranges embryo donations.

Outcomes of Donor Treatments

Insemination treatments with donor sperm have doubled in the past five years to nearly 4,000 cycles. The treatment outcomes of AID treatments have so far been disappointing. Since 2022, AID treatments have been documented in the **German Register for Inseminations (DERI)**, with only data from DERI centers being evaluated. Nearly 400 children have been born as a result of these treatments (Hammel et al. 2024). The birth rate, even among younger women up to age 34, is only a maximum of 16% (Hammel et al. 2024). If repeated AID treatment is unsuccessful, a change of method to IVF or ICSI treatment often follows. These have more than doubled from 1,129 cycles in 2018 to 2,610 cycles in 2022 (D·I·R Annual Report 2024, □ Fig. 6.8). In addition, there are patients, e.g., with a tubal factor, who opt primarily for IVF treatment. Since cryopreserved sperm cells show reduced motility after thawing and there may be an increased risk of fertilization failure, some patients choose ICSI over IVF. Fertilization failure in IVF treatment with donor sperm is probably more likely

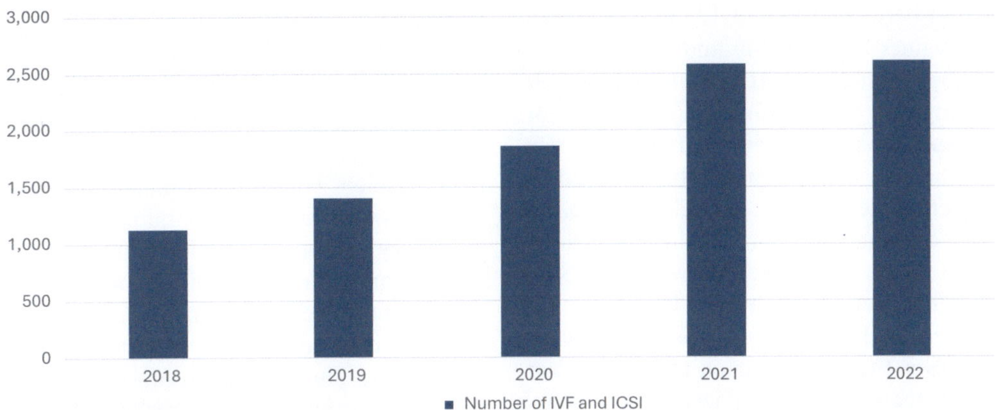

Fig. 6.8 Increase in the number of IVF and ICSI cycles with donor sperm from 2018 to 2022. (According to D·I·R (2024) Annual Report 2023)

due to a previously unknown oocyte factor rather than sperm quality after thawing. Some sperm banks, for this reason, only release their donor samples for ICSI treatments. In 2022, 2,610 heterologous IVF or ICSI treatments were performed with a pregnancy rate of 26.8%. These resulted in 520 births (D·I·R Annual Report 2023). Thus, pregnancy rates for donor treatments are also lower for these ART therapies compared to homologous treatments at 31% in the same period.

Safety of Therapy

The goal of an IVF treatment with hormone therapy, follicle puncture, and embryo transfer in the "fresh cycle" is an ongoing singleton pregnancy resulting in the birth of a **healthy child** while taking into account the **woman's health**. The two most important **quality criteria** for IVF treatment are the live birth rate and the **rate of ovarian hyperstimulation**. Additional indicators include the number of oocytes retrieved, the frequency of cycle cancellation, clinical and ongoing pregnancy rates, miscarriage rate, and the incidence of ectopic pregnancies as well as **multiple pregnancies**.

Glucose Metabolism Disorder as a Maternal and Fetal Risk Factor

A spontaneous pregnancy leads to massive changes in a woman's body. In order for a pregnancy to occur at all, women must be healthy enough for pregnancy. For example, for a **woman with diabetes** to be healthy enough for pregnancy, she should be adjusted to the **target values** for pregnancy already **three months before conception** (Table 6.12). Glucose levels must be measured capillary with a hand-held device calibrated for capillary plasma for pregnancy, or venously with a citrate-prepared Monovette (gray S-Monovette® GlucoEXACT from Sarstedt). With optimal management of a woman with diabetes mellitus, a rapid conception and a more favorable course of pregnancy can be expected.

Metabolic Disorders in Women Seeking Fertility Treatment

Many women seeking fertility treatment today are **overweight** or **obese** and thus often no longer healthy enough for uncomplicated conception and pregnancy, as they more frequently already have **impaired glucose tolerance** with fasting blood glucose values between 100 and 125 and postprandial values between 140 and 199 after a 75 g glucose challenge. It is therefore not surprising that obese women repeatedly report unexpected pregnancies and their **"Ozempic" babies** on social media, having used the diabetes medication semaglutide (Ozempic® or Wegovy®) for weight loss (Nadarajah 2025). Many women with PCOS are also overweight or obese. However, lean women with PCOS are also at risk, as **PCOS** is the **most common metabolic disorder in the reproductive phase** of a woman's life. While women with diabetes mellitus are prepared for pregnancy in terms of their health, this is not the case for women seeking fertility treatment. These women should also receive diabetological care and achieve the target values for pregnancy even before conception. Otherwise, women seeking fertility treatment are at a disadvantage compared to women with diabetes in preparing for pregnancy (◘ Table 6.12). For if women already have impaired glucose tolerance before pregnancy, a diagnosis of **gestational diabetes** would be made during pregnancy (Bals-Pratsch and Fill Malfertheiner 2017). Untreated glucose tolerance disorder is not only a factor in infertility, but also a **risk factor for miscarriage**.

◘ **Table 6.12**   Target blood glucose values in pregnancy

Time	mg/dl	mmol/l
Fasting (preprandial)	65–95	3.3–5.0
1 hour postprandial	<140	<7.7
2 hours postprandial	<120	<6.6

Source: Diabetes and Pregnancy S2e Guideline 2021 (2022) ► https://register.awmf.org/assets/guidelines/057-023l_S2e_Diabetes_und_Schwangerschaft_2022-01.pdf Last accessed 30.3.2025

Metabolic Disorders in the ART Cycle and Early Pregnancy

Every diabetologist knows that in women with diabetes, glucose levels rise at the onset of pregnancy and diabetes therapy must be intensified. Hormonal stimulation for an **IVF treatment** hormonally mimics an **early pregnancy** through polyfollicular oocyte maturation with **excessively elevated estrogen** and **progesterone levels**. In patients with already impaired glucose tolerance, further increases in glucose levels during hormone therapy can trigger diabetes mellitus. **Hyperglycemia** is **toxic** and can damage oocytes, thereby impairing fertilization, implantation, and the development of an ongoing pregnancy. If a pregnancy does occur despite metabolic imbalance, there is an increased risk of severe **malformations** of the **heart** and brain, which are attributable to harmful influences during the calculated fifth and sixth weeks of pregnancy (Bals-Pratsch et al. 2020). Such severe malformations are also known in women with diabetes who were not managed according to therapeutic targets in early pregnancy. Other **maternal** and **fetal risks** associated with metabolic disorders include stillbirth, preterm birth, increased cesarean section rate, and infants with fetal microsomia (growth restriction) or macrosomia (increased birth weight).

Ovarian Hyperstimulation Syndrome (OHSS)

Severe OHSS is a serious and life-threatening complication of controlled ovarian stimulation (COS). Fortunately, the risk of severe OHSS was calculated at only 0.2% per initiated stimulation cycle in the 2023 Annual Report of the German IVF Registry (D·I·R Annual Report 2023). However, it is possible that OHSS cases are not fully reported.

Risk Factors for OHSS

Young patients with many antral follicles or patients with PCOS are particularly at risk of developing OHSS after COS (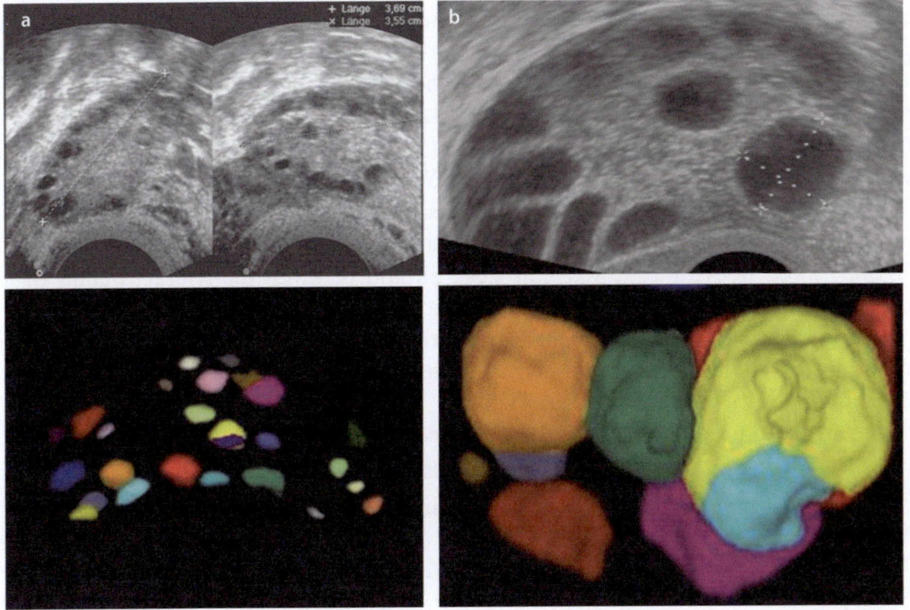 Fig. 6.9), as they usually respond to a standard FSH dose of 150–225 IU with excessive follicular maturation. More than 15 oocytes are often retrieved during follicle puncture. These patients are also referred to as **"high responders"**. When preparing for IVF treatment, prognostic criteria for a "high response" should be assessed to avoid endangering the health of **"high responder"** patients (◩ Table 6.13). This includes, in particular, the biomarkers anti-Müllerian hormone (AMH) and antral follicle count (AFC) (see ▶ Chap. 4). In at-risk patients, individualized stimulation in the antagonist protocol is indicated. In this protocol, ovulation can be triggered with a GnRH agonist to protect

◩ **Fig. 6.9** PCOS ovaries as a risk factor for OHSS before and during stimulation. **a:** polycystic ovary before stimulation in 2D ultrasound (top) and 3D ultrasound (bottom); **b:** stimulated polycystic ovary in 2D ultrasound (top) and 3D ultrasound with automated measurement of follicle size (bottom)

◩ **Table 6.13**   Prognostic factors for "high response" and "low response" in COS

Prognostic factors	High response	Low response
Age	<30 years	>39 years
Clinical findings	PCOS, polyfollicular ovaries	Ovarian surgery, ovarian endometriosis
Number of oocytes in previous follicle punctures	>15 oocytes	≤3 oocytes
Antral follicle count (AFC)	>15	<5–7
Anti-Müllerian hormone (AMH)	>3.5	<1.1 ng/ml

▣ Table 6.14   OHSS classification according to Rizk and Aboulghar (1991)

Severity		Findings
moderate		Ascites and enlarged ovaries
severe	Grade A	enlarged ovaries and marked ascites, normal biochemical profile
	Grade B	Additionally, tense ascites, severe dyspnea, increased hematocrit, creatinine, and liver values
	Grade C	Additionally, complications such as respiratory distress (ARDS), renal failure, and thrombosis

the patient's health if the ovaries respond unexpectedly strongly despite an adjusted stimulation dose. The oocytes obtained can be cryopreserved after fertilization for a deferred transfer in a subsequent cycle. In principle, every COS treatment carries a risk of OHSS, as individual factors may be more decisive than prognostic factors. Thus, in rare cases, even a "low responder" patient with only three oocytes retrieved can develop severe OHSS (▣ Table 6.13).

A distinction is made between early (**"early onset"**) and late (**"late onset"**) **OHSS**. Early OHSS is caused by hCG for inducing ovulation as a **trigger** for **OHSS**. The trigger for late OHSS is the hCG produced by the syncytiotrophoblast after successful implantation. If two or three embryos implant, endogenous hCG production from the respective syncytiotrophoblasts can be several times higher. As a result, the severity of late OHSS can be even greater.

OHSS Symptoms

Patients with severe OHSS complain of **typical symptoms** such as **rapid weight gain** with **massive fluid retention** of more than four to five kg. Fluid accumulates mainly in the abdominal cavity (**ascites**), but in more severe cases also in the chest cavity (**pleural effusion**) and pericardium (**pericardial effusion**). Heart rate then increases (**tachycardia**) and blood pressure drops (**hypoten-

sion**). In addition, there may be a decrease in urine output (oliguria) and **renal failure**, respiratory distress (**ARDS**), and **thrombosis**. Treatment of OHSS patients should take place in experienced inpatient facilities with the possibility of intensive care. With appropriate therapy, it is usually possible to stabilize and control the course. As a precaution, all patients undergoing COS should be given the contact details of such a facility. Severe OHSS is classified into three grades, A to C, according to the severity of clinical changes (▣ Table 6.14).

Mandatory Reporting to the Paul-Ehrlich-Institut (PEI)

If severe OHSS occurs with **hospitalization** of the patient and/or other **serious events** during the retrieval, processing, or preservation of tissues, a report must be submitted to the Paul-Ehrlich-Institut (PEI) in accordance with the Medicinal Products Act using the forms "Form G1b" (suspected serious **adverse reaction**) or "Form G1c" (reporting a serious **adverse event**) (Appendices 6.3 and 6.4). The form for reporting OHSS (adverse reaction) is, for example, already integrated in the IVF software MediTex, which is used by most fertility centers. The reporting deadline is 15 days after the fertility center becomes aware of a severe OHSS. The **report** is **mandatory,** and failure to comply with the reporting obligation will result in a **fine**.

Case Study

A 31-year-old **PCOS** patient with renewed desire for a child requested further treatment with IVF. Three previous stimulated IUI cycles had been unsuccessful. Two years earlier, she had given birth to a child after ovarian stimulation and IUI. She was informed that, due to her PCOS, she had an increased risk of OHSS with IVF treatment. For this reason, oocyte maturation was performed in the antagonist protocol with an adjusted low-dose LH-FSH stimulation using an FSH dose of 75–87.5 IU (Fig. 6.10). Ovulation was triggered with hCG, as the patient desired a fresh cycle transfer. Eleven mature oocytes were retrieved for IVF, of which only four were normally fertilized. No transfer could be performed because the fertilized oocytes did not develop into embryos. Due to the poor fertilization rate, the method was changed to ICSI in the following cycle. In addition, the stimulation was repeated with a **slightly higher dose** of 87.5–112.5 IU FSH, as the physician treating this cycle also wanted to retrieve more oocytes for fertilization. Ovulation was again triggered with hCG. Twenty-two mature oocytes were retrieved, of which 17 were normally fertilized by ICSI. The patient was admitted to a clinic with OHSS expertise one day after follicular puncture due to early-onset severe **OHSS**. Therefore, all oocytes were cryopreserved at the pronuclear stage. Fortunately, the patient was able to be discharged after four days. The transfer was postponed to a later cycle. The report to the PEI was made within the 15-day deadline.

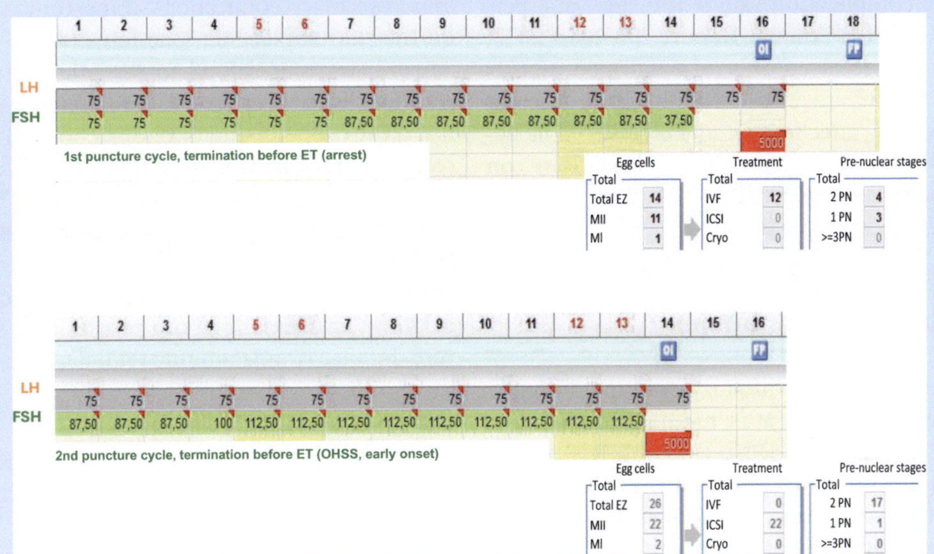

Fig. 6.10 Case study: ovarian stimulation in the antagonist protocol and "early-onset" OHSS after a slight increase in FSH dose in the second of two consecutive cycles

Case Study OHSS (Commentary)

Retrospectively, in the case study, increasing the stimulation dose to obtain a higher number of oocytes was unnecessary, as simply switching to the ICSI method had already resulted in a high fertilization rate and thus a sufficient number of fertilized oocytes. As the case study shows, ovarian stimulation for IVF or ICSI in a patient with **PCOS** is a balancing act, as the risks of both ineffective treatment and severe OHSS are high.

Complications During Oocyte Retrieval

Vaginal follicle puncture to retrieve oocytes for IVF is a low-risk surgical procedure. Vaginal bleeding can usually be managed on an outpatient basis without difficulty. The complication rate is less than one percent (D·I·R Annual Report 2023). In 2022, the PEI received only 24 confirmed reports of serious adverse events such as **internal bleeding**, **infections**, and **abscesses**. The reports are available in the "Newsroom" on the PEI website (Tissue Vigilance Report 2022, ▶ www.pei.de).

Multiple Pregnancies

The frequency of monozygotic and dizygotic twin pregnancies after natural conception is 1.2%, and for triplets it is 0.01%. Risks associated with multiple pregnancies include **prematurity**, **bleeding**, **gestational diabetes**, and **preeclampsia**. In addition, multiple pregnancies are known to have an **increased rate of malformations**, which may be related to the higher risk of gestational diabetes (GDM), as GDM can manifest early in pregnancy without being initially detected. Hyperglycemia is toxic and can lead to major malformations during the early embryonic period.

The transfer of a single embryo is generally sufficient to achieve the goal of a singleton pregnancy. Fortunately, the transfer of only one embryo, especially in younger women with a good prognosis, is becoming increasingly common, without significantly lowering pregnancy rates. The top DIR centers for pregnancy rates also include those that transfer an average of only 1.1 embryos.

Monozygotic Multiple Pregnancy

Even after the transfer of a single embryo, a subsequent division can result in a multiple pregnancy. The frequency of such a monozygotic multiple pregnancy is low, at 1.5% per transfer (D·I·R Annual Report 2023). Couples seeking fertility treatment should be informed about the risk of additional monozygotic pregnancies prior to IVF treatment. Monozygotic multiple pregnancies carry an additional risk for the so-called **feto-fetal transfusion syndrome**, abbreviated as **FFTS**. Due to abnormal vascular connections (anastomoses) on the shared placenta, one fetus (**donor** or "giver") transfers blood to the other fetus, resulting in poorer supply. This fetus does not grow properly and develops poorly. The recipient (**recipient**) is oversupplied and often produces too much amniotic fluid. This can lead to polyhydramnios, causing painful symptoms for the pregnant woman. If left untreated, severe cases can result in circulatory problems for both fetuses and severe damage or intrauterine fetal death.

Dizygotic Multiple Pregnancy

As documented in the D·I·R Annual Report 2023, the probability of a live birth after **transfer** of **two embryos** increases by only a factor of 1.07. At the same time, however, the probability of a multiple birth increases by a factor of 17.5 (D·I·R Annual Report 2023). This dramatic increase in the multiple birth rate is difficult to justify. It leads to an increase in **prematurity** from 18% to 86.2% in twins and to 100% in triplets (◻ Table 6.15). In triplets, very early preterm births with low birth weight are particularly common, resulting in a very high risk to child health (D·I·R Annual

◻ Table 6.15   Children born (singletons and multiples) depending on gestational week after IVF and ICSI (according to D·I·R Annual Report 2023)

Ongoing gestational week	20–26	27–31	32–37	38–41	42	% of total
Singleton (%)	0.5	1.3	16.3	81.2	0.8	78.8
Twin (%)	2.9	6.7	76.5	13.8	0.1	20.5
Triplet (%)	14.8	59.3	25.9	–	–	0.7

Report 2023). The most important risks of prematurity are **respiratory distress syndrome**, a typical intestinal disease of preterm infants (**necrotizing enterocolitis**), and **brain damage**.

🏠 Learning Objectives

- Know uterine malformations and their significance for involuntary childlessness
- Understand the effectiveness of ovarian stimulation treatment, ovulation induction, and controlled ovarian stimulation (COS) for ART procedures
- Know the timeline of an IVF cycle from preparation to pregnancy test
- Be able to explain the principle of frozen embryo transfer (FET) cycles (synchronizing the "age" of the developed oocyte and endometrium)
- Know measures to improve semen quality
- Be informed about surgical sperm retrieval, including testicular biopsy and TESE
- Know the key regulations in the SaRegG for donors, donor children, recipients, and fertility centers
- Have knowledge of measures to improve the safety of IVF treatment for maternal and child health

In fertility treatment, assisted reproductive technologies (ART) are central for both female and male causes. Surgical therapy is performed in cases of extensive endometriosis, for reversal of sterilization, and for uterine abnormalities. In cases of ovarian dysfunction, ovulation can be induced by ovarian stimulation treatment (OI). Stimulation is also performed in women who ovulate to increase fertility. The most important stimulation medication is FSH. For IVF or ICSI treatment, controlled ovarian stimulation (COS) is performed. Additional medications suppress premature ovulation. Surplus oocytes at the pronuclear stage can be cryopreserved and thawed and transferred in subsequent cycles (thaw treatment). The principle of a thaw treatment is the synchronization of endometrial development with that of the embryo at the time of transfer. In male infertility, the woman is usually treated within the framework of ART, as semen quality in men can only rarely be improved. In cases of azoospermia, surgical retrieval of sperm from testicular tissue is usually successful. If no sperm cells are found during testicular sperm extraction (TESE) for ICSI treatment, donor sperm treatment is possible. The fundamental right to knowledge of one's own parentage for donor children has been implemented in the Sperm Donor Registry Act. Treatments with donor sperm are increasingly being performed in same-sex couples and single women. The goal of fertility treatment is a singleton pregnancy resulting in the full-term birth of a healthy child.

Below is the link to the electronic supplementary material.

References

Aljubran A, Safar O, Elatreisy A (2022) Factors predicting successful sperm retrieval in men with non-obstructive Azoospermia: A single center perspective. Health Sci Rep 5:e727. ► https://doi.org/10.1002/hsr2.727

AWMF S2k-Leitlinie Weibliche genitale Fehlbildungen (2020) ► https://register.awmf.org/assets/guidelines/015-052l_S1_Weibliche_genitale_Fehlbildungen_2020-06.pdf. Zuletzt 21.5.2025

Bals-Pratsch M, Eder A, Gutknecht D (2020) Gestational Diabetes as a Maternal Risk Factor. Dtsch Arztebl Int. 117:421–422. ► https://doi.org/10.3238/arztebl.2020.0421b

Bals-Pratsch M, Fill Malfertheiner S (2017) Glukosestoffwechsel und assistierte Reproduktion. Gynäkologische Endokrinologie 15:108–115. ► https://doi.org/10.1007/s10304-017-0134-2

Beckers NG, Macklon NS, Eijkemans MJ et al (2003) Nonsupplemented luteal phase characteristics after the administration of recombinant human chorionic gonadotropin, recombinant luteinizing hormone, or gonadotropin-releasing hormone (GnRH) agonist to induce final oocyte maturation in in vitro fertilization patients after ovarian stimulation with recombinant follicle-stimulating hormone and GnRH antagonist cotreatment. J Clin Endocrinol Metab 88:4186–92. ► https://doi.org/10.1210/jc.2002-021953

Bhattacharya S, Harrild K, Mollison J et al (2008) Clomifene citrate or unstimulated intrauterine insemination compared with expectant management for unexplained infertility: pragmatic randomised controlled trial. BMJ 337:a716. ► https://doi.org/10.1136/bmj.a716

Casarramona G, Lalmahomed T, Lemmen C (2022) The efficacy and safety of luteal phase support with progesterone following ovarian stimulation and intrauterine insemination: A systematic review and meta-analysis. Front Endocrinol (Lausanne) 13:960393. ► https://doi.org/10.3389/fendo.2022.960393

Damke E, Kurscheidt FA, Irie MMT et al (2018) Male Partners of Infertile Couples With Seminal Positivity for Markers of Bacterial Vaginosis Have Impaired Fertility. Am J Mens Health 12:2104-2115. ► https://doi.org/10.1177/1557988318794522

D·I·R (2023). Jahrbuch 2022. J Reproduktionsmed Endokrinol 20 (Sonderheft 1), 1–60

D·I·R (2024). Jahrbuch 2023. J Reproduktionsmed Endokrinol 21 (Sonderheft 4), 1–64

Epelboin S, Labrosse J, De Mouzon J et al (2023) Higher risk of pre-eclampsia and other vascular disorders with artificial cycle for frozen-thawed embryo transfer compared to ovulatory cycle or to fresh embryo transfer following in vitro fertilization. Front Endocrinol (Lausanne). 14:1182148. ► https://doi.org/10.3389/fendo.2023.1182148

Franik S, Le QK, Kremer JA et al (2022) Aromatase inhibitors (letrozole) for ovulation induction in infertile women with polycystic ovary syndrome. Cochrane Database Syst Rev. 9:CD010287. ► https://doi.org/10.1002/14651858.CD010287.pub4

Grimbizis GF, Gordts S, Di Spiezio Sardo A, et al (2013) The ESHRE/ESGE consensus on the classification of female genital tract congenital anomalies. Hum Reprod 28:2032–44. ► https://doi.org/10.1093/humrep/det098

Goulart ACX, Farnezi HCM, França JPBM et al (2020) HIV, HPV and Chlamydia trachomatis: impacts on male fertility. JBRA Assist Reprod. 24:492–497. ► https://doi.org/10.5935/1518-0557.20200020

Hammel A Bleichrodt C Thorn P Klym K (2024) Deutsches Register für Insemination (DERI). In: D·I·R (ed) Jahrbuch 2023. J Reproduktionsmed Endokrinol 21:49–51

Itskovitz-Eldor J, Kol S, Mannaerts B (2000) Use of a single bolus of GnRH agonist triptorelin to trigger ovulation after GnRH antagonist ganirelix treatment in women undergoing ovarian stimulation for assisted reproduction, with special reference to the prevention of ovarian hyperstimulation syndrome: preliminary report: short communication. Hum Reprod 15:1965–8. ► https://doi.org/10.1093/humrep/15.9.1965

Lunenfeld B (1963) Treatment of anovulation by human gonadotrophins. J Int Fedn Gynecol Obstet 1,153

Müller MD, Hohl MK (2020) Die praktische Bedeutung der Müllerschen Fehlbildungen. Fachheilkunde aktuell 2:1–10 ► https://frauenheilkunde-aktuell.ch/de/fachmagazin/ausgaben/2020-02/die-praktische-bedeutung-der-muellerschen-fehlbildungen/frauenheilkunde-aktuell-2020-02-die-praktische-bedeutung-der-muellerschen-fehlbildungen.pdf?highlight=m%C3%BCller-gang. Zuletzt 21.5.2025

Nadarajah S (2025) Ozempic babies: are weight loss drugs leading to unintended pregnancies? BMJ 388:q2440. ► https://doi.org/10.1136/bmj.q2440

Rizk B, Aboulghar M (1991) Modern management of ovarian hyperstimulation syndrome. Hum Reprod 6:1082–7. ► https://doi.org/10.1093/oxfordjournals.humrep.a137488

Schoysman R, Vanderzwalmen P, Nijs M (1993) Pregnancy after fertilisation with human testicular spermatozoa. Lancet 342:1237. ► https://doi.org/10.1016/0140-6736(93)92217-h

Wessel JA, Danhof NA, van Eekelen R et al (2022) Ovarian stimulation strategies for intrauterine insemination in couples with unexplained infertility: a systematic review and individual participant data meta-analysis. Hum Reprod Update 28:733–746. ► https://doi.org/10.1093/humupd/dmac021

Zitzmann M, Nieschlag E (2004) Rauchende Männer—ein Fertilitätsrisiko. Reproduktionsmed. Endokrinol 1, 9–12

Early Pregnancy

Contents

Gestational Age and Embryonic Period

Embryology deals with the development of the fertilized egg cell (pronuclear stage) and the resulting embryo. From an **embryological perspective**, gestational age is given as the **developmental week** after fertilization. According to this calculation, a pregnancy lasts **38 weeks or 266 days**. In clinical practice, however, gestational age is not calculated from the time of "**conception**" (**post conceptionem**, abbreviated as **p.c.**), but from the **first day of the last menstrual period** (**post menstruationem**, abbreviated as **p.m.**), since the exact time of fertilization is often not precisely determinable in natural conception. With this **clinical calculation**, a pregnancy lasts **40 weeks or 280 days** (◘ Table 7.1). Conception usually occurs 14 days after the start of menstruation, so mathematically, the pregnancy is already incorrectly considered two weeks old at the time of fertilization, and with the missed period, it is incorrectly considered four weeks old instead of just two. For the calculation of gestational weeks (GW), the due date, and the determination of maternity protection periods, the clinical approach starting from the last menstrual period is decisive. The **calculated due date (EDD)** is the day of completion of the 38th GW **p.c.** or the 40th GW **p.m.**

Clinically, pregnancy is divided into three **developmental phases** (gestational weeks according to p.m.):

I. Trimester 1st–13th GW, II. Trimester 14th–26th GW, III. Trimester 27th–40th GW. The **first trimester** covers the 8-week period from fertilization (p.c.). This developmental phase is the **embryonic period**. The first three weeks are referred to as the early developmental phase, during which the basic body plan is formed. From the 3rd GW p.c., organogenesis with organ development begins. After the embryonic period, the **fetal period** follows. The **second** and **third trimesters** are mainly characterized by fetal growth. For a **mature infant** to be born, delivery should not occur before the completed 37th GW p.m. A **term birth** is defined as the birth of a child from the **38th GW p.m.** up to the 42nd GW, and a **preterm birth** is when a child is born before the completion of the **37th GW p.m.** The health risks for preterm infants are severe. From the end of the second trimester (26th GW p.m.), they have a good chance of survival with neonatal intensive care.

> Preterm birth: Birth of a child before the completion of the calculated 37th GW.

The **organogenesis** begins at the time of the missed menstrual period. At this point, women are often not yet aware of their pregnancy. During this developmental phase, an embryo is particularly susceptible to harmful factors. Most **malformations**, such as heart defects and brain malformations, arise during this critical phase. Noxae

◘ Table 7.1 Calculation of gestational age

Time of calculation	Start of pregnancy	GW*	Pregnancy duration**	Embryonic period
post menstruationem (p.m.)	Fertilization minus 14 days	40	280	1st–10th GW* (Organogenesis 5th–10th GW)
post conceptionem (p.c.)	Time of fertilization	38	266	1st–8th GW* (Organogenesis 3rd–8th GW)

*GW = gestational weeks, **Pregnancy duration (days)

include harmful substances (including nicotine and alcohol), but also toxic hyperglycemia when glycemic targets are exceeded in gestational diabetes or diabetes mellitus.

Implantation and Multiple Pregnancies

A viable blastocyst implants into the endometrium around the sixth day of development (see ▶ Chap. 2). The outer trophoblast cells (**syncytiotrophoblast**) penetrate further into the endometrium and begin to produce **hCG** (◘ Fig. 7.1). The placenta later develops from the inner and outer trophoblast. Due to hCG stimulation of the corpus luteum, menstruation is suppressed. As early as the 9th day of development, the embryoblast (inner cell mass) differentiates into the bilaminar embryonic disc (epiblast and hypoblast) with the amniotic cavity. From these two germ layers, the basic body plan of the embryo is formed (see ▶ Chap. 2). Around the 12th day of development

p.c., the **chorionic cavity** forms between the trophoblast and the embryo. This is usually visible on ultrasound from the fifth GW p.c. The **amniotic cavity** can only be visualized later on ultrasound. It enlarges progressively until the end of the third month of pregnancy. In contrast, the chorionic cavity becomes increasingly narrow until the amniotic and chorionic membranes come into contact and the chorionic cavity obliterates.

If more than one embryo has implanted, each embryo normally forms its own chorionic and amniotic cavity and its own placenta. About 90% of twin pregnancies are dizygotic. If the placentas are close together, they can fuse. The two chorionic cavities can also merge into a single chorionic cavity, mimicking a monozygotic twin pregnancy with separation at the blastocyst stage. In this case, vascular connections can develop between the two placentas. Thus, in rare cases, the dreaded feto-fetal transfusion syndrome (FFTS) can also occur in dizygotic twin pregnancies (see ▶ Chap. 6).

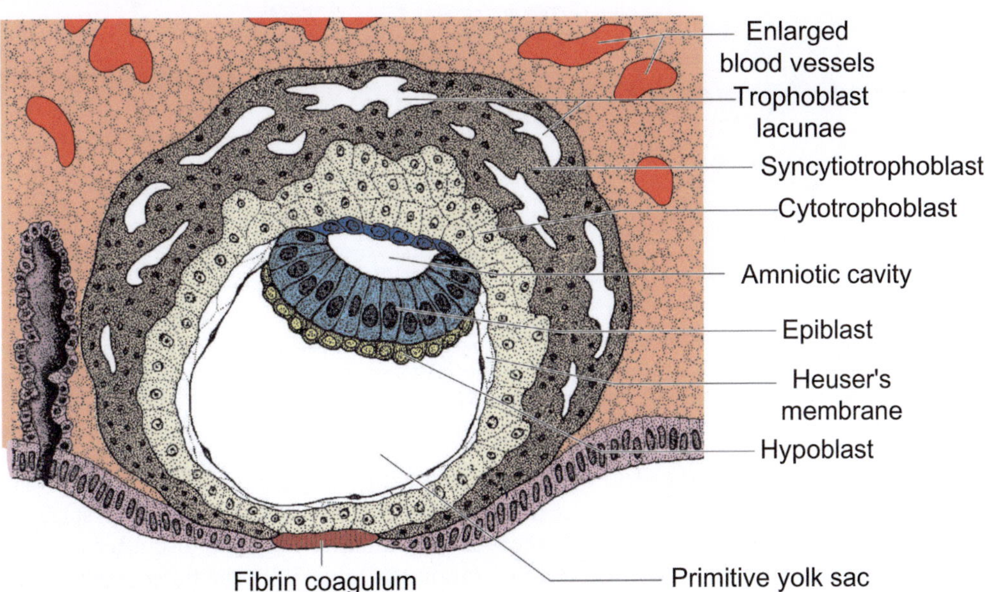

◘ **Fig. 7.1**   Bilaminar embryonic disc. 9-day-old blastocyst after successful implantation. Reproduced with permission from: Sadler TW (2014a, b)

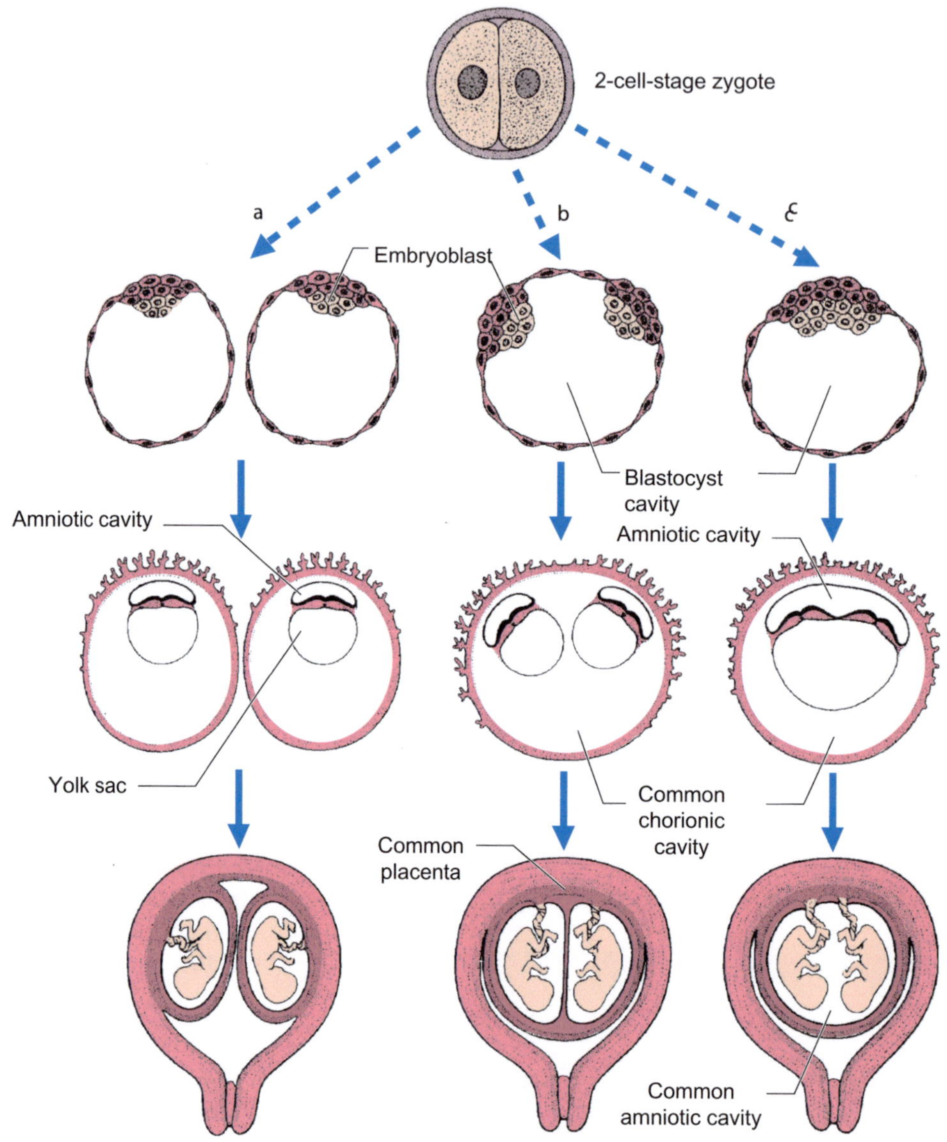

⬛ Fig. 7.2 Monozygotic twins, fetal membranes (chorionic and amniotic cavities) in three possibilities of twin formation. **a** Division at the two-cell stage **b** Division at the blastocyst stage **c** Division after implantation, bilaminar embryonic disc. Reproduced with permission from: Sadler TW (2014a, b)

In **monozygotic twins**, the development of the chorionic cavities and placentas depends on the developmental stage at the time of separation (⬛ Fig. 7.2). There are **three possibilities for twin formation**: separation at the two-cell stage, at the blastocyst stage with complete division of the embryoblast, and at the developmental stage of the bilaminar embryonic disc after implantation (⬛ Table 7.2). The most common origin of monozygotic twins is constriction at the blastocyst stage. Monozygotic twins

◘ Table 7.2   Dizygotic and monozygotic twins, fetal membranes and placentas

Twins	Time of separation	Chorionic cavity	Amniotic cavity	Placenta
dizygotic	–	2	2	2
monozygotic	a: two-cell stage	2	2	2
	b: blastocyst stage	1	2	1
	c: bilaminar embryonic disc	1	1	1

have a significantly increased risk of FFTS at 15% (see ▶ Chap. 6). The uneven blood flows are caused by vascular connections in the shared placenta. These harmful vascular connections can usually be ablated prenatally by laser therapy in the uterus. Intrauterine laser therapy can save the affected children in about 70% of cases. Without treatment, the probability that both children will die in utero is about 90%.

It is assumed that only about 30% of established twin pregnancies actually result in the birth of twins. Frequently, one twin disappears during the first and at the beginning of the second trimester. Either it regresses or, more rarely, the twin becomes mummified (fetus papyraceus). If a twin dies and regresses, this is referred to as a "**vanishing twin**".

Endocrinology of Early Pregnancy, Pregnancy Test

By the end of the second GW p.c., enough human chorionic gonadotropin (hCG) is produced that hCG can be detected in a blood sample. The pregnancy test is negative if the measured hCG value is <5 IU/L. The determination is not exact. Even with modern measurement methods, the measurement inaccuracy is still around 5%. HCG is produced in the early placenta and initially serves to maintain the corpus luteum. As a result, there is no drop in hormones, but rather a pregnancy-related increase in

progesterone and estradiol. HCG consists of two subunits, alpha (α) and beta (β). The β-subunit is crucial for the specific effects of hCG in pregnancy. From the fourth month of pregnancy, the placenta itself produces sufficient estradiol and progesterone. The corpus luteum in the ovary then regresses.

The **hCG** values approximately double every two days in early pregnancy up to a peak, then decrease with the third month of pregnancy and stabilize at a high level. If hCG values do not rise adequately, there is suspicion of a disturbed early pregnancy and an impending **spontaneous abortion**. In **ectopic pregnancies (EP)** as well, the values usually do not rise adequately. In these cases, bleeding typically occurs along with a further increase in hCG values. High hCG values may indicate a **multiple pregnancy**. In cases of massively elevated hCG values, a serious pregnancy disorder such as a **hydatidiform mole** or a choriocarcinoma should also be considered.

Ultrasound in Early Pregnancy

Sonographic confirmation of pregnancy is usually performed around the seventh week p.m. If a **chorionic cavity** can be visualized within the uterine cavity, a normally established pregnancy is clinically confirmed (◘ Fig. 7.3). The chorionic cavity is also referred to as the gestational sac. By the seventh to eighth GW p.m., an embryo is usually visible. The **crown-rump length** can be

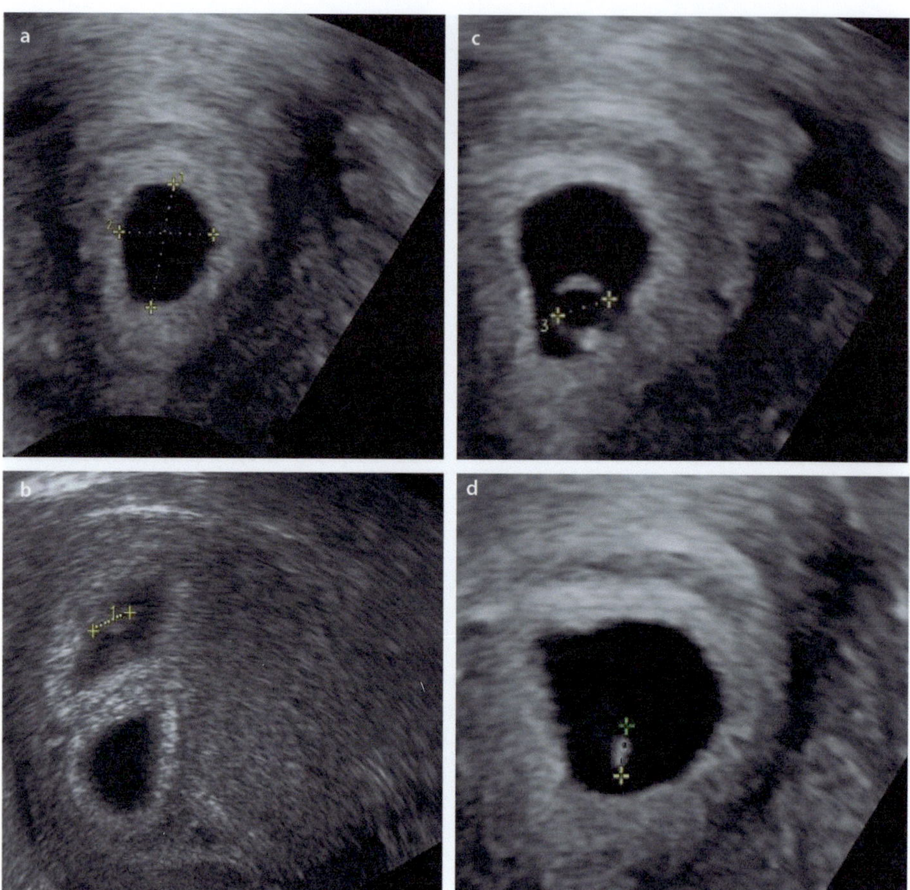

Fig. 7.3   Ultrasound in early pregnancy. **a** Chorionic cavity **b** 2 chorionic cavities (dizygotic twins) **c** Chorionic cavity with yolk sac **d** Chorionic cavity with embryonic structure

measured and the **cardiac activity** detected. This examination is usually performed transvaginally. On ultrasound, a chorionic cavity appears as a round structure with an echogenic rim ("bagel sign", see below). It is usually well visualized at hCG values of 1,000–2,000 IU/L. It must be distinguished from a pseudogestational sac. Such a cavity is often seen in ectopic pregnancy. However, the distinction from a pseudogestational sac is only certain if the **yolk sac** as an embryonic structure can also be visualized within the chorionic cavity. This develops approximately after about two weeks p.c. below the embryonic disc and normally measures up to 5 mm. It is probably important for the nutrition of an early embryo. In addition, it is also required for the provision of primordial germ cells before their later migration to the gonadal ridges.

In addition, the location of the chorionic cavity in the uterus must be determined sonographically. If two or more chorionic cavities are detected, a multizygotic **multiple pregnancy** is present. The chorionic cavities must be examined very carefully to determine whether two embryos may be present in one chorionic cavity, as this would indicate a monozygotic twin pregnancy. The outcome of an IVF treatment is documented in the German IVF Register (D·I·R) as a clinical pregnancy if one or more chorionic cavities can be detected.

Disorders of Early Pregnancy

Early miscarriages occur in 10 to 15% of all clinically confirmed pregnancies. For the women affected, the unfavorable pregnancy outcome is often psychologically very stressful. The psychological exceptional situation should be given sufficient attention. If there is no emergency situation, the full range of therapeutic options for miscarriage should be explained and offered. This also applies to suspected extrauterine (ectopic) pregnancy, with the options of expectant management, medical treatment, and surgical therapy. In about half of all early miscarriages, the location of the pregnancy is unclear. A pregnancy with unclear localization is referred to as a "pregnancy of unknown location" (PUL).

Early Miscarriage

A non-viable pregnancy within the first 12 weeks of gestation (GW) post conception with an empty chorionic cavity or a chorionic cavity containing an embryo without cardiac activity, located either inside or outside the uterus, is defined as an early miscarriage or early pregnancy loss (Guideline on disturbed early pregnancy 2025).

Pregnancy ultrasound should ideally be performed no later than the eighth to ninth week of gestation post menstruation. Eight types of miscarriage are distinguished (◘ Table 7.3). However, an **abortus imminens** does not yet represent a lost pregnancy, but rather a threatened miscarriage. Many pregnancies with threatened miscarriage have a good prognosis for ongoing

◘ **Table 7.3** Types of miscarriage up to 12th week of gestation

Miscarriage	Symptoms	Measures
Very early miscarriage (biochemical pregnancy)	Positive pregnancy test	none
Threatened miscarriage (abortus imminens)	Usually painless bleeding, often retrochorionic hematoma	Conservative
Incipient miscarriage (abortus incipiens)	Cervix open, bleeding, chorionic cavity in cervical canal	Expectant vs. medical vs. surgical management
Incomplete miscarriage (abortus incompletus)	Cervix open, bleeding, pain	Expectant vs. medical vs. surgical management
Complete miscarriage (abortus completus)	Uterine cavity empty after expulsion of chorionic cavity, previous clinical confirmation of pregnancy	none
Missed abortion	Embryo without cardiac activity, no bleeding or pain	Expectant vs. medical vs. surgical management
Septic miscarriage	Ongoing miscarriage with fever >39 degrees, painful uterus	Emergency: anti-infective therapy, including repeat curettage of retained pregnancy tissue
Blighted ovum	Empty and growing gestational sac without embryonic components	Curettage

pregnancy and delivery with conservative management. In cases of bleeding during pregnancy, **Rh prophylaxis** should be performed in Rh-negative pregnant women. According to the current guideline on disturbed early pregnancy in the first trimester (2025), routine administration of anti-D immunoglobulin to Rh (RhD)-negative women with symptoms of abortus imminens is not recommended, as there is little evidence that women become sensitized after uterine bleeding in the first 12 weeks of pregnancy if the pregnancy continues. However, it may be advisable to administer anti-D immunoglobulin if the bleeding is heavy, recurrent, or associated with lower abdominal pain, especially as the pregnancy approaches the 12th week.

> **Very early miscarriages**, also known as biochemical pregnancies, are defined as pregnancy losses before, during, or shortly after implantation.

Very early miscarriages are associated with delayed and heavier bleeding. Such pregnancies are usually not perceived by women as miscarriages. Very early miscarriages are often diagnosed after fertility treatment, as the pregnancy test with hCG determination is usually performed about 15 days after ovulation or follicle puncture and fertilization. A very early miscarriage is detected during planned hCG monitoring or in the event of bleeding. In cases of **abortus incipiens** or **incompletus** or a missed miscarriage (**missed abortion**), expectant management vs. medical management (Cytotec®) vs. surgical management (suction curettage, possibly with cytogenetics) can be discussed with the patient. The prerequisite, however, is that there is no emergency situation such as severe or life-threatening bleeding. A **septic miscarriage** is defined as a non-viable intrauterine pregnancy complicated by **infection**

of the pregnancy, endometrium and myometrium, as well as the adnexa with peritonitis. This can lead to life-threatening sepsis with possible septic shock and multi-organ failure. After initiation of high-dose antibiotics, curettage is performed to remove pregnancy tissue. In a **blighted ovum**, no embryonic structure can be visualized in the chorionic cavity. This is a placental development disorder, usually of genetic origin. Only paternal genes are present, maternal genes are absent. Therapy consists of suction curettage with histology and cytogenetics to distinguish from other, mostly benign, molar pregnancies and to detect chromosomal abnormalities. In general, the risk of Asherman's syndrome must be considered with curettage, especially after repeat curettage for retained pregnancy tissue (residuals), where the risk is particularly high.

Extrauterine (Ectopic) Pregnancy

In an ectopic pregnancy (EP), implantation of a fertilized egg occurs outside the uterine cavity. The **rupture** of a tubal pregnancy is a feared complication. Such an event leads to internal bleeding. This can result in a life-threatening **emergency situation** requiring immediate surgical intervention. The incidence of such an extrauterine pregnancy is one to two percent. Tubal pregnancy is the most common form of ectopic pregnancy. Implantation usually occurs at the end of the fallopian tube in the ampullary region. Ectopic pregnancies can also rarely occur interstitially/cornually (uterine wall/tubal angle), cervically (cervix), in a cesarean scar, abdominally (abdominal cavity), and in abdominal organs (e.g., liver). **Heterotopic pregnancies** are very rare. This refers to the simultaneous occurrence of an intrauterine and an extrauterine pregnancy. The incidence is significantly higher with ART if at least two embryos are transferred. Risk factors for EP include a previous ectopic pregnancy, known tubal pathology, adnexitis, tubal surgery (e.g., tubal reconstruction), intrauterine device (IUD), infertility, as well as nicotine abuse and advanced reproductive age >35 years.

Symptoms of an ectopic pregnancy include secondary amenorrhea, bleeding, and lower abdominal pain. Diagnosis of an ectopic pregnancy is made by clinical examination, serial hCG measurements, and transvaginal sonography. In hCG monitoring, the value does not rise appropriately. In about 90% of cases, an ectopic pregnancy can be localized by ultrasound. A typical sign is the "**bagel sign**," an echogenic ring of variable thickness surrounding a unilocular, round, central or eccentric cyst (◘ Fig. 7.4). A yolk sac can also often be visualized. In some cases, an intact pregnancy with an embryo with cardiac activity can even be seen. If a tubal pregnancy can be localized with high certainty by ultrasound, it is usually treated surgically.

In the **treatment** of tubal pregnancy, a tube-preserving approach is preferred if future fertility is desired. In this procedure, the fallopian tube is longitudinally incised over the ectopic pregnancy and the pregnancy tissue is removed (**salpingotomy**). However, there is an increased risk of recurrence for another ectopic pregnancy. After a salpingotomy, regular postoperative hCG monitoring must be performed until negativity, as in 4 to 15% of cases, further treatment of residual pregnancy tissue in the tube is required (Taran et al. 2015). **Salpingectomy** (removal of the fallopian tube) is primarily preferred in cases of recurrence, a damaged tube, or completed family planning. In consultation with the patient, this can also be performed bilaterally. **Medical treatment of EP** is performed with the cytostatic agent methotrexate. This treatment may extend over several weeks. hCG monitoring in blood samples must be continued until hCG is no longer detectable. If treatment fails, surgical therapy is usually necessary. In summary, the decision between removal of the fallopian tube (salpingectomy) and a tube-preserving approach (salpingotomy) depends on the clinical situation and risk of recurrence, the patient's history, and her wishes.

Recurrent Miscarriages

> Recurrent miscarriages (WSA, RSA): at least two consecutive miscarriages (definition varies).

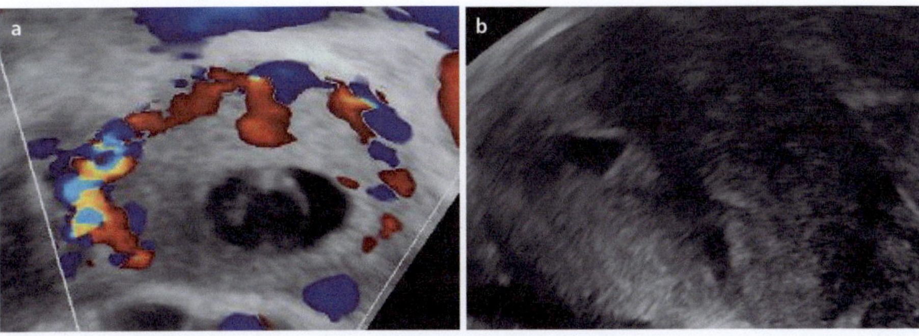

◘ **Fig. 7.4** Tubal pregnancy. **a** Tubal pregnancy, chorionic cavity with yolk sac, "bagel sign," color Doppler **b** Pseudogestational sac intrauterine (not round, without embryonic structures)

Miscarriages can occur repeatedly. If there are at least two consecutive miscarriages, the diagnosis of recurrent miscarriage is made according to the American Society for Reproductive Medicine (ASRM). Recurrent miscarriages are also referred to as **recurrent spontaneous abortions** (abbreviated as **RSA**). The definition is not used uniformly. According to the AWMF guideline "Diagnosis and treatment of women with repeated spontaneous abortions" (2022) and the WHO definition, the diagnosis is only made after three or more consecutive miscarriages. This includes not only early miscarriages up to the 12th week of gestation post conception, but also the rarer late miscarriages up to the 22nd week of gestation post conception with a fetal weight <500 g. The incidence of recurrent miscarriages, according to the ASRM definition, is up to five percent.

The treatment of RSA patients, who often experience significant psychological distress, is a diagnostic and therapeutic challenge. Only a few causes are known, and in the majority of affected women, no risk factor can be identified. An overview of risk factors for recurrent miscarriages is shown in ◘ Table 7.4. The most common cause of spontaneous miscarriages, accounting for 50 to 60%, is **chromosomal abnormalities**. During fertilization, meiotic errors often occur in the oocytes, which usually have no further prognostic significance for the affected women. However, in RSA, balanced chromosomal aberrations can be detected in one partner in four to five percent of cases. These so-called translocations often lead to chromosomal imbalances during fertilization and are therefore causative for miscarriage. **Malformations** of the **uterus** such as septate uterus or bicornuate uterus, and changes such as submucosal **myomas** or **endometrial defects** can impair implantation and further development of an embryo or fetus. **Thrombophilias** (tendency to form blood clots) have been associated with an increased risk of miscarriage. The most common inherited thrombophilia is the **factor V Leiden mutation**. It has been hypothesized that untreated thrombophilia leads to thrombosis in the **uteroplacental circulation**, which begins as early as the 11th to 12th day post conception. This would impair the growth of the embryo or fetus and the placenta. For this reason, treatment with heparin was recommended. However, the effectiveness of heparin treatment could not be demonstrated (Quenby et al. 2023). It is possible that the tendency to miscarry is also individually related to general health, as patients with thrombophilia also have a higher risk of **thrombosis** or **embolism**. In such cases, guideline-based **heparin therapy** should be administered during pregnancy from the first trimester. Risk factors include, among others, obesity, nicotine abuse, age >35 years, and ART treatment (Bates et al. 2016).

◘ **Table 7.4** Risk factors for recurrent miscarriages

Risk factors	Explanation
Chromosomal abnormality	e.g., translocations
Uterine causes	Malformations, including submucosal myomas
Immunological causes	Antiphospholipid syndrome and autoimmune diseases
Hormonal disorders	Thyroid disease
Metabolic disorders	Obesity, polycystic ovary syndrome (PCOS) and insulin resistance (IR)

A rare coagulation disorder is **antiphospholipid syndrome (APS)**. This is an **autoimmune disease** that requires interdisciplinary management together with experienced rheumatologists. **Endocrine causes** of miscarriage include **thyroid diseases**. Severe thyroid dysfunction should be managed by specialist internist endocrinologists or radiologists. Luteal phase deficiency is not primarily considered a risk factor for miscarriage. However, it can indirectly promote miscarriage. Due to a deficiency in corpus luteum hormone, a threatened miscarriage (abortus imminens) may occur with the formation of hematomas, which can also spread under a chorionic cavity. Bleeding can fundamentally lead to pregnancy loss. For this reason, the AWMF guideline on repeated spontaneous abortions (2022) recommends **miscarriage prophylaxis** with **progesterone**. In RSA patients with **PCOS** or **obesity, metabolic disorders** are usually present. Preconceptionally, these include especially glucose tolerance disorders and insulin resistance. If pregnancy occurs, gestational diabetes can be diagnosed in over 50% of cases. If left untreated, toxic hyperglycemia can repeatedly lead to miscarriage (Sick 2018).

Learning Objectives
- Knowledge of early pregnancy
- Presentation of possible developmental disorders in this phase
- Presentation of the particularities of multiple pregnancies
- Knowledge of recurrent miscarriages

The embryonic period comprises the first eight weeks after fertilization, during which the organs are formed. In this vulnerable phase, the organs are sensitive to harmful influences that can lead to malformations. From an embryological perspective, gestational age is calculated from the time of fertilization. It is given in developmental days or weeks. A blastocyst implants into the endometrium around the sixth day of development. The amniotic cavity and chorionic cavity are formed. In monozygotic twins, separation of an embryo occurs within the first two weeks of development. hCG is produced by the early placenta. It stimulates the corpus luteum, so that rising progesterone and estrogen levels maintain the pregnancy. hCG is already measurable at the end of the second week of development. In pregnancy ultrasound, from the fifth to the ninth week of development, the chorionic cavity with the yolk sac and the embryo with cardiac activity should be visible. Clinically, gestational age is calculated from the first day of the last menstrual period, so that, arithmetically, the pregnancy is two weeks older compared to the embryological age. If a child is born before the calculated 38th week of gestation, it is considered a preterm birth. Ten to fifteen percent of pregnancies end in miscarriage. Implantation outside the uterine cavity is referred to as ectopic pregnancy (EP). Most often, this is a pregnancy in the fallopian tube (tubal pregnancy), especially if the tubes are damaged. If two or three miscarriages occur in succession, this is referred to as recurrent spontaneous abortions (RSA).

References

Bates SM, Middeldorp S, Rodger M (2016) Guidance for the treatment and prevention of obstetric-associated venous thromboembolism. J Thromb Thrombolysis. 41:92–128. ▸ https://doi.org/10.1007/s11239-015-1309-0

Diagnostik und Therapie von Frauen mit wiederholten Spontanaborten (2022) S2k Leitlinie. ▸ https://register.awmf.org/assets/guidelines/015-050l_S2k_Diagnostik-Therapie-wiederholte-Spontanaborte_2022-08.pdf Zuletzt am 6.4.2025

Gestörte Frühgravidität im 1. Trimenon (2025) S. 128 ► https://register.awmf.org/assets/guidelines/015-076l_S2k_Frueher-Schwangerschaftsverlust-im-1-Trimenon_2025-01.pdf Zuletzt am 4.4.2025

Quenby S, Booth K, Hiller L et al. (2023) ALIFE2 Block Writing Committee; ALIFE2 Investigators. Heparin for women with recurrent miscarriage and inherited thrombophilia (ALIFE2): an international open-label, randomised controlled trial. Lancet 402(10395):54–61. ► https://doi.org/10.1016/S0140-6736(23)00693-1

Sick MMU (2018) Frauen mit habituellen Aborten: Analyse des präkonzeptionellen Glukose- und Insulinstoffwechsels, Gestationsdiabetes sowie Schwangerschaftsoutcome. ► https://epub.uni-regensburg.de/37405/1/E-Version%20%2813.06.2018%29.pdf Zuletzt am 6.4.2025

Taran F-A, Kagan K-O, Hübner M et al (2015) The Diagnosis and Treatment of Ectopic Pregnancy. Dtsch Arztebl Int 112: 693–704; ► https://doi.org/10.3238/arztebl.2015.0693 Zuletzt am 6.4.2025

Sadler TW (2014a) Zweischichtige Keimscheibe (2. Woche). In: Sadler TW (ed) Taschenlehrbuch Embryologie, 12th edn. Thieme-Verlag, Stuttgart, p 79–90

Sadler TW (2014b) Entwicklung der Eihäute und der Plazenta. In: Sadler TW (ed) Taschenlehrbuch Embryologie, 12th edn. Thieme-Verlag, Stuttgart, p 156–179

7

Fertility Preservation

Contents

Supplementary Information The online version contains supplementary material available at
► https://doi.org/10.1007/978-3-662-73035-5_8.

Strategies and Technologies for Fertility Preservation

Severe damage to the germinal epithelium caused by chemotherapeutic agents or radiation leads to temporary or permanent **infertility**. The clinical symptom is **amenorrhea** in women and **azoospermia** in men. In men, chemotherapy generally results in permanent azoospermia. This risk is only lower with chemotherapies using the drugs Adriamycin, Thiotepa, Cytarabine, and Vinblastine (Meistrich 2013). The preservation of fertility through the **cryopreservation** of gametes and germ cell tissue is referred to as fertility preservation. Oocytes and sperm as well as ovarian and testicular tissue can be cryopreserved. Advances in cancer treatment have significantly increased long-term survival among cancer patients. In oncology, fertility preservation is considered a supportive adjunct therapy for young cancer patients. The **quality of life** of patients can thus be improved. After overcoming cancer, young people often wish to have their own child. According to the guideline on **fertility preservation** in oncological diseases (2017), there is consensus that counseling on fertility preservation concepts, taking into account life circumstances, the recommended oncological therapy, and the individual risk profile, should be an integral part of oncological treatment for female and male patients.

Fertility preservation is now performed not only in malignant diseases but, in exceptional cases, also in **benign diseases**. The prerequisite is the need for germ cell-damaging therapies, such as extensive surgical interventions for endometriosis or drug therapy with cytostatics like cyclophosphamide in inflammatory-rheumatological diseases.

Measures for fertility preservation in women have gained significant importance over the past 20 years. More and more young women today have not yet completed their family planning at the time of cancer diagnosis. The age of first-time mothers has increased (see ▸ Chap. 3). Most women now have their first child at age 30 or older. However, it is especially the new strategies and technologies that have led to an increase in fertility preservation measures. On the one hand, surgical interventions in young female cancer patients are performed as fertility-sparing as possible, preserving the uterus so that patients can carry a pregnancy after overcoming cancer. On the other hand, it was only with the development of **vitrification** ("glassification") that cryopreservation of oocytes with good "revival rates" became possible. In contrast, fertility preservation through cryopreservation of sperm using the established standard method, so-called slow freezing ("**slow freezing**"), has been possible for many decades, as sperm are more resistant than oocytes to the cell-damaging sharp ice crystals that form during "slow freezing" (see ▸ Chap. 6). Ovarian and testicular tissue are usually also frozen using the "slow freezing" protocol, similar to sperm.

Germ Cell-Damaging Cancer Therapies

In women, cancer therapy damages the germinal epithelium in the ovary. Not only the maturing oocytes but also a large proportion of the **primordial follicles** (see ▸ Chap. 2) as the oocyte reserve are lost. With timely planning, there is usually enough time in cancer cases to freeze oocytes before starting cancer treatment. For a stimulation treatment with oocyte retrieval, a **time window** of two to three weeks is required (◘ Table 8.1). However, the extent of oocyte damage also depends on the patient's age, the drugs used, and the dosage. Young women generally have such a good ovarian reserve that, in exceptional cases, even after high-dose chemotherapy, the germinal epithelium is not completely and permanently

□ Table 8.1 Time windows for fertility-preserving measures in women and men

Measure Cryopreservation	Woman	Man
GnRH agonists	max. 1 week	Not meaningful
Transposition of the gonads	max. 1 week	Not meaningful
Ovarian tissue*/Testicular tissue*	max. 1 week	max. 1 week
Oocytes**/Sperm*	approx. 2 weeks	same day up to 3 days
Repeat cryopreservation of oocytes**/sperm*	approx. 4 weeks	approx. 2 to 5 days
Combination ovarian tissue*/testicular tissue* and oocytes**/sperm*	approx. 3 weeks	max. 1 week

*"slow freezing"; **"ultrar-apid freezing" (vitrification)

damaged. In rare cases, spontaneous pregnancies can still occur. **Chemotherapy** drugs are classified according to their damaging effect on germ cells as high risk (**"high risk"**), medium risk (**"medium risk"**), and low risk (**"low risk"**). The damaging effect is considered more toxic to gonadal tissue the more frequently secondary amenorrhea occurs, i.e., permanent absence of menstruation (Liedtke and Kiesel 2012). For example, breast cancer drugs such as cyclophosphamide (Endoxan®) have a high risk, docetaxel (Taxotere®) a medium risk, and methotrexate a low risk. The latter drug is also used for the medical treatment of ectopic pregnancies.

Medical Counseling Session

The content of a medical counseling session at a fertility center regarding fertility preservation primarily includes information about the risks, practical implementation, and technical aspects (□ Fig. 8.1). The **time**

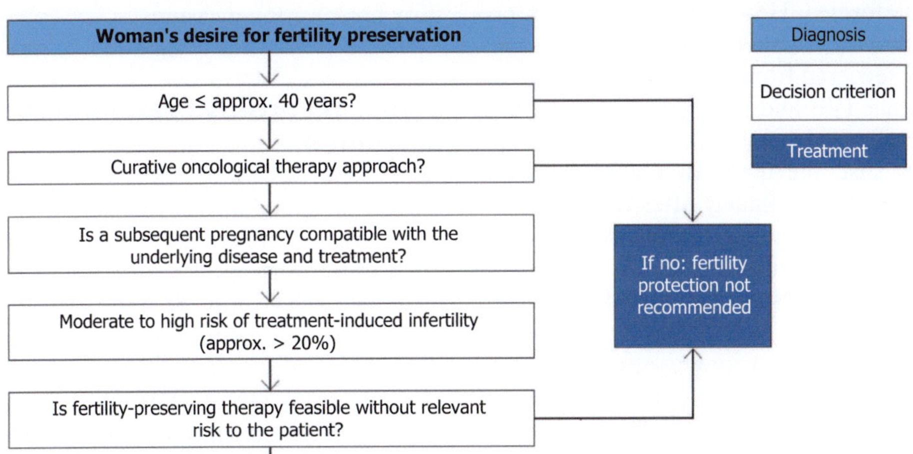

□ Fig. 8.1 Indication and implementation of fertility-protective measures in oncological and non-oncological diseases. (With kind permission from: Von Wolff M, Nawroth F (2020))

window for each fertility-preserving measure must be discussed. Before starting treatment, it is important to determine ovarian reserve. In women with a very low ovarian reserve ("low responder"), fertility preservation measures usually do not appear sensible or promising (see below). In men, cryopreservation may also not be meaningful or possible. This is the case if only immotile or no sperm are found in the ejaculate.

In addition, it must be discussed which **methods** can be used to obtain oocytes and sperm. For oocyte retrieval, hormonal stimulation and the **surgical retrieval of oocytes** via vaginal follicle puncture are necessary. **Ovarian tissue retrieval** is usually performed as part of a **laparoscopy** under general anesthesia. These two methods can also be combined (see below). In men, fertility preservation measures are generally straightforward to perform (◘ Table 8.1), as there are usually sufficient and suitable **sperm** available for **cryopreservation**. If the semen quality is not reliably sufficient for cryopreservation, ejaculates can be collected and cryopreserved on several consecutive days. If cryopreservation of sperm is not possible, **surgical retrieval of sperm** via testicular biopsy with cryopreservation can be performed. However, it is uncertain preoperatively whether sperm can be successfully retrieved from the testicular tissue and whether IVF and ICSI treatment can later be performed (see ▶ Chap. 6). Therefore, in every case, the tissue should be examined for sperm immediately after removal (fresh TESE), and histology should be performed to assess spermatogenesis. A cryo-reserve of sperm can also be enlarged by **combining** repeated semen collections and a testicular biopsy with cryopreservation, so that all options for future fertility treatment are exhausted in cases of severely impaired semen quality (see below).

Apart from cryopreservation of ovarian tissue, a **future fertility treatment** after fertility preservation measures should generally be performed using IVF and ICSI. Simpler methods such as insemination after thawing cryopreserved semen samples are not sufficiently effective, as the number of cryopreserved samples is limited ("uniques") and cannot be replaced. Even if amenorrhea or azoospermia does not occur after cancer therapy, continued **long-term storage** of the samples is recommended, as there is a risk of cancer recurrence. In such cases, fertility preservation measures may be considered again. Cancer therapy can also damage genetic material, leading to **DNA strand breaks**. This affects the quality of oocytes and sperm. For example, fertilization, embryo development, and implantation may be impaired or disrupted, reducing the chances of having a biological child.

If the **risk** of **future infertility** due to planned gonadotoxic therapy is low (<20%), the necessity of a fertility-preserving measure should be carefully **weighed** by considering the **advantages and disadvantages**. Especially in women, fertility preservation is associated with both oocyte retrieval following stimulation treatment and ovarian tissue removal, which are surgical procedures with known risks. After medical counseling, patients should be given time to consider and then decide for or against fertility preservation measures.

Limits of Fertility Preservation in Women

During the initial medical consultation with the oncologist, oncological aspects regarding a future **pregnancy** should be discussed in detail (◘ Fig. 8.1). It must also be assessed whether a future pregnancy is compatible with the underlying disease, as the goal of fertility preservation is a subsequent ongoing pregnancy resulting in the birth of a healthy child. Examination findings must be evaluated to determine whether fertility preservation is justifiable based on the **clinical situation**. For example, if chemotherapy for leukemia must begin immediately, there is no time for oocyte retrieval. If young female cancer patients already have an **advanced cancer** and cure is unlikely, fertility preservation measures do not appear meaningful. For example, there is no curative approach for advanced and metastatic breast cancer.

Before fertility preservation, **prognostic factors** must be assessed to determine whether fertility-preserving measures can be effectively performed. If AFC and AMH values are low (■ Table 6.13), it is questionable whether the **ovarian reserve** is sufficient to obtain enough oocytes for future fertilization and embryo transfer, or whether enough primordial follicles will be present in the ovarian tissue for ovarian function after transplantation. Patients must also be counseled about the likelihood of a future ongoing pregnancy and live birth based on their age. **Women** aged **40 years and older** have a very low chance of having a biological child, as usually only a few oocytes can be retrieved. In subsequent fertilization, there is an increased rate of non-viable oocytes. Age-related chromosomal abnormalities are more common in oocytes, and fertilization is more likely to result in **chromosomal missegregation**.

Transposition of the Ovaries Prior to Radiation

Ovarian damage from radiation therapy is severe. Even a low dose of 2 Gy reduces follicle density by 50%. The extent of damage is age-dependent and lower in younger women. If radiation therapy is planned and the ovaries are within or near the radiation field, they can usually be surgically transposed out of the pelvis during a **laparoscopy**. However, this operation is not a routine procedure, and experience is limited. The repositioning of the ovaries must be tension-free to avoid circulatory disturbances and thus damage to the ovarian follicles. The ovaries should be positioned with a safety margin of 4 cm above the pelvic brim. The transposition of the ovaries out of the radiation field is called **ovarian transposition** or ovariopexy. In cervical cancer, Ewing's sarcoma (bone cancer, especially in children and adolescents), Hodgkin's and non-Hodgkin's lymphomas, and anal and rectal cancer, the pelvis may be within the radiation field. Therefore, ovarian transposition should be considered in these cancers. The treatment is effective, as ovarian function is preserved in about 70% of cases (Mossa et al. 2015).

Damage to the **uterus** must also be considered if it is within or near the radiation field. There is no standard procedure for fertility preservation of the uterus. It cannot be transposed as easily as the ovaries. For example, if the uterus is within or immediately adjacent to the radiation field, as in rectal cancer, the endometrium is usually permanently damaged. Even at a distance of 10 cm, a radiation dose is still 10% effective. As a result of radiation therapy, the endometrium may no longer be able to build up adequately during preparation for embryo transfer. Thus, embryo implantation is generally no longer possible. After surviving cancer, patients are therefore unlikely to be able to carry a pregnancy themselves, and uterine transplantation does not appear promising in these cases.

"Suppression" of the Ovaries by Medication

Treatment with **GnRH agonists** (see ▶ Chap. 6) is frequently performed, as it can be easily implemented by administering depot preparations at monthly intervals during chemotherapy. GnRH agonists should be given one week before the start of chemotherapy due to the initial "flare-up effect" and continued for one to two weeks after the last chemotherapy cycle. Alternatively, treatment with GnRH antagonists, which do not have a "flare-up effect" (off-label use), is possible. **Downregulation** during GnRH therapy leads to hormonal withdrawal symptoms such as hot flashes and sleep disturbances. These symptoms are already expected from chemotherapy, as follicular cell damage leads to cessation of estrogen production. Long-term use of GnRH agonists (>6 months) can also lead to osteoporosis with increased fracture risk due to estrogen deficiency. However, the duration of chemotherapy rarely exceeds the critical period of six months.

Therapy with GnRH agonists, which leads to **functional suppression** and **reduced blood flow** to the ovarian tissue, is intended to protect primordial follicles from the toxicity of chemotherapy. Primary follicles that have already begun the one-year developmental process toward mature oocytes are not protected (◨ Fig. 2.3). Primordial follicles can also enter the process of oocyte maturation during GnRH agonist therapy, as this begins independently of LH and FSH. Naturally, GnRH agonists are not indicated in children, and the hormonal efficacy in adolescents is questionable. The **effectiveness of therapy** with GnRH agonists is **not reliably proven**. To assess this more accurately, studies should document and evaluate not only amenorrhea but also FSH and AMH levels. Therefore, GnRH administration should not be performed as the sole intervention for fertility preservation. Hormonal therapy is only recommended in addition to effective fertility preservation measures such as cryopreservation of oocytes or ovarian tissue.

Freezing of Oocytes

The freezing of unfertilized and fertilized oocytes (◨ Fig. 1.2) has become an established and standardized technique over the past 20 years. The **vitrification** method has been instrumental in this develop-

ment. With this technique, harmful ice crystal formation within the cells is avoided, as the cells are frozen with a very high cooling rate after the addition of so-called cryoprotectants. This method is also referred to as "**ultra-rapid freezing**" (Trounson et al. 1987). The oocytes are transferred into an amorphous, glass-like state. Preparation and execution of oocyte retrieval for vitrification takes about two to three weeks. If fertility preservation is integrated into treatment planning from the time of cancer diagnosis, there is usually sufficient time for oocyte cryopreservation.

For vitrification, oocytes must be completely freed from the surrounding granulosa cells. This allows assessment of oocyte maturity under the microscope. Oocytes must be mature (**MII oocytes**) for cryopreservation and subsequent fertilization. Only mature oocytes can be fertilized. After thawing, depending on age, between 70 and 95% of **oocytes are viable**, and of these, 70 to 85% can be **fertilized** (Walker et al. 2022). Thus, not every retrieved oocyte can be vitrified, successfully thawed, and fertilized. This information is also important for patients when deciding for or against oocyte cryopreservation.

Stimulation is performed as controlled ovarian stimulation (**COS**) using the **antagonist protocol** (see ▶ Chap. 6). Stimulation can begin at any phase of the cycle (early follicular phase to luteal phase). In practice, this stimulation start is referred to as "**random-start stimulation**." Only in the case of a large leading follicle (≥13 mm) in the late follicular phase is ovulation induction with hCG or a GnRH agonist initially recommended. Stimulation starts about two days later, directly after ovulation. Standard treatment involves gonadotropin stimulation. Before follicle puncture, ovulation is triggered with a **GnRH agonist** and not with an hCG preparation (◨ Fig. 8.2). This can drastically reduce the risk of ovarian hyperstimulation syndrome

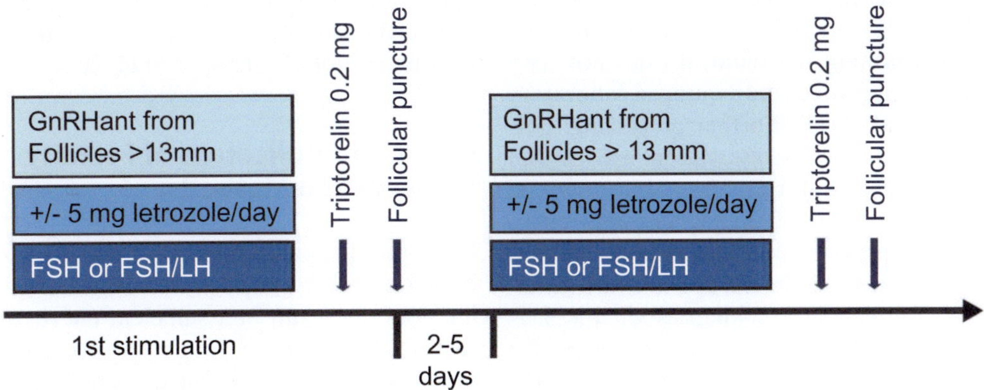

Fig. 8.2 Modified ovarian stimulation for fertility preservation and double stimulation. Double stimulation antagonist protocol: Triggering ovulation with the GnRH agonist (Triptorelin®) after the first stimulation, start of the second stimulation after follicle puncture. GnRHant: GnRH antagonist. (With kind permission from: Germeyer and von Wolff (2020))

(OHSS) (<0.2%), but not completely eliminate it (Germeyer and von Wolff 2020). In hormone receptor-positive breast cancer, additional administration of letrozole (aromatase inhibitor) should be used for ovarian stimulation.

If, during a later thawing procedure, one or more embryo transfers can be performed consecutively, one or more pregnancies and births may result. The number of live-born children per woman is referred to as the **cumulative live birth rate (CLBR)**. In women **over 35 years**, a maximum CLBR of about **35%** can be achieved (Cobo et al. 2016). In women **up to 35 years**, a CLBR of **85%** can be achieved with 15 oocytes. In these women, each additional oocyte increases the CLBR by 8.4%, whereas in women aged 36 and older, the increase is only 4.9% per additional oocyte. However, the CLBR cannot be further increased by additional mature oocytes if 15 oocytes are available for women up to 35 years and 11 oocytes for women aged 36 and older. Thus, **repeated stimulations** to obtain additional oocytes do not increase the chances of a live birth in these groups. **Thawing rates** also differ between the two **age groups**. In women up to 35 years, the thawing rate is about 95%, while in women aged 36 and older, it is only 82%.

Freezing of Ovarian Tissue

In contrast to the cryopreservation of oocytes, the cryopreservation of ovarian tissue for later transplantation was not previously considered a standard procedure. Coverage of costs by statutory health insurance (GKV) is currently provided, but is still regularly reviewed by the Federal Joint Committee (G-BA). **Cryopreservation of ovarian tissue** is recommended when the **time window** for oocyte cryopreservation is **less than two weeks**. This method also has its place in girls before completion of puberty or in cases of intact virginity. The tissue is removed under anesthesia via laparoscopy. This can be combined with a tubal patency test. To maximize the chances of spontaneous pregnancy, the ovarian tissue should later be transplanted on the side with a patent fallopian tube. Usually, the procedure is performed unilaterally and half an ovary is removed. The tissue must be immediately transferred into a pre-cooled transport medium. Overnight cooled transport to a highly specialized laboratory for further processing of the ovarian tissue is possible. This option is often used if the facility performing the removal does not have its own approved and equipped laboratory (Lotz et al. 2022). Further processing, portioning, and cryopreservation are carried out in the laboratory.

Initial results of pregnancies and births after approximately 500 **transplantations** of ovarian tissue in Europe are now available. In the registry analysis of the *FertiPROTEKT* Network e.V. (Network for Fertility-Protective Measures), 64 of the 196 transplanted patients became pregnant (32.7%). Fifty-two children were born alive. Only 9 women **aged 35 and older**, but 43 women **under 35 years** had a child (**birth rate 16.7%** versus **28.2%**). Thus, the chance of having one's own child after age 35 is 11.5% lower than under 35. The live birth rate in the *Ferti*PROTEKT registry data is confirmed in other publications. In another data analysis of 285 transplanted women from 5 European centers, 75 children born were documented (Dolmans et al. 2021). Thus, **one in four women** had a **child** after transplantation. Two-thirds of these women conceived **spontaneously**, one-third with **IVF treatment**. In this analysis as well, the pregnancy rate after transplantation was significantly higher in younger women. Even after gonadotoxic therapy for autoimmune diseases and other non-malignant conditions, about one in four women has a child after transplantation (Finkelstein et al. 2024).

The **birth rate** after **IVF treatment** was 21% (Dolmans et al. 2021). However, embryo transfer could only be performed in 50% of IVF cycles. The possible reason for this is reduced oocyte quality after transplantation. These data also show that **spontaneous pregnancies** are highly possible in transplanted patients. In principle, pregnancies after transplantation are also possible **from** the **remaining ovarian tissue** if this tissue still has residual function. Interestingly, data from Australia support this theory, as pregnancy rates after trans-

plantation of cryopreserved ovarian tissue were demonstrably not higher than without transplantation (Finkelstein et al. 2024).

Modified Application of Fertility Preservation Methods

Cryopreservation of sperm and oocytes can be performed repeatedly if a single freezing does not result in a sufficient **oocyte** or **sperm cell reserve** for future fertility treatment (◘ Table 8.1). Repeated cryopreservation of ejaculates can be performed at short notice. **Repeat cryopreservation** should be recommended if only a very small amount of ejaculate with limited quality could be frozen, or if the quality was borderline sufficient for a later ICSI treatment (see above). It is helpful for counseling and decision-making if a sample is thawed immediately after cryopreservation and the **revival rate (WBR)** of the sperm is determined. If the WBR is reduced, repeat cryopreservation should be recommended.

If the **oocyte reserve** is not sufficient after cryopreservation, a repeat stimulation can be performed if there is a sufficiently large time window before the start of tumor therapy. In practice, in this so-called **double stimulation**, stimulation is started again two to five days after follicle puncture (◘ Fig. 8.2). At the start of stimulation, there should ideally not be too many cystic corpora lutea or follicular cysts present. For this reason, GnRH antagonists are often administered from the first follicle puncture until the renewed start of stimulation before a planned double stimulation. GnRH antagonists should be started again when follicles reach a size of 13 mm. Ovulation is triggered as in the first stimulation with a GnRH agonist.

If repeated cryopreservation of oocytes and sperm still does **not result in a sufficient reserve** for future fertility treatment, depending on the time window for fertility preservation, a testicular biopsy or ovarian tissue removal for germ cell retrieval is also possible.

Even with these additional surgical measures, a sufficient reserve is not guaranteed. Germ cell retrieval and germ cell tissue removal can also be performed in **combination** (Table 8.1). **Cryopreservation** of **sperm cells** and performing a **testicular biopsy** are possible independently of each other in terms of timing. However, the combination of **oocyte retrieval** and removal of **ovarian tissue** must be planned. In practice, removal of ovarian tissue followed by stimulation treatment has proven effective, as the quality of ovarian tissue is not as good after follicle puncture as it is before stimulation (Fig. 8.3).

Patients without a sufficient reserve of oocytes and sperm are likely to be women and men whose infertility would have become apparent during a fertility workup due to reduced ovarian reserve or impaired semen quality. However, in men with testicular tumors, semen quality is usually impaired due to the disease itself.

Coverage of Costs for Fertility Preservation Measures

Since 2021, highly technical reproductive medicine measures for fertility preservation have become benefits covered by statutory health insurance (GKV) (Federal Joint Committee (G-BA) 2021). The scope of benefits is regulated in the "Directive of the Federal Joint Committee on Cryopreservation of Oocytes or Sperm or Germ Cell Tissue and Corresponding Medical Measures Due to Germ Cell-Damaging Therapy (**"Cryo-RL"**)" (Appendix 8.1). Germ cell-damaging treatments include surgical removal of the gonads, radiation therapy, and chemotherapy. For **entitlement to benefits**, the necessity of germ cell-damaging therapy must be certified on a **form** by a **specialist** who has diagnosed or is treating the underlying disease (Appendix 8.2). This specialist must also certify that he or she has established the **indication** for **reproductive medical treatment** and has provided an **initial consultation** on this. Subsequently, the **reproductive medicine specialist** with advanced training or the **andrologist** with the additional qualification must document his or her **counseling** on the prospects of success and risks of the possible measures and any psychosocial burdens on the form. **Eligible** are female patients up to their 40th birthday and male patients up to their 50th birthday.

The first version of the "Cryo-RL" included cryopreservation of unfertilized oocytes, sperm, and testicular tissue. Accord-

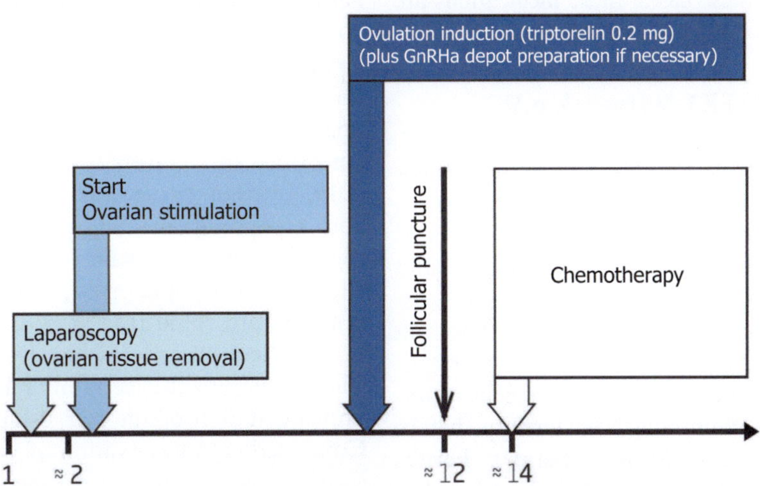

Fig. 8.3 Combined retrieval of oocytes and ovarian tissue. GnRHa: GnRH agonist. (Reproduced with permission from: Germeyer and von Wolff (2020))

ingly, the services were included with billing codes in the uniform fee schedule for statutory health insurance physicians (EBM). Previously, the expensive medical services plus the costs for the necessary high-priced medications and storage costs had to be paid privately by the affected patients. In 2022, the "Cryo-RL" was expanded to include **cryopreservation of ovarian tissue** including surgical services (laparoscopy, in exceptional cases laparotomy) with the corresponding billing codes. Eligible for ovarian tissue retrieval are children and adolescents no earlier than after the onset of menarche and women up to their 40th birthday. A **review** of cost coverage for cryopreservation of ovarian tissue by the G-BA is planned after two years.

Implementation of the "Cryo-RL" is still **not sufficiently regulated** for the **storage costs** of germ cells and germ cell tissue. Most storage facilities, even if located in close proximity to fertility centers, are not run by physicians and can only bill storage costs privately. Storage costs can only be billed through the Association of Statutory Health Insurance Physicians by qualified and approved physicians. The prescription of medications for ovarian stimulation is also not regulated in the "Cryo-RL" for **hormone receptor-positive tumors**. In these cases, these **medications** are contraindicated (**off-label use**).

*Ferti*PROTEKT Network e.V.

The network was founded by **university women's clinics** in 2006 and has been a registered **non-profit association** since 2015. It now includes more than 160 university and non-university member centers in Germany, Austria, and Switzerland. The aim of the association is to ensure that every patient of reproductive age can receive comprehensive counseling on fertility before undergoing gonadotoxic therapy. Fertility-preserving therapies should be offered in a standardized manner and their effectiveness should be regularly evaluated through scientific analysis. Furthermore, the effects of applied chemotherapies on fertility should continue to be investigated in order to be able to use less gonadotoxic drugs in cancer treatment in the long term, if possible. The implementation of fertility preservation is an **interdisciplinary task**. Involved are specialists in gynecological endocrinology and reproductive medicine, oncologists of all specialties including pediatric oncologists, human geneticists, as well as reproductive biologists and psychologists. Fertility-preserving measures in men are not yet recorded by the network. The network " **Androprotect** " is additionally committed to preserving **male fertility**, especially in **boys** before puberty. This scientifically oriented network was founded in 2012 by the Center for Reproductive Medicine and Andrology (CeRA) at the University Hospital Münster. It includes physicians from various specialties as well as biologists.

Consultations on fertility preservation, possibly with subsequent interventions, are mainly conducted for breast cancer (43%), followed by malignant lymphomas (22.3%), other malignancies (25.5%), and benign diseases (*Ferti*PROTEKT 2024). The number of consultations has doubled in the last 10 years from about 1,000 to about 2,000. **Cryopreservation** of oocytes is mainly performed at private fertility centers, while cryopreservation of ovarian tissue is mainly performed at university hospitals. Until 2019, ovarian tissue was mostly removed and cryopreserved. Since 2020, for fertility preservation, **mainly oocytes** are retrieved and cryopreserved, with a continuing upward trend (■ Fig. 8.4). The number of these procedures has even doubled. This development is certainly related to the implementation of the "Cryo-RL" in 2021. Combined cryopreservation of oocytes and ovarian tissue is rarely performed.

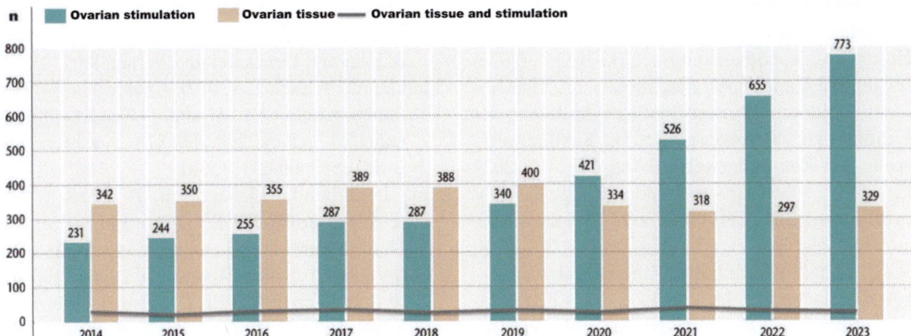

Fig. 8.4 Ovarian stimulations and cryopreservations of ovarian tissue 2014–2023. (Reproduced with permission from: *Ferti*PROTEKT (2024))

Learning Objectives

- Convey knowledge about the effects of gonadotoxic therapies on fertility
- Presentation of the limitations and possibilities of fertility-protective measures

Fertility preservation refers to the cryopreservation of oocytes and sperm as well as ovarian and testicular tissue prior to germ cell-damaging therapies. These therapies include chemotherapy or radiation therapy or complete or extensive removal of ovarian and testicular tissue. In men, fertility preservation has been common practice for many decades. In women, fertility preservation with oocytes has only been possible since the availability of vitrification as a gentle method of cryopreservation. However, there are limits to successful or responsible cryopreservation: for example, if the oocyte reserve is low or if the underlying disease has a poor prognosis. GnRH agonists induce ovarian quiescence and can be used in addition to the effective methods of cryopreservation of germ cells and tissues. Oocyte and sperm retrieval for cryopreservation can be repeated if the cryo-reserve is borderline small. Usually, there is sufficient time for fertility-preserving measures before tumor therapy if fertility preservation is considered during therapy planning. In principle, after fertility-preserving measures, fertility treatment should be performed using the ICSI method in order to achieve the best possible pregnancy rates with the limited number of cryopreserved samples. However, ART is not routinely recommended after transplantation of ovarian tissue, as spontaneous pregnancies often occur. The *Ferti*PROTEKT and AndroProtect networks have been established to provide optimal care for affected patients.

Below is the link to the electronic supplementary material.

References

Gemeinsamer Bundesausschuss (G-BA) (2021) Richtlinie des Gemeinsamen Bundesausschusses zur Kryokonservierung von Ei- oder Samenzellen oder Keimzellgewebe sowie entsprechende medizinische Maßnahmen wegen keimzellschädigender Therapie (Kryo-RL). BAnz AT 19.02.2021 B7: 1–4. ▶ https://www.bundesanzeiger.de/pub/publication/6Lgl9NcpzhoCi0en3V0/content/6Lgl9NcpzhoCi0en3V0/BAnz%20AT%2019.02.2021%20B7. pdf?inline. Zuletzt 15.4.2024

Gemeinsamer Bundesausschuss (G-BA) (2022) Bekanntmachung eines Beschlusses des Gemeinsamen Bundesausschusses über eine Änderung der Richtlinie zur Kryokonservierung: Kryokonservierung von Keimzellgewebe. BAnz AT 14.11.2022 B2: 1–3. ► https://www.bundesanzeiger.de/pub/publication/uBGEHcNpHfzwT7revKw/content/uBGEHcNpHfzwT7revKw/BAnz%20AT%2014.11.2022%20B2.pdf?inline Zuletzt 15.4.2024

Cobo A, García-Velasco JA, Coello A et al (2016) Oocyte vitrification as an efficient option for elective fertility preservation. Fertil Steril105:755–764.e8. ► https://doi.org/10.1016/j.fertnstert.2015.11.027. Epub 2015 Dec 10. PMID: 26688429

Dolmans MM, von Wolff M, Poirot C et al (2021) Transplantation of cryopreserved ovarian tissue in a series of 285 women: a review of five leading European centers. Fertil Steril 115(5):1102–1115. ► https://doi.org/10.1016/j.fertnstert.2021.03.008

Fertilitätserhalt bei onkologischen Erkrankungen. S2k Leitlinie (2017) S. 41. ► https://register.awmf.org/assets/guidelines/015-082l_S2k_Fertilitaetserhaltung-bei-onkologischen-Therapien_2017-12-verlaengert.pdf Zuletzt 16.4.2024

*Ferti*PROTEKT (2024). In: D·I·R (2024) Jahrbuch 2023. J Reproduktionsmed Endokrinol 21 (Sonderheft 4): 45–48

Finkelstein T, Zhang Y, Vollenhoven B et al (2024) Successful pregnancy rates amongst patients undergoing ovarian tissue cryopreservation for non-malignant indications: A systematic review and meta-analysis. Eur J Obstet Gynecol Reprod Biol. 292:30–39. ► https://doi.org/10.1016/j.ejogrb.2023.11.004

Germeyer A, von Wolff M (2020) Ovarielle Stimulation. In: Von Wolff M, Nawroth F (ed) Indikationsstellung. Indikation und Durchführung fertilitätsprotektiver Maßnahmen bei onkologischen und nicht-onkologischen Erkrankungen, Schmidt & Klaunig, Druckerei und Verlag, Kiel, 215–227

Liedtke C, Kiesel L (2012) Chemotherapy-Induced Amenorrhea—An Update. Geburtshilfe Frauenheilkd. Sep;72(9):809–818. ► https://doi.org/10.1055/s-0032-1315361

Lotz L, J Bender-Liebenthron, R Dittrich, L et al. (2022) FertiPROTEKT (Transplantation group), Determinants of transplantation success with cryopreserved ovarian tissue: data from 196 women of the FertiPROTEKT network, Human Reproduction, 37(12):2787–2796. ► https://doi.org/10.1093/humrep/deac225

Meistrich ML (2013) Effects of chemotherapy and radiotherapy on spermatogenesis in humans. Fertil Steril 100(5):1180–6. ► https://doi.org/10.1016/j.fertnstert.2013.08.010

Mossa B, Schimberni M, Di Benedetto L et al (2015) Ovarian transposition in young women and fertility sparing. Eur Rev Med Pharmacol Sci 9:3418–25

Trounson A, Peura A, Kirby C (1987) Ultrarapid freezing: a new low-cost and effective method of embryo cryopreservation. Fertil Steril 48(5):843–50. ► https://doi.org/10.1016/s0015-0282(16)59542-9

Von Wolff M, Nawroth F (2020) Indikationsstellung. In: Von Wolff M, Nawroth F (ed) Indikation und Durchführung fertilitätsprotektiver Maßnahmen bei onkologischen und nicht-onkologischen Erkrankungen. Schmidt & Klaunig, Druckerei und Verlag, Kiel, 28–35

Walker Z Lanes A Ginsberg Elizabeth (2022) Oocyte cryopreservation review: outcomes of medical oocyte cryopreservation and planned oocyte cryopreservation. ► Reproductive Biology and Endocrinology volume 20,1–14. ► https://doi.org/10.1186/s12958-021-00884-0 Zuletzt 12.4.2024

Basics of the IVF Laboratory

Contents

Supplementary Information The online version contains supplementary material available at ▶ https://doi.org/10.1007/978-3-662-73035-5_9.

Sperm Preparation for IUI, IVF, ICSI

IVF treatment was introduced more than 40 years ago as a therapeutic option for tubal infertility. In connection with this ground-breaking new therapy, new in vitro techniques were developed. These also include methods for sperm preparation, which have triggered a transformation in the way insemination treatment is performed.

Introduction to Sperm Preparation

As part of assisted reproductive technologies (ART), the ejaculate must be processed. The sperm cells are separated from the seminal fluid and the fertilization-competent sperm are selected. In natural fertilization, nature's protective mechanisms ensure that only competent sperm reach the fallopian tube and are able to fertilize an egg cell. The seminal fluid also contains prostaglandins, which, in the case of **intrauterine insemination (IUI)** with ejaculate, can trigger cramps in the woman. Many semen samples contain microbes, which also poses an infection risk. For this reason, insemina-

tions were previously performed only intra-vaginally or into the cervix. In both **intravaginal (IVI)** and **intracervical insemination (ICI)**, the cervix acts as a natural filter for the ejaculate. The sperm are naturally separated from the seminal plasma, so that only motile sperm can actively pass through the cervix during IVI or ICI. With the new methods of sperm preparation, prostaglandins can be effectively removed from the seminal fluid, microbial contamination reduced, and the concentration of motile sperm increased many times over. This makes it possible to transfer the prepared sperm directly into the uterine cavity using a catheter. After bypassing the cervix with an insemination catheter, the sperm can reach the fallopian tube without further obstacles to fertilization. With these preparation techniques, IUI can be performed with minimal risk.

The prerequisites for a sperm's fertilization capability are maturity and motility, as well as good "external qualities" (normal morphology) and good "internal qualities" (DNA integrity). Sperm preparation makes it possible to isolate and concentrate the normally shaped, mature, motile, and functional sperm from the seminal fluid for fer-

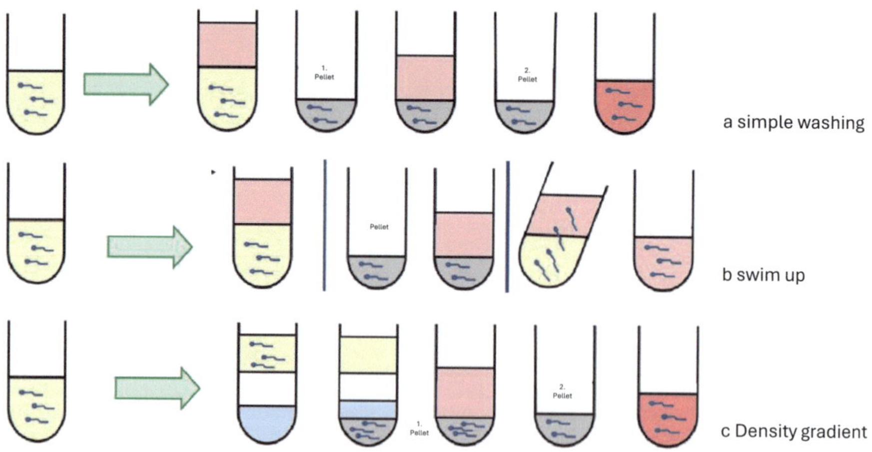

Fig. 9.1 Standard methods of sperm preparation: **a** simple washing **b** swim up **c** density gradient (two-layer). (Adapted from Baston-Büst D (Specialization Qualification in Reproductive Medicine))

tilization (◨ Fig. 5.3). During preparation, the specially composed culture medium initiates **capacitation**, so that the sperm become capable of fertilization after ejaculation (see ▶ Chap. 2). This process increases the permeability of the sperm to calcium. The motility of the sperm is enhanced, and the important acrosome reaction required for fertilization of the egg cell at the end of the fallopian tube is triggered. There are different methods of sperm preparation (◨ Fig. 9.1). Depending on the semen quality in the diagnostic **pre-semen analysis**, the individually appropriate preparation method is selected.

Standard Methods for Sperm Preparation

Simple Washing

After liquefaction, the ejaculate is layered 1:1 with a standard culture medium (**medium**), mixed, and centrifuged. This causes the sperm to be forced to the bottom of the tube, forming a **pellet**. The supernatant is discarded and the cells are resuspended in a wash medium (first wash step). After another **centrifugation**, the sperm are again forced to the bottom of the tube (second pellet). The supernatant is again discarded. Finally, the pellet is resuspended in culture medium (second wash step) and can be used for ART treatment. This method can also be used in cases of severely impaired semen quality.

Swim Up

The ejaculate is layered with medium, mixed, and centrifuged as in simple washing. The pellet is then overlaid with culture medium and incubated at a **45-degree** angle in the **incubator** at 37 degrees for **one hour**. The highly motile sperm migrate from the pellet into the overlaid culture medium. Finally, the supernatant containing the motile sperm is pipetted off. This method can be used when semen quality is good.

Density Gradient

Two media with different densities are layered in a tube, with the higher-density medium at the bottom. This **gradient** is overlaid with the ejaculate. The tube is centrifuged. Immotile and non-viable sperm, as well as other cells and microbes, unlike mature and functional sperm, cannot pass through the gradient. After centrifugation, only the mature, motile, and functional sperm have reached the bottom of the tube. The supernatant, consisting of the remaining seminal plasma and the two-layer gradient, is discarded. The pellet is resuspended in a wash medium and, after a wash step, used for fertility treatment. This preparation method is also suitable for impaired semen quality.

Preparation Methods for Selecting Sperm with Intact DNA

With the advancement of ART techniques, there are now additional preparation methods, some of which may become standard procedures in the future. These methods must prove to be effective, time- and cost-efficient. In particular, the new methods aim to better select the best sperm with intact DNA for ART treatment, since sperm DNA integrity, along with motility and morphology, is an important quality criterion. Sperm with fragmented DNA are associated with lower fertilization rates, impaired embryo development, and higher miscarriage rates. Patients with an increased proportion of sperm with DNA fragmentation can already be identified through an extended pre-semen analysis. The **Sperm Chromatin Structure Assay (SCSA)** is considered the "gold standard" in diagnostics for assessing DNA integrity and detecting strand breaks (see ▶ Chap. 5). Some "sperm sorting" methods are suitable for IVF and ICSI treatment, others only for ICSI (◨ Table 9.1).

◨ Table 9.1   Sperm preparation for selection of sperm with intact DNA

Method	Technical Requirements	Outcome
*MACS: Magnetic-activated cell sorting	e.g., MiniMACS™ device	Miscarriage rate ↓, PR ↑, LBR ↑
*MSS: microfluidic sperm sorting	ZyMōt™ chamber (consumable)	Miscarriage rate ↓, PR ↑
**IMSI: intracytoplasmic morphologically selected sperm injection	Adaptation of microscope equipment	Miscarriage rate →, LBR →
**PICSI: physiological ICSI	PICSI® dish (consumable)	Miscarriage rate ↓, embryo quality ↑, PR ↑

PR: pregnancy rate, LBR: live birth rate, *suitable for IVF and ICSI, **suitable for ICSI

Among the extended therapeutic semen analyses for examining sperm DNA and preparation is the **Magnetic-Activated Cell Sorting (MACS)** test (Pacheco et al. 2020). Sperm with strand breaks can be labeled with magnetic microparticles and then successfully separated from sperm with intact DNA using magnetic fields. The sperm with intact DNA are then used for IVF or ICSI treatment. This method can reduce the miscarriage rate and increase pregnancy and live birth rates. Sperm with intact DNA can also be isolated using a **Microfluidic Sperm Sorting** (MSS) system. In this microfluidic sperm sorting, motile sperm must actively pass through a barrier with small openings. Sperm with insufficient progressive motility are already held back by the barrier. Sperm with good motility must actively and independently, in a process akin to natural selection, swim through the openings into a separate chamber, where they accumulate. For IVF or ICSI treatment, sperm from this separate chamber are used. As far as is known, this method can improve pregnancy rates (Parrella et al. 2019; Zaha et al. 2023). In patients with a conspicuously high DNA fragmentation index (DFI), embryo development can be improved just as well with sperm selected by an MSS system as with testicular sperm obtained after testicular biopsy (Hunkler et al. 2024).

With **IMSI (intracytoplasmic morphologically selected sperm injection)**, it is possible, by optically enhancing the ICSI microscope (≥ 6,000x), to specifically select sperm for ICSI based on their detailed morphology and inject them into the egg cell. Sperm with **vacuoles** are an indication of incipient degeneration and thus DNA fragmentation. Such non-functional sperm can be identified and excluded from ICSI. However, it has not yet been demonstrated that IMSI leads to a lower miscarriage rate or a higher birth rate (Duran-Retamal et al. 2020). Another option for selecting the best sperm is the **physiological ICSI (PICSI)** method. This utilizes the ability of mature sperm to bind to hyaluronan, which naturally surrounds the egg cell with the cumulus cells. Only mature sperm with good genetic integrity bind to hyaluronan. In contrast, motile but immature sperm do not bind. Various studies have shown that PICSI can increase both the fertilization rate and the proportion of embryos with good quality (Novoselsky Persky et al. 2021). At the same time, pregnancy rates were higher in older patients (West et al. 2022) and miscarriage rates were reduced (Kirkman-Brown et al. 2019). Overall, the success of the PICSI method remains controversial.

Testicular sperm are almost immotile, so that vital and non-vital sperm cannot initially be distinguished for ICSI treatment. The active agent **theophylline** is a cell activator, so that viable sperm are activated and become motile. By adding theophylline to the medium, it is possible to improve fertilization and achieve pregnancy by injecting activated motile sperm.

Procedure of IVF and ICSI Treatment

Additional Equipment in the ART Laboratory for ICSI

The term ART treatment encompasses all types of artificial reproduction, including IUI, but especially oocyte treatment with IVF and ICSI. An ICSI treatment is a specialized procedure within IVF treatment. While IVF was originally developed for patients with tubal damage, the ICSI technique is an advanced IVF method for patients with severely reduced semen quality (see ▶ Chap. 5) or for couples after fertilization failure. Oocyte treatment with ICSI is also necessary for other ART procedures such as preimplantation genetic diagnosis (PGD). For this specialized oocyte treatment, the ART laboratory must be equipped with a microscope with higher magnification (200–400x), as well as a micromanipulator and a heated microscope stage. The heated microscope stage is necessary because oocytes, which are sensitive to changes in temperature and pH, must remain outside the incubator for a longer period due to the additional microinjection. ICSI treatment is time- and labor-intensive and can only be performed safely by highly qualified and trained personnel (◻ Fig. 6.3). An oocyte is about 0.1 mm in size, while a sperm head is only about 0.005 mm (◻ Table 2.1). The time for oocyte handling outside the incubator should be kept as short as possible to ensure good pregnancy outcomes after ICSI.

Preparation of Culture Dishes and Media the Day Before

Already one day before an ART treatment, the culture media for sperm preparation and the ART procedure must be prepared. The time in the incubator for pre-warming the media and adjusting the pH value takes several hours. The culture dishes for **IVF** and **ICSI** are prepared differently. Therefore, the treatment method must be determined no later than one day before oocyte retrieval so that the culture dishes are ready for the chosen oocyte treatment. This also applies to many **additional procedures** that must be appropriately prepared for the day of oocyte retrieval. For example, device-specific culture dishes ("slides") for time-lapse incubators must be prepared with medium. These special incubators allow time-lapse monitoring of embryo development from the moment of fertilization (see below). There are no additional time buffers for incubating the media on the day of oocyte retrieval, because the "trigger shot" (hCG) sets the natural chronological sequence of the subsequent fertilization steps. In ICSI treatment, approximately 40 hours after ovulation induction, a sperm should be injected into each oocyte. If the **natural timing** of the **fertilization process** is deviated from, the fertilization results become uncertain.

Procedure of IVF and ICSI Treatment on the Day of Oocyte Retrieval in the ART Laboratory

On the day of oocyte retrieval, sperm collection and preparation are performed first to prepare for oocyte treatment (see above). At the time of follicular puncture, it should already be certain that fertilizable sperm are available for ART treatment. First, a **therapeutic semen analysis** is performed to determine sperm concentration and motility. This is followed by preparation of the ejaculate using the previously determined method. For insemination of oocytes in

IVF, a second semen analysis is performed after preparation. The volume and absolute concentration of the prepared sperm cells for insemination are documented. In ICSI, a second semen analysis after preparation is not required. However, it must be documented whether sperm cells are available for ICSI treatment. The main differences in the procedures for IVF and ICSI treatment in the ART laboratory are summarized in ◘ Table 9.2.

In a standard **IVF treatment**, oocytes and sperm are combined in a culture dish. The sperm must find their own way into the oocyte. On the day of oocyte retrieval, the oocytes are immediately selected from the aspirates, which consist of follicular fluid and blood admixtures. This step is called **oocyte isolation**. For fertilization, 100,000 to 1 million sperm/ml are added to the oocytes up to four hours later. The sperm must penetrate the **cumulus-oocyte complex** (COC) and bind to the zona pellucida in order to enter the oocyte (◘ Fig. 2.6). The next morning, fertilization is checked, the so-called "PN check." Both the female and male pronuclei must have formed, and the second polar body must have been extruded (◘ Fig. 1.2).

In **ICSI treatment** as well, oocytes are isolated from the follicular aspirate as in IVF. The main differences between IVF and ICSI are summarized in ◘ Table 9.2. For ICSI, the cumulus complex must be removed from the oocytes before fertilization. In technical terms, this process is called **denudation**. The maturity of the oocytes is determined, as only mature oocytes (MII oocytes) can be fertilized by ICSI. The "naked" oocytes are injected with a single sperm each under the ICSI microscope. The time window of up to four hours after retrieval should be observed in ICSI to avoid disrupting the natural fertilization process. Otherwise, fertilization failure or abnormal development of the fertilized oocytes may occur. In standard treatment, after sperm preparation, motile sperm with normal morphology are selected for ICSI. Under the ICSI microscope, the selected sperm are immobilized by tapping the tail with the injection pipette and then drawn tail-first into the ICSI pipette. Injection into the oocyte is performed head-first (◘ Fig. 6.3). The sperm do not have to find their own way to or into the oocyte. The next morning, as in IVF, fertilization is checked.

◘ **Table 9.2**   Differences in the Procedure of IVF and ICSI Treatment in the ART Laboratory

	IVF	ICSI
Technical Equipment	Standard microscope	Specially equipped microscope with higher magnification, micromanipulator, heated microscope stage
Follicular puncture (Day 0)	Oocyte isolation	Oocyte isolation
Sperm preparation	100,000 to 1 million sperm/ml	Selection by motility and morphology, one sperm per oocyte
Preparation of oocyte treatment	Cumulus-oocyte complex (COC) remains	Removal of cumulus, assessment of oocyte maturity
Fertilization method (Day 0)	Insemination	Microinjection
Fertilization check (Day 1)	Removal of cumulus Assessment of oocyte maturity PN check	PN check

Fertilization Check One Day After Retrieval and Fertilization Errors

To determine the maturity of the oocytes and the signs of fertilization ("PN check"), in IVF the oocytes must first be denuded. In ICSI, the oocytes are already "naked" because denudation was performed before ICSI the previous day. In a normal **fertilization**, two **pronuclei** are visible in the oocyte at the "PN check" 20 to 24 hours after oocyte treatment (Fig. 9.2). The formation of both pronuclei indicates that the oocyte is activated. Activation leads to increased metabolic activity in the oocyte and initiates the fertilization cascade, followed by embryo development. One pronucleus comes from the oocyte, the other from the sperm (Fig. 1.2). However, normal fertilization does not always occur. Only fertilized oocytes can develop into a competent embryo and result in the birth of a child. **Fertilization errors** are identified by the presence of **no pronucleus**, only **one pronucleus**, or **more than two pronuclei** in the oocyte (Fig. 9.2, Table 9.3). The cause may lie in oocyte quality (oocyte factor) or sperm quality (**sperm factor**). If no pronucleus forms, in IVF the sperm may be unable to pene-

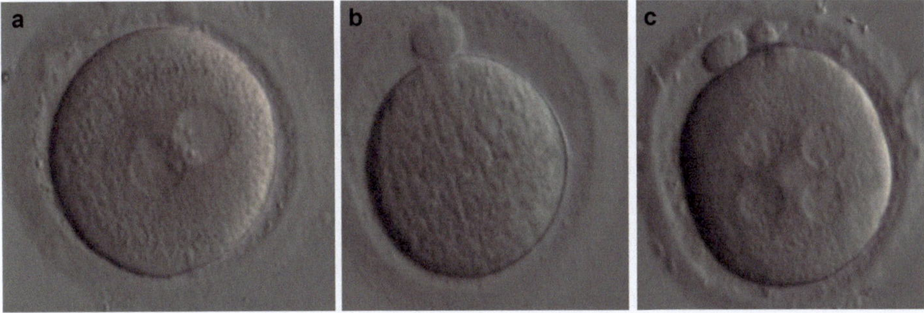

 Fig. 9.2 Normal and abnormal fertilization in IVF and ICSI treatment. **a**: Normal fertilization: 2 pronuclei; **b**: no pronucleus, no fertilization; **c**: 6 pronuclei (4 visible in the image plane), abnormal fertilization. (Adapted from Gutknecht D (Specialization in Reproductive Medicine))

 Table 9.3 Fertilization errors after IVF and ICSI treatment

Level of disturbance	Sperm factor	Oocyte factor
Cumulus*	No penetration	n.s.
Zona*	Zona binding does not work	n.s.
Oocyte*	No penetration	n.s.
Sperm-zona block does not work*	n.s.	≥ 3 pronuclei
Oocyte immature	n.s.	No polar body
No oocyte activation	e.g., DNA fragmentation	No pronucleus
All chromosomes extruded into 2nd polar body	n.s.	1 pronucleus
> 1 chromosome set in the oocyte	n.s.	3 pronuclei

*Disturbance only in oocyte treatment with IVF method

trate the cumulus cells surrounding the oocyte, fail to bind to the zona, fail to enter the oocyte, or fail to trigger the fertilization cascade. The sperm factor can usually be overcome by ICSI. If pronucleus formation fails after ICSI, the sperm DNA may no longer be intact (fragmented). Fertilization failure may also be due to the oocyte. An **oocyte factor** exists, for example, if the oocyte is of poor quality or immature. Immature oocytes have not yet extruded a polar body and are identified and excluded from treatment before ICSI. Fertilization disorders can also result if the zona pellucida reaction does not function. In this oocyte defect, sperm bind to the zona pellucida, but multiple sperm can enter the oocyte and form multiple pronuclei (**polyspermy**, ◘ Fig. 9.2). Such abnormally fertilized oocytes may not be cultured according to the guidelines of the German Medical Association. If, during fertilization, all chromosomes are extruded into the second polar body or if extrusion of the second polar body fails and the chromosomes remain in the oocyte, only one (**monoploidy**) or three pronuclei (**triploidy**) may form.

Temperature Control for Quality Assurance

The oocyte completes meiosis only upon fertilization by a sperm. The proper separation of chromosomes is organized by the **spindle apparatus**, which is stable only at **37 degrees**. To ensure correct chromosome distribution during meiosis and subsequent cell divisions, temperature must be strictly controlled during fertilization. Abnormally fertilized oocytes are usually detected during fertilization control ("PN check") and must not be cultured. **Chromosome missegregation** during subsequent cell divisions can lead to **developmental arrest**, **implantation failure**, or **miscarriage**. To preserve the spindle apparatus and thus the developmental competence of embryos, the temperature for oocytes in the ART laboratory must be strictly maintained at 37 degrees. This means that all surfaces in contact with oocytes must be at 37 degrees. This concept of a so-called **heat chain** must be implemented seamlessly from oocyte retrieval to embryo transfer (◘ Fig. 9.3). This also includes pre-warming the tubes used to

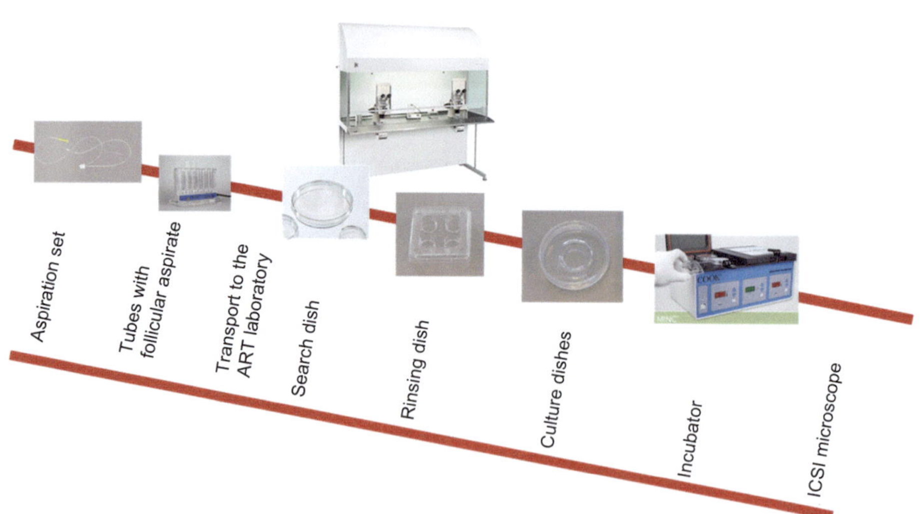

◘ **Fig. 9.3** Heat chain from oocyte retrieval to embryo transfer. (Adapted from Gutknecht D (Specialization in Reproductive Medicine))

collect follicular fluid and maintaining the temperature in the culture dishes. At every station of the heat chain, the temperature must be regularly checked and monitored for cold spots.

Additional Procedures (PICSI, Calcium Ionophore, Assisted Hatching)

During IVF or ICSI treatment, additional procedures can be performed that may improve pregnancy and birth rates. Important additional procedures include PICSI, the addition of a calcium ionophore to the medium, and assisted hatching. Decisions regarding additional treatments are made individually during the medical consultation.

Additional procedures are performed at different times during oocyte culture and may overlap with additional procedures during sperm preparation.

In **physiological ICSI (PICSI)**, the ability of sperm to bind to **hyaluronan** (hyaluronic acid) is used to select the best sperm for ICSI (◘ Table 9.1). The cumulus-oocyte complex contains a high proportion of hyaluronan, and only mature and functional sperm have a receptor for this component. Immature sperm or those with DNA fragmentation and early apoptosis (programmed cell death) lack a receptor for hyaluronan. If this receptor is missing, the sperm cannot bind and therefore cannot fertilize an oocyte. This natural selection process for mature and intact sperm for ICSI is utilized in the PICSI procedure. The aim is primarily to improve embryo quality and reduce miscarriage rates (see above). On the day of oocyte retrieval, sperm are selected directly from the PICSI® dish for ICSI. The central area of this dish is coated with hyaluronan. Mature, bound sperm can be identified for ICSI because they display characteristic **rotational movement** (◘ Fig. 9.4). In the standard ICSI procedure, by contrast, sperm are selected only by morphology and motility, not by "intrinsic qualities." The alternative to the PICSI®

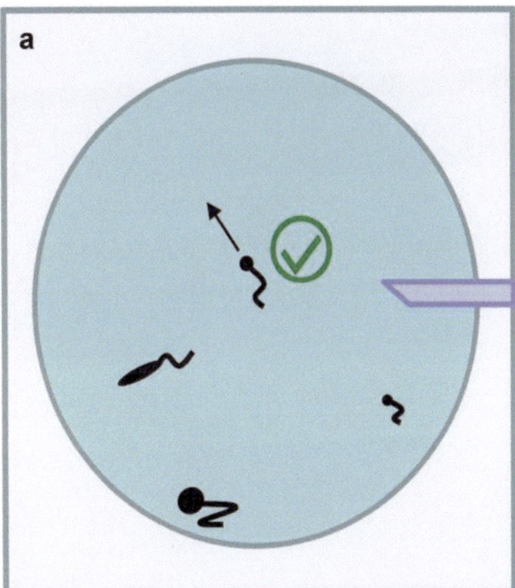
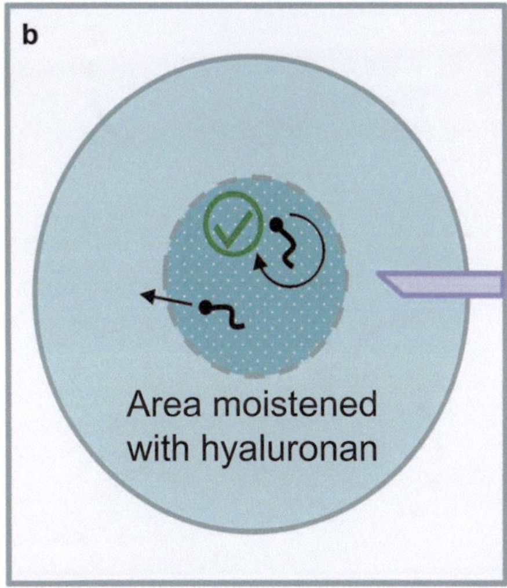

◘ **Fig. 9.4** Sperm selection with physiological ICSI (PICSI). **a:** ICSI dish for sperm injection. Selection of sperm by motility and morphology; **b:** PICSI® dish for sperm injection. Selection of sperm by binding to hyaluronan, "rotational movement," motility, and morphology. (Adapted from Trapphoff T (Specialization in Reproductive Medicine))

dish is SpermSlow®. This hyaluronan-containing medium is added to an ICSI dish. Intact sperm with the hyaluronan receptor **swim more slowly**. Sperm selection is based on morphology and additionally on the modified motility of the sperm.

During fertilization in the oocyte, **calcium currents** play an important role. The mature oocyte (MII oocyte) has stored calcium in the endoplasmic reticulum (ER) for the fertilization process. The signal for calcium release is the entry of the sperm into the oocyte. This activates the oocyte and releases the stored calcium. The second meiotic division (meiosis II) is triggered. After completion of meiosis II, the female and male pronuclei have formed, and the second polar body has been extruded (Fig. 9.5). Activation of oocytes can be enhanced chemically by adding a **Ca-ionophore**. This is a molecule that transports calcium across a cell membrane. A Ca-ionophore is used after fertilization failure, due to a low fertilization rate of < 30%, or in cases of reduced embryo quality to activate the oo-

cyte. In addition, this treatment is recommended for ICSI with testicular sperm. In this chemical oocyte activation, calcium is released within the oocyte and calcium also flows in from outside. This is intended to facilitate fertilization with completion of meiosis II. In practice, additional oocyte treatment with a Ca-ionophore is usually performed immediately after ICSI on the day of oocyte retrieval. The oocytes are incubated for about 15 minutes in a culture medium supplemented with Ca-ionophore. Current data show that artificial activation of oocytes can increase fertilization rate, embryo quality, implantation rate, and live birth rate (Tejera et al. 2021; Chen et al. 2022; Shan et al. 2022). No negative impact on child health has been observed. Since the exact timing of fertilization is not known in IVF, Ca-ionophore treatment cannot be used with this fertilization method.

Thinning or opening of the zona pellucida (egg shell) is referred to as "assisted hatching" or "laser treatment." This oocyte

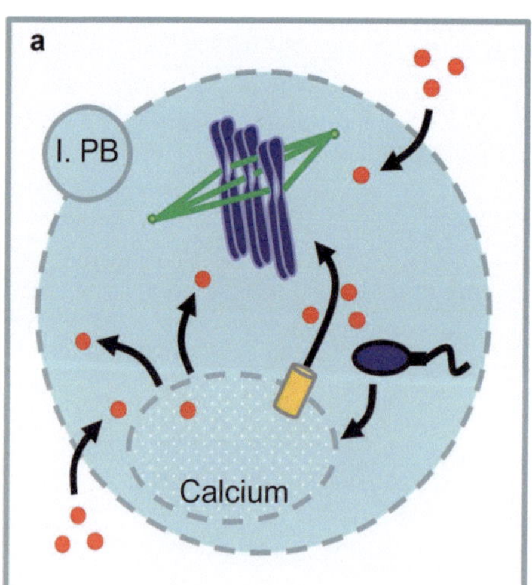

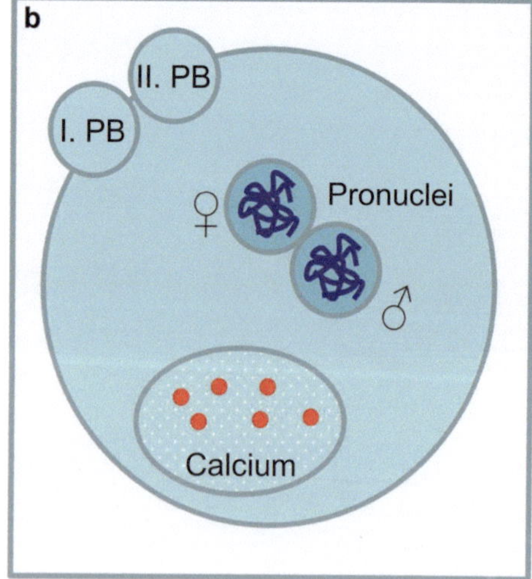

Fig. 9.5 Activation of the oocyte with Ca-ionophore. **a**: Addition of Ca-ionophore causes calcium influx in addition to release of calcium from the intracellular calcium store, activation of the oocyte, and initiation of meiosis II. **b**: Completion of meiosis II, extrusion of the second polar body, formation of pronuclei, and onset of embryonic development. (Adapted from Trapphoff T (Specialization in Reproductive Medicine))

treatment is usually performed shortly before transfer, regardless of the day of development. Assisted hatching is therefore performed on days two to five of development, depending on the timing of transfer. Thinning of the zona pellucida is performed with a laser that can be set with micrometer precision. This allows the laser treatment to be performed without any apparent risk of injury to the embryo. The laser treatment is intended to facilitate the natural hatching of an embryo from the egg shell on days 5 to 6 of development. Successful hatching of an embryo is a prerequisite for implantation. From an embryological perspective, assisted hatching can be recommended for embryo transfer after thawing, as cryopreservation can cause hardening of the zona pellucida. However, the benefit of this procedure is not clearly proven due to conflicting data (ASRM guideline 2022). Live birth rates are not demonstrably higher in either fresh or FET cycles. However, hatching through the laser opening does not increase the risk of monozygotic twins.

Fundamentals of Embryology

The **embryonic period** refers to the time span from the development of the fertilized egg (pronuclear stage) to the embryo (see ▶ Chap. 7). This period begins with early development from the moment of fertilization and ends with the completion of organ formation in the 8th week of development (calculated as the 10th week of pregnancy). In the early phase up to the 2nd week of development, the miscarriage rate is high. However, many women are unaware of their pregnancy during this phase. Menstruation occurs as expected or is only a few days late. The next phase of the embryonic period is characterized by **organogenesis**. Each organ system has its own sensitive phase. By the time a pregnancy is detected by a positive test, **brain** and **heart** are already forming. In this critical phase, teratogenic influences therefore mainly lead to brain and heart defects.

Fertilization

Fertilization (fertilization) naturally takes place in the fallopian tube (see ▶ Chap. 2, ◘ Fig. 2.6). A mature oocyte has completed meiosis I and is referred to as a metaphase II oocyte, abbreviated as **MII oocyte**. The first polar body has been extruded from the oocyte and lies between the cell membrane and the zona pellucida (◘ Figs. 1.2 and 9.2). ◘ Table 9.4 contains the **chronological sequence** of the individual steps of fertilization and subsequent development up to the blastocyst. Successful penetration by a sperm activates the oocyte, completing meiosis II (◘ Fig. 9.5). The second polar body is extruded, and the **female** and **male pronuclei** are formed. On day 1, 16 to 20 hours after insemination of the oocytes or after microinjection, the so-called **"PN check"** (see above) is performed to determine whether two **pronuclei** have formed. If only one pronucleus or three pronuclei are

◘ **Table 9.4** Timetable of early embryonic development

	Day 0	Day 1		Day 2	Day 3	Day 4	Day 5
Stage	MII oocyte	2-PN stage	2-cell stage	4-cell stage	8-cell stage	Morula	Blastocyst
Hours after insemination	0	16–20	26–29	42–44	66–70	90–100	114–120

visible, this likely indicates irregular fertilization in the sense of monoploidy or triploidy. Such cells may not be cultured according to professional regulations. If **two pronuclei** are visible, the oocyte is considered **normally** fertilized. However, fertilization is only properly completed with the first cell division. This begins, in the case of timely development, about 26 hours after insemination of the oocytes. First, the pronuclei dissolve, and immediately thereafter the first **cleavage division** to form the **2-cell stage** begins. Meiotic errors in the oocyte, a disturbed zona pellucida reaction, and translocations (see below) lead to **misdistribution** of individual chromosomes (monosomies and trisomies) or to loss or gain of entire chromosome sets (monoploidies and triploidies).

Embryo Morphology and Division

On day 1 after insemination of the oocytes or after microinjection, the first cell division occurs immediately after completion of fertilization. The two cells formed by constriction (**cleavage**) are also referred to as **blastomeres**. One day later, on day 2, the next cell division to the **4-cell stage** occurs, and on day 3 to the **8-cell stage**. These divisions also occur by cleavage. These cleavage divisions by constriction are synchronous and do not lead to an increase in embryo size. Up to day 3 of development, maternal genes primarily control development. From day four onward, paternal genes also regulate further developmental steps. The cells adhere closely together, so that cell boundaries are no longer clearly visible. This process is called **compaction**. Due to the large number of cleavages, a sphere densely packed with cells forms. This stage consists of about 16 cells and is referred to as the **morula**. From day 5 onward, the cells have already differentiated into outer trophoblast and inner embryoblast cells, and fluid accumulates, forming a cavity. This stage

is called the **blastocyst**. The inner cell mass (embryoblast cells) will later form the child, and the outer trophoblast cells will form the placenta. After hatching from the zona pellucida, the embryos can implant.

Time Lapse

During in vitro culture of human germ cells, the **developmental potential** must be assessed. Typically, the developmental potential of oocytes or embryos is checked up to four times during culture. For this purpose, they are removed from the incubator to be evaluated under the microscope using "**snapshots**." In general, the environmental conditions outside the incubator are less favorable for oocytes and embryos than inside. Therefore, the time spent outside the incubator must be kept to a minimum. When assessing the developmental potential of an embryo using "snapshots," the main focus is on the cell morphology of the developmental stages from the oocyte to the blastocyst. The assessment criteria in the cleavage stage are the **number of blastomeres**, the degree of fragmentation (proportion of detached cell fragments), and the multinucleation of the blastomeres. If the number of blastomeres is odd and a high **fragmentation index** (> 50%) is observed, there is suspicion of chromosomal abnormalities and a high risk of low developmental competence. "**Multinucleation**" of embryonic cells also indicates chromosomal abnormalities, caused by segregation errors during meiosis (Yazdani et al. 2024).

A detailed observation of oocytes and embryos without disturbing the culture conditions is only possible in a special incubator with a built-in camera and integrated time-lapse recording technology (**time-lapse incubator**). With this equipment, it is possible to study the temporal morphological development of a fertilized oocyte up to the blastocyst. In combination with artificial intelligence (AI) we may be at a turning point for selecting a developmentally competent blastocyst for embryo transfer (Giménez et al. 2023). It can be assumed that mature, objective assessment criteria for the **developmental competence** of an **embryo** to support embryologists will soon be available. Even now, there are preliminary data for culture in a time-lapse incubator showing an improved cumulative live birth rate and a shortened interval to live birth (Reignier et al. 2021). However, the acquisition costs, including necessary maintenance, for a time-lapse incubator are usually in the six-figure range. In addition, the special consumables such as culture dishes ("slides") are expensive.

If oocytes and fertilization processes are also to be assessed, the surrounding cumulus cells must be removed for an unobstructed view of the oocytes. However, "naked" oocytes can no longer be fertilized by IVF treatment (see above). Therefore, the ICSI method is necessary for fertilization. In a time-lapse incubator, usually **6** to **12 images** per **hour** are taken per oocyte or developmental stage. This provides a wealth of additional information during all developmental steps from the oocyte to the morula and blastocyst. Critical developmental events can be assessed more reliably, as developmental disorders that occur before or after the snapshots in standard culture cannot be detected without a time-lapse incubator. This is especially true for assessing whether fertilization has occurred normally and whether cell divisions proceed regularly. Regular "binary divisions" and a timely developmental course indicate a high developmental potential of the fertilized oocytes. **Erroneous** developmental steps such as **trichotomous division** of cells, **cell fusions**, excessively rapid cell divisions, or prolonged **time intervals** until cell division indicate reduced or absent **developmental potential**. Such critical developmental errors cannot be detected with conventional assessment.

Fundamentals of Genetics

Humans have approximately 20,000 genes arranged on 46 chromosomes. Each **chromosome** is present twice, so every somatic cell has a double (**diploid**) set of chromosomes. 44 of the chromosomes are called autosomes, the other two are gonosomes, the sex chromosomes X and Y. Women have two X chromosomes, and men have one X chromosome and a much shorter Y chromosome. The autosomes form 22 pairs of chromosomes, each consisting of one maternal and one paternal chromosome. The sex chromosomes in women, with two X chromosomes, are also paired. In men, the two dissimilar chromosomes X and Y are also referred to as a pair. For the **karyotype**, the notation **46,XX** is used for women and **46,XY** for men. For human reproduction, cell divisions (mitoses) and maturation or reduction divisions (meiosis) are important (◘ Fig. 9.6). In mitosis, identical daughter cells with a female or male karyotype are produced. After completion of the two-stage meiosis, mature oocytes and spermatids with a single, so-called **haploid** set of chromosomes are formed. The karyotype formulas are **23,X** for oocytes and **23,X** and **23,Y** for sperm cells.

Mitosis and Meiosis

In the **resting phase** before cell division, the chromosomes are decondensed. They carry genetic information and consist mainly of DNA (deoxyribonucleic acids). The genetic information is encoded by the different sequence of the four **nucleic bases** adenine, thymine, guanine, and cytosine in the DNA. Shortly before cell division, the DNA synthesis phase begins. The chromosomes double their DNA content, which is

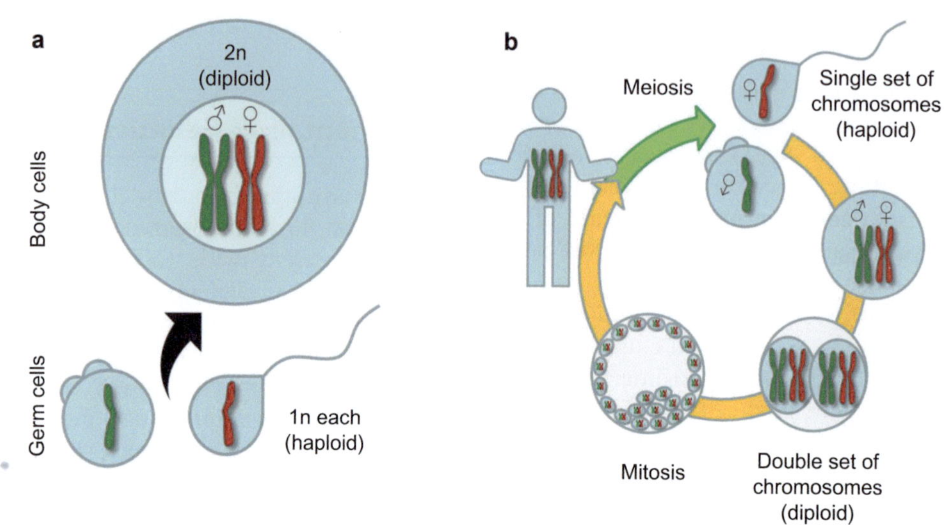

◘ **Fig. 9.6** Haploid and diploid chromosome sets after meiosis and mitosis. **a**: haploid chromosome set in germ cells and diploid chromosome set in somatic cells; **b**: haploid chromosome set after meiosis (germ cells), diploid chromosome set after mitosis (somatic cells). (Adapted from Trapphoff T (Specialization Qualification Reproductive Medicine))

spatially organized as a **double helix**. The two strands are unwound, separated, and replaced complementarily by pairing of the four nucleic bases. As a result, two identical DNA strands are formed from one DNA strand. This means that a chromosome now consists of two **daughter chromosomes (chromatids)**. The two chromatids are held together by the **centromere**. It divides the chromatids into two arms, which are usually of different lengths. The typical X structure of the chromosomes with the two chromatids is formed by the centromere. Errors during DNA duplication, also referred to as **replication**, can lead to mutations.

A cell division occurs in four phases and begins with the **prophase**. The chromosomes contract and condense. After preparation, the chromosomes can be visualized as slender threads under the light microscope. The DNA content has doubled in the preceding synthesis phase, so that each chromosome consists of two daughter chromosomes. Microscopically, the two daughter chromosomes cannot be distinguished. The formation of the spindle apparatus also begins. The two centrioles migrate to the two poles of the cell and serve as the organizational centers for the **spindle apparatus**. This ensures the regular distribution of chromosomes. In the subsequent prometaphase, the fibers of the spindle apparatus attach to the **centromere**. The chromosomes become visible as compact rods as they contract and condense even further. In the **metaphase**, they align at the equatorial plane. The two daughter chromosomes are separated longitudinally, with the centromere also being divided. In the **anaphase**, the two daughter chromosomes are moved by the spindle apparatus to opposite poles of the cell. In the **telophase**, the migration of the daughter chromosomes to the opposite cell poles is complete, and the chromosomes de-spiral again. They are then no longer visible under the light microscope. The cell begins to constrict into two daughter cells. This completes cell division, resulting in two daughter cells, each with 46 chromosomes.

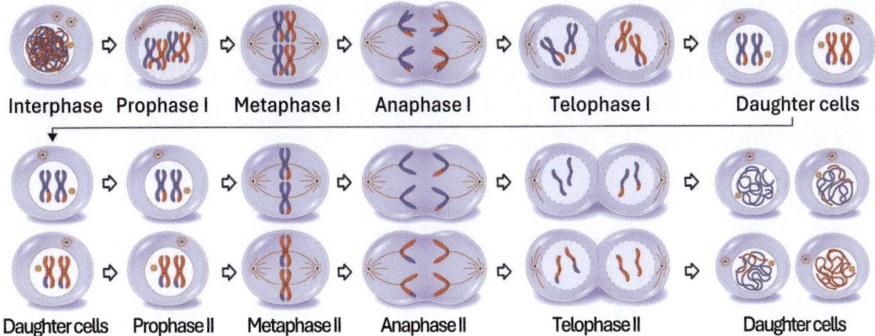

Fig. 9.7 Crossover and separation of chromosomes in meiosis I and II. Meiosis I (top): diploid cell with two pairs of chromosomes, each forming a chiasma in prophase and distribution of homologous chromosomes to two daughter cells, each with a haploid set of chromosomes; meiosis II (bottom): two daughter cells with the altered maternal and paternal chromosomes. The two daughter chromatids are distributed to two daughter cells each

In the division of somatic cells (**mitosis**), the daughter chromosomes of the paired paternal and maternal chromosomes are distributed to the two daughter cells. **Meiosis** (**■** Figs. 2.2 and 9.7) is also referred to as maturation division or reduction division. Here, germ cells (oocytes and sperm) are formed from stem cells (oogonia and spermatogonia). The oogonia and spermatogonia first develop into **primary oocytes** and **spermatocytes**, which enter meiosis. This occurs in two stages, called meiosis I and meiosis II. At the end of meiosis, oocytes and sperm cells each have only 23 chromosomes and thus a single (haploid) set of chromosomes. Unlike mitosis, in **meiosis I** the maternal and paternal chromosomes, each consisting of two daughter chromosomes, first pair up. These lie parallel to each other and exchange gene segments by breaking at one or more points. This genetic phenomenon is called "**crossover**." The daughter chromosomes of the maternal and paternal homologous chromosomes cross over at the exchange points, which initially remain attached. This crossover stage is called a **chiasma**. The exchange of genetic material between homologous chromosomes takes time, so the first phase (prophase) of meiosis I is pro-

longed. Due to the exchange of genetic material, the chromosomes are no longer identical to the original maternal and paternal chromosomes. As meiosis progresses, the homologous chromosome pairs migrate to the center of the cell (equatorial plane) and align on the spindle with the attachment points facing outward. As they move apart to the two opposite cell poles, the homologous chromosomes separate. At the end of meiosis I, the **secondary oocytes** and **spermatocytes** are formed from the primary oocytes and primary spermatocytes, each with only 23 chromosomes. The distribution of the homologous maternally and paternally inherited chromosomes is random, increasing genetic diversity. This is followed by **meiosis II**, which proceeds like a normal cell division (mitosis). The 23 chromosomes, each consisting of their two daughter chromatids, align at the equatorial plane on the spindle. These chromosomes split longitudinally, and the two daughter chromatids move to opposite cell poles. After completion of meiosis I and II, mature oocytes and spermatids are formed, each with a single, haploid set of 23 chromosomes. Uniquely, only **one mature oocyte** is produced from a primary oocyte, as in both cell divisions one set of chromosomes or one daughter chromosome is extruded into the 1st or 2nd polar body. In contrast, four spermatids develop from one primary spermatocyte (◼ Fig. 2.2). However, only after undergoing spermiogenesis do four **mature sperm cells** arise from the four spermatids (◼ Fig. 2.5).

Genotype and Phenotype

The determination of genotype began with the groundbreaking discovery of the "secret of life" by Franklin as well as Crick and Watson in 1953. With their joint discovery of the **double helix structure** of DNA, they uncovered the blueprint of life and its significance for cell division. The genetic information, also called the **genome**, was decoded as part of the international Human Genome Project (HGP) starting in 1990. Since 2021, human DNA is considered to be fully decoded. Every person has a **genotype** with individual genetic information. These are encoded in approximately 20,000 genes. The new possibility of DNA sequencing, determining the order of the four nucleic acid bases, was a revolution for the biological sciences. This method is used in the diagnosis of hereditary diseases and in cancer research. Today, there are **genome databases** that also contain data from private individuals, for example in genealogy. Donor-conceived children use such DNA databases when searching for their genetic father or half-siblings (see ▶ Chap. 6). The search is, at least for half-siblings, almost always successful.

In reproductive medicine, genome sequencing of patients is not performed in routine clinical practice. However, genetic tests such as chromosome analysis are often ordered as part of preliminary diagnostics. In addition, genetic diagnostics are performed as part of **preimplantation genetic diagnosis** on polar bodies or trophectoderm cells. For a **chromosome analysis** to determine the karyotype, a blood sample is taken. **Gene analyses** are performed in symptomatic women, for example with primary amenorrhea, or in symptomatic men, for example with azoospermia. In these cases, testing is usually done for Fragile X syndrome (FraX) or for the most common mutations in cystic fibrosis (CFTR gene). If, in the case of suspected hereditary disease, further counseling and molecular genetic diagnostics with sequencing are necessary, this extended diagnostics should be carried out in cooperation with a human genetics center. Such cooperation is also undertaken for polar body diagnosis or preimplantation genetic diagnosis (see below). The genotype can be used to infer the external appearance. However, there are exceptions, for example in the expression of sex, which are referred to as "**disorders of sexual development**" (DSD). For instance, there are men with the karyotype 46,XX and women with the karyotype 46,XY. The determining factor for the development of male sex characteristics is the sex-determining gene **SRY** (sex determining region of Y gene), which, during meiosis in the **XX male**, has been transferred from the Y chromosome to an X chromosome. Men with a 46,XX karyotype are infertile, similar to patients with Klinefelter syndrome (47,XXY). In **XY females**, on the other hand, there is a complete **androgen receptor defect** (complete androgen insensitivity syndrome, abbreviated CAIS). Therefore, androgens are ineffective in the development of the male phenotype, resulting in a complete absence of sexual hair. Abdominal or inguinal testes occur, patients have uterine aplasia and a blind-ending vagina. The mutation is located on an X chromosome.

The term **phenotype** refers to the appearance of an organism with its actual morphological and physiological characteristics. These include, for example, blood group, eye and hair color, body height, as well as female and male sex organs. In a chromosome pair, the **dominant** hereditary traits, such as dark hair color on one parental chromosome, and not the **recessive** traits on the other parental chromosome, are expressed. Features of a phenotype can, for example in Down syndrome (47,XX + 21 or 47,XY + 21), be expressed differently and individually variable despite identical genetic information. The **range** of physical **stigmata** is very broad. Intellectual disability can also vary greatly in severity. Social integration, upbringing, education, vocational training, and integration are achieved with varying success depending on the individual. These depend on support and the extent of physical and intellectual disabilities. Apart from syndromes, malformations are typically not genetic but are caused by biological, physical, or chemical factors. These so-called **teratogens** usually include medications, bacteria, viruses, radiation, maternal diabetes, and obesity. In metabolic disorders, toxic hyperglycemia during pregnancy can more frequently lead to neural tube defects and heart defects. Such severe malformations may possibly be prevented by intensified blood glucose control (Sadler 2014). In summary, the phenotype does not necessarily allow conclusions to be drawn about the genotype.

Epigenetics

Epigenetics is a subfield of biology that deals with changes in gene activity that are not caused by changes in the DNA sequence itself. The **expression of genes** can be modified during critical pre- and postnatal developmental phases by factors such as environmental influences, hormones, nutritional factors, or maternal diseases and behaviors. As a result, the function of organs and organ systems can be permanently shaped. The term **imprinting** is also used for this. For example, later insulin resistance and obesity in children of obese mothers and fathers can already be preprogrammed by **fetal programming** (Brandt and Wabitsch 2017). IVF or ICSI treatment takes place during the particularly vulnerable phase of fertilization and the early phase of embryonic development. In these phases, external influences during each cell division with DNA duplication can lead to faulty modification of histones, which serve as "packaging material" for DNA, or of the DNA itself. This can result in the unintended activation or deactivation of genes encoded on it. External influences discussed as causes of epigenetic changes include hormone stimulation, in vitro culture, and cryopreservation in the context of IVF or ICSI treatment. **Beckwith-Wiedemann syndrome**, **Prader-Willi syndrome**, and **Angelman syndrome** are based on such epigenetic disturbances. These are very rare diseases with a frequency of 1:10,000–1:15,000. The association between ART treatment and such epigenetic changes is unproven and the discussions are controversial.

Chromosomal Anomalies (Numerical, Structural)

For reproductive medicine consultations, both numerical and structural chromosomal aberrations are relevant. Human **somatic cells** normally have 46 and human **germ cells** (gametes) have 23 chromosomes (◨ Fig. 9.6). All chromosomes are referred to as **autosomes** if they are not **gonosomes** (sex chromosomes) (see above). Chromosomes are paired (diploid or 2n) in somatic cells and present as single copies in germ cells (haploid or 1n). The term "euploid" means that a complete set of chromosomes is present. If one or more chromosomes are present in an abnormal number, this is called an **aneuploidy**. If each chromosome is present in duplicate as normal, this is called a **disomy**. If a single chromosome is missing, this is called a **monosomy**. If only one homologous chromosome is present in addition, this is called a **trisomy**. Numerical aneuploidies usually arise from missegregation of chromosomes during meiosis. Most often, missegregation occurs in oocytes and less frequently in sperm cells. The risk of **trisomies** increases with maternal age, as oocytes begin meiosis before birth, and aging processes in the cells can lead to missegregation of chromosomes. In contrast to trisomies, a **triploidy** is present when not just one chromosome, but the entire set of chromosomes is present three times (see above). Either two of the three chromosome sets come from the father or from the mother. The cause may be fertilization of an egg cell by two sperm or failure to expel the first polar body. Structural chromosomal aberrations include **translocations** (relocation of chromosome segments), as well as **deletions** (loss of chromosome segments) or **insertions** (gain of chromosome segments). Structural anomalies arise after chromosome breaks affecting one or more chromosomes. What happens to the fragments is crucial. If only insignificant segments are lost or gained, the total amount of genetic material remains unchanged (**balanced**). If significant chromosome segments are lost or gained, the genetic material is **unbalanced**, usually with serious consequences.

Numerical Chromosomal Aberrations

Common numerical chromosomal aberrations include trisomies 21 (Down syndrome), 18 (Edwards syndrome), and 13 (Patau syndrome). With a risk of 1:500, **trisomy 21 (Down syndrome)** is the most common form. About 30% of these pregnancies result in miscarriage. Children with Down syndrome are born with a heart defect in 50% of cases. People with Down syndrome are short in stature, tend to have weak muscles and loose connective tissue (e.g., joints can be hyperextended). They also have a round face, a flat back of the head, and usually slightly upward-slanting eyes. The hands are broad with short fingers and often have a single transverse palmar crease. The second most common trisomy is **Edwards syndrome (trisomy 18)**. The incidence in live births is about 1:6,000. The rate of miscarriage and stillbirth is significantly increased. Severe malformations of the heart, skull, face, brain, abdomen, and limbs are usually already detectable by prenatal ultrasound. 80% have heart defects. Only 5 to 10% of children born survive beyond one year. **Trisomy 13 (Patau syndrome)** ranks third and occurs with a risk of 1:8,000. These fetuses also usually present in prenatal ultrasound with a severe malformation syndrome. Miscarriages are common and 80% have a heart defect. The life expectancy of children born with this condition is about 90 days. 90% of children die within the first year of life.

The most common numerical chromosomal aberrations of the sex chromosomes (gonosomes) are, in women, **Ullrich-Turner syndrome** (UTS) and in men, Klinefelter syndrome (see ▶ Chap. 5). UTS is a monosomy X. The cells have only one X chromosome (**45,X0**). The cause is usually a mitotic or meiotic error in the sperm cells before fertilization. The division of the two sex chromosomes into two daughter cells fails, and both sex chromosomes migrate into one cell. The failure of the two members of a homologous chromosome pair to separate is called **non-disjunction**. This results in one sperm with 24 (24,XY) and one sperm with only 22 chromosomes (22,0). Normally, two sperm with 23 chromosomes would be produced (23,X or 23,Y). Fertilization of an egg after regular separation of the sex chromosomes (23,X) with a sperm after irregular separation of the sex chromosomes with only 22 chromosomes (22,0) leads to a female karyotype with monosomy X (45,X0). Typical **stigmata** in UTS are especially short stature, neck folds, and heart and kidney malformations. The women are generally **infertile** because the ovaries are not properly developed. Puberty usually does not occur. However, the women are of average intelligence and usually have a normal life expectancy.

In (**Klinefelter syndrome, 47,XXY**) or (Triple X syndrome, 47,XXX), there is a trisomy of the sex chromosomes. The extra X chromosome, as in UTS, results from a failure of the sex chromosomes to separate. This segregation error before fertilization occurs about equally often during oocyte and sperm maturation. In mothers over 40 years of age, non-disjunction of the gonosomes occurs more frequently. Overall, meiosis produces oocytes and sperm with 24 chromosomes each (24,XX and 24,XY) and those with only 22 chromosomes each (22,0). Fertilization of a sperm after regular separation of the sex chromosomes (23,X or 23,Y) with an oocyte after irregular separation of the sex chromosomes (24,XX) leads to a gonosomal trisomy for the sex chromosomes, either with a male or female karyotype. The frequency of Klinefelter syndrome (47,XXY) is about 1:500 to 1:1,000 and for **Triple X syndrome** (47,XXX) about 1:1,000. Men with Klinefelter syndrome are generally **infertile** (see ▶ Chap. 5). Women with Triple X syndrome are mostly unremarkable and therefore usually not diagnosed. In some cases, however, there may be premature ovarian failure (premature ovarian insufficiency) and thus infertility.

Structural Anomalies

After chromosome breaks, fragments can attach to other chromosomes. This situation is called a **translocation**. These most commonly occur between chromosomes 13, 14, 15, 21, and 22. Translocations are **balanced** if there is neither a loss nor a gain of significant genetic material. In this case, there are no changes in the phenotype and the affected individuals are clinically unremarkable. However, if translocations are **unbalanced**, miscarriages or syndromes with malformations often occur. There are two different types of translocations: the **reciprocal translocation** with a mutual (reciprocal) exchange of fragments, and the **Robertsonian translocation** with the fusion (merging) of two chromosomes into a **translocation chromosome**. Down syndrome can also be caused by an unbalanced translocation. This cause of Down syndrome is hereditary and accounts for only about 5% of all Down syndrome cases, as in about 95% there is a so called free trisomy, which arises from a segregation error during meiosis.

Prenatal Diagnostics

Polar body diagnosis (PBD), like preimplantation genetic diagnosis (PGD), is classified as **prenatal diagnostics (PND)**. PBD is performed on unfertilized oocytes up to the pronuclear stage, while PGD is performed on fertilized oocytes from the cleavage to the blastocyst stage. Thus, PBD and PGD are investigative procedures on oocytes and embryos before the onset of successful implantation and pregnancy. In diagnostic procedures during **pregnancy**, the **ultrasound examination** of the fetus is central, supplemented by the analysis of **fetal cells** from amniotic fluid, placental tissue cells, and fetal or maternal blood. In contrast, PBD examines genetic material from an oocyte before fertilization is complete. Only maternal genes are analyzed, and this is done indirectly via the 1st and 2nd polar bodies of meiosis I and II, as the polar bodies indirectly reflect the chromosomes in the oocyte nucleus. With **preimplantation genetic diagnosis** after fertilization and the onset of embryonic development, both maternal and paternal genes can be directly analyzed in the sampled cells. PGD is preferably performed at the blastocyst stage on day five of development. In Germany, PBD was initially practiced as an alternative to PGD before the latter was legally regulated for exceptions in 2011 and implemented in 2013. The removal of polar bodies or embryonic cells for PBD or PGD must be performed under sterile conditions in the ART laboratory. Otherwise, there is a high risk of contamination of the genetic material to be analyzed, rendering the genetic findings unreliable.

Polar Body Diagnosis (PBD)

Until 2013, polar body diagnosis was used both for genetic testing of hereditary diseases and for cytogenetic diagnosis of chromosomal abnormalities in cases of translocations or increased risk of aneuploidies. Women of advanced reproductive age have an increased risk of aneuploidy. Polar bodies are only fragments of a cell nucleus with very little and unstable genetic material. Nature expels and discards them as a "**waste product**." In contrast to PBD, PGD examines several cells with stable genetic material. Therefore, polar body diagnosis is particularly demanding and also carries a high risk of oocyte loss during testing. Both the biopsy and the genetic analysis had to be completed within a small **time window** of 25 hours after ICSI, according to the conservative interpretation of the German Embryo Protection Act (ESchG). This also meant that within this time window, oocytes with normal test results had to be selected for embryo transfer, and abnormal oocytes discarded. Any delay would have resulted in the formation of an embryo, making PBD no longer legally permissible, as the pronuclei dissolve and the first cell division—and thus embryonic development—occurs after 26 to 29 hours. If the PBD time window is exceeded, selection would no longer be performed on oocytes but on embryos. Selection of embryos based on the PBD result would have been prohibited.

Performing PBD for Hereditary Diseases and Aneuploidies

For **testing for hereditary diseases**, the **1st and 2nd polar bodies** must be sequentially removed and genetically analyzed. This determines whether the altered gene remains in the oocyte or has been expelled with the 1st or 2nd polar body. The 2nd polar body is extruded about 15 hours after ICSI. Therefore, the 1st polar body is usually biopsied 1 hour after ICSI, and the 2nd polar body after it is expelled from the oocyte. Due to the tight time window, genetic analysis was started immediately after the staggered removal of each polar body. In PBD, all mature oocytes must be biopsied and analyzed, as it is not yet known at the time of biopsy which oocytes will fertilize normally. Only about 70–80% of oocytes can be fertilized, and of these, only 30 to 50% develop into a blastocyst. Thus, only one in four oocytes results in a viable blastocyst. Therefore, polar body diagnosis for hereditary diseases was very time- and labor-intensive. Today, polar body diagnosis still has clinical relevance for **testing** an age-related increased risk of **aneuploidies**, in cases of miscarriage due to trisomy or implantation failure. For the gain or loss of genetic material, it is sufficient to biopsy the **1st** and **2nd polar bodies together** up to 15 hours after ICSI. However, no pregnancy benefit has been demonstrated for aneuploidy testing with PBD, making it difficult to justify the high costs of this complex diagnostic procedure (Verpoest et al. 2018).

Preimplantation Genetic Diagnosis (PGD)

The performance of preimplantation genetic diagnosis (PGD) is regulated in **§ 3a ESchG** (Appendix 9.1). This paragraph was added to the law in 2011. It states that PGD may only be performed in exceptional cases. Prerequisites for performing PGD include counseling and information on the medical, psychological, and social consequences.

In addition, a **positive vote** from an interdisciplinary **ethics committee** is required. PGD may only be performed in approved centers for preimplantation genetic diagnosis that have the necessary personnel, diagnostic, medical, and technical resources. Exceptions allowing PGD include genetic disposition in the woman and/or man if there is a **high risk** of a serious hereditary disease in the offspring of **at least 25%**. Another exception is the detection of a serious impairment of an embryo (e.g., in cases of parental translocation carriers) that is highly likely to result in stillbirth or miscarriage. Further details for the implementation of § 3a ESchG have been specified by the federal government in the so-called **Preimplantation Genetic Diagnosis Ordinance (PIDV)** (Appendix 9.2). The federal states are responsible for approving PGD centers and establishing an ethics committee. The central office for documentation of PGD treatments was established at the federal **Paul-Ehrlich-Institute (PEI)**. PGD centers must report their treatment data annually to the PEI. The federal government's PGD reports, which must be prepared every four years, include the analysis of all registry data, including treatment outcomes. The third **report of the federal government** on experiences with preimplantation genetic diagnosis was published in 2024. This report is available in the "Newsroom" on the PEI website (▶ www.pei.de).

Ethics Committees

There are five ethics committees nationwide (▣ Table 9.5). The federal states of Bavaria, Berlin, and North Rhine-Westphalia each have their own ethics committee, while the remaining northern and southern states have established joint committees. Only Saxony-Anhalt does not yet have an ethics committee. One will be established as soon as an application for approval as a PGD center is submitted. The application to perform PGD must be submitted in the federal state where the **approved human genetics center for preimplantation genetic diagnosis (PGD center)** is located. This center may cooperate with several reproductive medicine facilities. Thus, an approved PGD

▣ **Table 9.5** Ethics committees for preimplantation genetic diagnosis

Committee	Federal States	Location	Fees and Expenses	Approved human genetics PGD centers
North	Brandenburg, Free Hanseatic City of Bremen, Free and Hanseatic City of Hamburg, Mecklenburg-Western Pomerania, Lower Saxony, Schleswig-Holstein	Hamburg Medical Association	€1,500 to €3,000	2
South	Baden-Württemberg, Hesse, Rhineland-Palatinate, Saarland, Saxony, Thuringia	Baden-Württemberg State Medical Association	€1,500 to €4,000	3
Bavaria	Bavaria	Bavarian State Ministry for Health and Care	€100 to €5,000	4
Berlin	Berlin	State Office for Health and Social Affairs	€1,500	0
North Rhine-Westphalia	North Rhine-Westphalia	North Rhine Medical Association	€1,300 to €3,000	1

center always consists of a human genetics center with one or more **reproductive medicine facilities**. These may also cooperate with another human genetics PGD center. Ethics committees are interdisciplinary, comprising four experts in medicine, two experts in ethics and law, and one representative each for the interests of patients and for the self-help of people with disabilities. The eight members must decide on applications by a two-thirds majority. Applicants are informed of the **decision** in writing: "Your application to perform preimplantation genetic diagnosis is **approved**" or "Your application to perform preimplantation genetic diagnosis is **rejected**." If an application is rejected, the affected couple can only pursue **legal action** before an administrative court. Such a lawsuit takes several years to reach a decision. In the past, the Bavarian Ethics Committee for Preimplantation Genetic Diagnosis in particular has repeatedly issued negative votes in cases of hereditary diseases. Special burdens such as pregnancy terminations in connection with a hereditary disease (Weiske et al. 2017) or pronounced symptoms of a hereditary disease in the partner were not taken into account by the ethics committee. Affected couples have taken legal action. The **administrative courts** in Regensburg (VG, judgment of 24.01.2019—RO 5 K 17.335) and, at the highest level, in Leipzig (Supreme Administrative Court, judgment of 05.11.2020—3 C 12.19) have overturned the respective decisions of the ethics committee.

> **Guiding Principles for Ethics Committee Decisions**
> 1. Ethics committees for preimplantation genetic diagnosis have no discretion regarding the existence of the prerequisites for a high risk of a serious hereditary disease.
> 2. The existence of the prerequisites for a high risk of a serious hereditary disease must be decided separately in each individual case. A hereditary disease is considered serious, in particular, if it is characterized by low life expectancy or severity of the clinical picture and poor treatability, and thus differs significantly from other hereditary diseases.
> 3. If it is unclear whether a hereditary disease should be classified as serious due to the expected manifestation of the disease in the offspring based on the genetic disposition of at least one parent, additional burdens associated with the genetic disposition for the affected woman or couple must also be taken into account.

The **rejection rate** for applications to perform PGD, in contrast to the national average, was 10 to 15% at the Bavarian Ethics Committee for Preimplantation Genetic Diagnosis before the Supreme Administrative Court's ruling in Leipzig in 2019. The approval practice has changed since the ruling, as the burdens on applicants can now be given greater consideration. Since then, the rejection rate of the Bavarian Ethics Committee has dropped to about 2% (German Bundestag 2024).

Performing PGD

Cell collection for PGD is carried out in a **reproductive medicine center** that cooperates with the **human genetics PGD center**. Both facilities must be **jointly approved** as a "tandem." The human genetics center acts as the lead, and the reproductive medicine facility as the partner that provides the cells for PGD. PGD may only be performed once the ethics committee's decision is available. In trophectoderm diagnosis, only viable fertilized oocytes at the blastocyst stage are examined. With timely development, the fertilized oocyte differentiates into a blastocyst on the fifth day of development. The outer trophectoderm cells, which can only further differentiate into chorionic villi, are

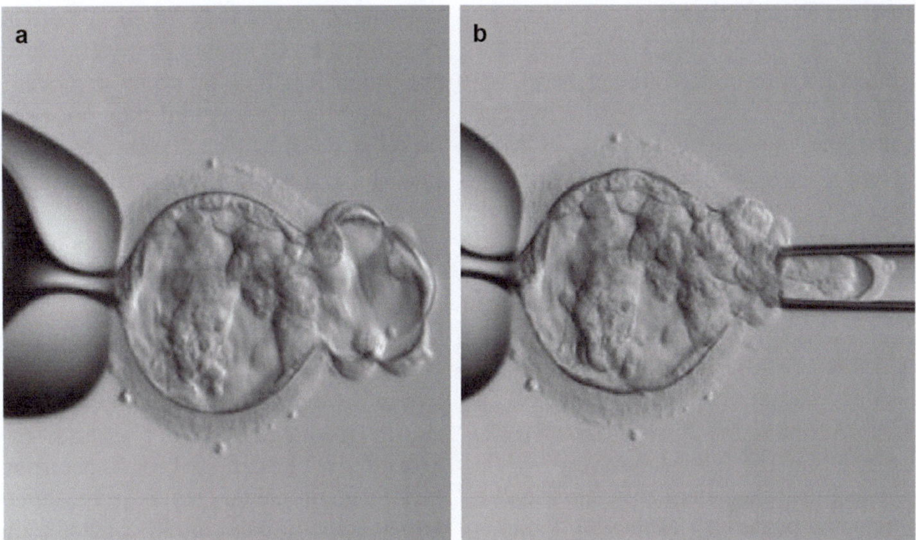

Fig. 9.8 Trophectoderm biopsy. **a** Trophectoderm cells begin to hatch from the zona pellucida; **b** Biopsy: 3–5 trophectoderm cells are aspirated into a glass pipette

biopsied (**Fig. 9.8**). The inner cells, from which the child will later develop, are not touched. During the biopsy, three to five cells are usually removed with a glass pipette for genetic analysis. After the biopsy, the blastocysts are frozen, and only the biopsy samples are transported to the human genetics PGD center. The result is usually available a few weeks later. The findings report is typically discussed with the patient by the treating reproductive medicine specialist. The thawing treatment is then planned. If no embryo is available for transfer, another PGD cycle is planned according to the individual situation.

Special Requirements for Hygiene

Contamination of an **oocyte culture** is highly feared, as it usually inhibits the growth of the cultured oocytes. If a culture in an incubator becomes contaminated, this contamination can also harm other cultures in the incubator (cross-contamination). The transfer of contaminated embryos is crit-ical, as the infection can be transmitted to the uterus and disrupt implantation. For this reason, strict hygiene must be maintained in the ART laboratory (Gutknecht et al. 2021). **Germs** are primarily present in the air, on the skin, in the vagina, in the intestines, and on the floor. Dust is a carrier of germs. Important sources of infection are staff and patients. In particular, the human armpit and scalp have a high density of germs. Hands also have a relatively high germ count. Ejaculates and follicular aspirates are always colonized with germs. Another infection risk is cardboard boxes in which goods for the IVF area are delivered. Therefore, it is very important to separate the **practice area** with consultation and examination rooms as well as administrative offices from the **area** for **outpatient surgery** including the **ART laboratory**. An appropriate **hygiene concept** is required by the Ordinance on the Manufacture of Medicinal Products and Active Substances (AMWHV) § 6 for the operation of a fertility center (see ▶ Chap. 1).

Infection Prophylaxis

For infection prevention, the general hygiene regulations according to the hygiene plan for the practice area, such as **hygienic hand disinfection** and wearing **practice clothing** and practice shoes, are sufficient (Fig. 9.9). Surfaces and equipment should be easy to clean, there should be sufficient walking areas and enough space for storage, access to sensitive areas must be restricted, dust collectors should be avoided, and cables should be organized, e.g., in channels. **Access to the operating room (OR)** area, including the **ART laboratory**, is via a **personnel airlock**, where **area-specific clothing** must be put on (Table 9.6). Patients are admitted to the patient rooms via a separate entrance and receive an OR gown and foot protection (e.g., socks). Technicians and maintenance staff must also wear area-specific clothing. In the OR area, **disposable caps** and a **mouth-nose protection (MNP)** are mandatory. For medical procedures, **surgical hand disinfection** including the forearms is required. When materials for the ART laboratory are delivered, the outer cartons must be removed before the area airlock, and the goods should be repacked into clean containers if possible. The storage of inner cartons should be avoided.

For **germ reduction**, **ejaculates** and **follicular aspirates** are processed. This is done by repeated washing steps and rinsing of the cells (Fig. 9.1). Germ reduction in ejaculate is, among other things, very effective in the density gradient. In addition, the culture media for sperm cells and for oocyte culture contain the broad-spectrum antibiotic gentamicin. Thanks to this effective **prophylaxis**, infections in oocyte culture are very rare. Gentamicin is used in human medicine for severe infections.

Cross-contamination refers to the transfer of germs, e.g., from a member of the laboratory staff to a couple's culture or between the cultures of different couples. Hygiene regulations must be strictly observed to minimize the risk of germ transfer. The

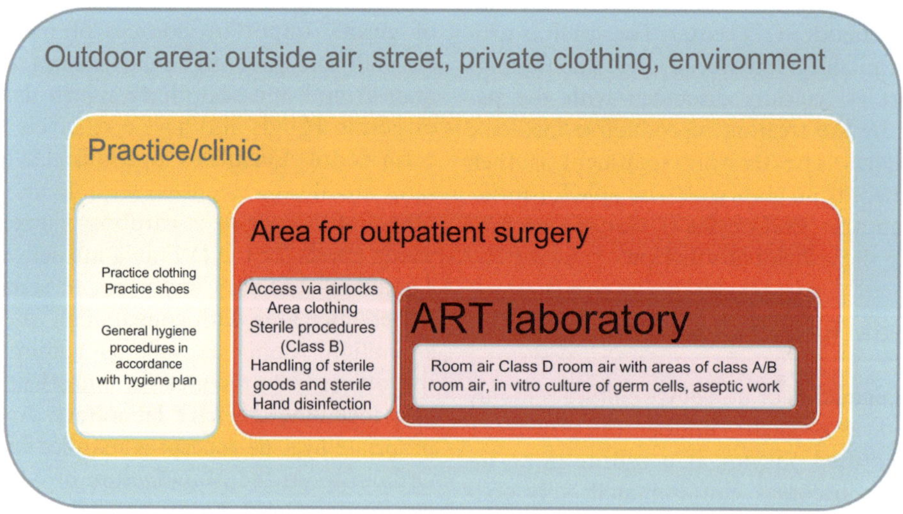

Fig. 9.9 Premises and hygiene requirements. With increasing cleanliness, additional hygiene measures are implemented according to the hygiene concept. Practice area/clinic (orange), area for outpatient surgery (red), and ART laboratory (dark red). (Adapted from Gutknecht D [Specialization Qualification in Reproductive Medicine])

Table 9.6 Measures for germ reduction in the ART laboratory

Measures	Explanation
Airlocks	Area-specific clothing for staff and technicians, removal of street clothes including shoes for patients, repacking of outer cartons before entering the OR area
Air filters	Fine dust filters for room air class D are required in the ART laboratory (requirement AMWHV § 36)
Washing steps and density gradient	Repeated washing and rinsing to reduce germs in ejaculate and follicular aspirate, massive germ reduction in ejaculate by density gradient
Germ inactivation	Culture media contain the broad-spectrum antibiotic gentamicin as a prophylactic
Disposable materials, workstation separation, disinfection	Prevention of cross-contamination between laboratory staff and patient cultures or between patient cultures
Disinfection	Alcohol is potentially harmful to embryos, quaternary ammonium compounds are recommended for surfaces and instruments, some preparations have been tested for embryo safety
Hygiene controls	Air samples, sedimentation plates, and contact samples (requirement AMWHV § 36)

risk can also be reduced by using sterile disposable materials and enforcing strict separation of workstations for each couple's culture. Additional surface and equipment disinfection is recommended.

Disinfectants

When using **disinfectants** in the **ART laboratory** and adjacent rooms in the procedure area, their **toxicity to germ cells** must be **considered**. One of the most effective disinfectants is **70% alcohol**. This is regularly used for hand disinfection. However, alcohol evaporates and can thus enter the culture vessels for germ cells and damage them. The same applies to **chlorine-containing disinfectants**, e.g., foam for disinfecting ultrasound probes (Tristel Duo ULT®). Therefore, the doors to the ART laboratory must be briefly closed during hand disinfection or during disinfection of ultrasound probes in the procedure area before or after outpatient procedures. For the ART laboratory, disinfect-

ants containing ammonium salts are preferable. These remain on surfaces and do not evaporate. Some brands have been proven to be harmless to embryos. However, there are also some brands that are combined with alcohol or fragrances. These should not be used in the ART laboratory. In summary, for surface and immersion disinfection in the ART laboratory, **quaternary ammonium compounds (QUADS)** are recommended. There are preparations such as Fermacidal D2® that have been tested and found to be safe for embryos. Preparations have different spectra of activity. Therefore, the use of **different preparations** in various rooms such as andrology, ART laboratory, and procedure area is recommended for a **broader spectrum of activity**. These products should also be rotated between rooms.

Room Air Class

The air in the ART laboratory must be filtered to keep the supply of fine dust (< 1 µm) such as bacteria, viruses, yeasts, pollen, and aerosols as low as possible. For this purpose, the rooms are equipped with **High Efficiency Particulate Air (HEPA) filters**. This ensures compliance with the legal requirements of AMWHV § 36. This regulation requires **class D room air** for the ART laboratory. This is considered a clean area for less critical steps in the production of sterile products. The **handling and processing of germ cells** takes place in workbenches under **laminar air flow conditions**. The legally required class A room air is not feasible, as this would endanger the safety and quality of the germ cells. For this reason, the AMWHV requirement can be deviated from. A procedure room is sufficient for operations with a low risk of wound infection, such as follicular punctures. For larger procedures such as laparoscopy, an operating room with appropriate room air technology (HVAC) that meets cleanroom conditions would be necessary.

Regular checks must be carried out and documented to ensure compliance with the **room air class in the ART laboratory**. This is legally binding as stipulated in the AMWHV. For this purpose, air samples are taken for active particle and germ count measurement, sedimentation plates for passive particle measurement, and contact plates during critical work steps. To meet class A or B room air, the number of "colony-forming units" (CFU) must be ≤ 1 or ≤ 5, respectively.

Learning Objectives

- Know the significance and methods for processing ejaculate
- Understand the importance of temperature control for oocyte culture
- Be able to explain the developmental steps of the oocyte from fertilization to the development of a blastocyst
- Know the significance of the embryonic period as a phase for organ malformations
- Be able to explain the difference between polar body and preimplantation genetic diagnosis
- Know the hygiene concept in a fertility center

In the IVF laboratory, oocytes and sperm cells are brought together in a culture dish with the goal of fertilization. For fertilization to be successful, the sperm must be processed. The sperm should be motile, normally shaped, mature, and intact. In IVF treatment, the sperm must reach and fertilize the oocytes on their own. In contrast, in ICSI treatment, a single sperm is injected into a mature oocyte. Fertilization errors can be caused by oocytes or sperm, but also by culture conditions. To minimize the risk of fertilization errors, a stable culture temperature of approximately 37°C is especially necessary. With time-lapse incubators (built-in camera), continuous and undisturbed monitoring of oocyte culture is possible. For example, blastocysts that are not capable of development can be identified and excluded from transfer. Chromosomes, as carriers of genetic information, consist mainly of DNA. This coils (condenses) during mitosis and meiosis. Sperm and oocytes have the haploid chromosome set (23,X or 23,Y), somatic cells have the diploid chromosome set (46,XX or 46,XY). Errors in distribution or new mutations can occur during the separation of chromosomes in meiosis or during DNA replication after cell divisions (mitoses). Preimplantation genetic diagnosis are only permitted in exceptional cases for known chromosomal disorders and hereditary diseases after a positive vote from an ethics committee. For safe oocyte culture, a hygiene concept for infection prophylaxis, including room air control, is necessary.

Below is the link to the electronic supplementary material.

References

Brandt S, Wabitsch M (2017) Bedeutung der mütterlichen Adipositas für die Gesundheit der Kinder. Gynäkologische Endokrinologie 15, 131–138. ► https://doi.org/10.1007/s10304-017-0132-4

Chen X, Zhao H, Lv J et al (2022) Calcium ionophore improves embryonic development and pregnancy outcomes in patients with previous developmental problems in ICSI cycles. BMC Pregnancy Childbirth 22:894. ► https://doi.org/10.1186/s12884-022-05228-3

Deutscher Bundestag (2024) Dritter Bericht der Bundesregierung über die Erfahrungen mit der Präimplantationsdiagnostik. Drucksache 20/10060. ► https://dserver.bundestag.de/btd/20/100/2010060.pdf. Zuletzt 30.4.2025.

Duran-Retamal M, Morris G, Achilli C et al (2020) Live birth and miscarriage rate following intracytoplasmic morphologically selected sperm injection vs intracytoplasmic sperm injection: An updated systematic review and meta-analysis. Acta Obstet Gynecol Scand 99:24–33. ► https://doi.org/10.1111/aogs.13703

Giménez C, Conversa L, Murria L et al (2023) Time-lapse imaging: Morphokinetic analysis of in vitro fertilization outcomes. Fertil Steril120:218-227. ► https://doi.org/10.1016/j.fertnstert.2023.06.015

Gutknecht D, Blumenauer V, Hauff B et al (2021) Leitlinie für die Führung und Einrichtung eines Labors für die Durchführung Assistierter Reproduktionstechnologien beim Menschen (ART-Labor) innerhalb einer reproduktionsmedizinischen Versorgungseinrichtung der Arbeitsgemeinschaft Reproduktionsbiologie des Menschen (AGRBM). ► https://www.agrbm.de/wp-content/uploads/AGRBM_Leitlinie_2021-05-21.pdf. Zuletzt 3.5.2025

Hunkler K, Dunn A J, Driver N (2024) Blastulation development rateswith Zymot Microfluidics Device and testicular sperm extraction in infertile couples with prior poor blastulation rates and elevated DNA Fragmentation. Fertil Steril 122: 4, Supplement e427October 2024. ► https://doi.org/10.1016/j.fertnstert.2024.08.283. ► https://www.fertstert.org/article/S0015-0282(24)01897-1/fulltext

Kirkman-Brown J, Pavitt S, Khalaf Y et al. (2019) Sperm selection for assisted reproduction by prior hyaluronan binding: the HABSelect RCT. Efficacy and mechanism evaluation 6. ► https://doi.org/10.3310/eme06010

Novoselsky Persky M, Hershko-Klement A, Solnica A et al (2021) Conventional ICSI vs. physiological selection of spermatozoa for ICSI (picsi) in sibling oocytes. Andrology. 9:873–877. ► https://doi.org/10.1111/andr.12982

Pacheco A, Blanco A, Bronet F et al (2020) Magnetic-Activated Cell Sorting (MACS): A Useful Sperm-Selection Technique in Cases of High Levels of Sperm DNA Fragmentation. J Clin Med 9:3976. ► https://doi.org/10.3390/jcm9123976

Parrella A, Keating D, Cheung S et al (2019) A treatment approach for couples with disrupted sperm DNA integrity and recurrent ART failure. J Assist Reprod Genet 36:2057–2066. ► https://doi.org/10.1007/s10815-019-01543-5

Reignier A, Lefebvre T, Loubersac S et al (2021) Time-lapse technology improves total cumulative live birth rate and shortens time to live birth as compared to conventional incubation system in couples undergoing ICSI. J Assist Reprod Genet 38:917–923. ► https://doi.org/10.1007/s10815-021-02099-z

Practice Committee of the American Society for Reproductive Medicine (2022) Electronic address: asrm@asrm.org. The role of assisted hatching in in vitro fertilization: a guideline. Fertil Steril 117:1177–1182. ► https://doi.org/10.1016/j.fertnstert.2022.02.020

Sadler TW (2014) Angeborene Fehlbildungen und pränatale Diagnostik. In: Sadler TW (ed) Taschenlehrbuch Embryologie 12. Auflage, Georg Thieme Verlag Stuttgart New York, 180–194

Shan Y, Zhao H, Zhao D et al (2022) Assisted Oocyte Activation With Calcium Ionophore Improves Pregnancy Outcomes and Offspring Safety in Infertile Patients: A Systematic Review and Meta-Analysis. Front Physiol 12:751905. ► https://doi.org/10.3389/fphys.2021.751905

Tejera A, Alegre Ferri L, Gamiz Izquierdo P et al (2021) Treatment with Calcium Ionophore Improves The Results in Patients with Previous Unsuccessful Attempts at The Fertilization: A Cohort Study. Int J Fertil Steril 15:286–293. ► https://doi.org/10.22074/IJFS.2021.136168.1013

Verpoest W, Staessen C, Bossuyt PM et al (2018) Pre-implantation genetic testing for aneuploidy by microarray analysis of polar bodies in advanced maternal age: a randomized clinical trial. Hum Reprod 33:1767–1776. ► https://doi.org/10.1093/humrep/dey262

Weiske K, Sauer T, Bals-Pratsch M (2017) PID in Deutschland: Die Instanz der Ethikkommissionen—Betrachtungen aus ethischer Perspektive. J. Reproduktionsmed. Endokrinol 14, 107–112

West R, Coomarasamy A, Frew L et al (2022) Sperm selection with hyaluronic acid improved live birth outcomes among older couples and was connected to sperm DNA quality, potentially affecting all treatment outcomes. Hum Reprod. 37:1106–1125. ► https://doi.org/10.1093/humrep/deac058

Yazdani A, Halvaei I, Boniface C et al (2024) Effect of cytoplasmic fragmentation on embryo development, quality, and pregnancy outcome: a systematic review of the literature. Reprod Biol Endocrinol. 22–55. ► https://doi.org/10.1186/s12958-024-01217-7

Zaha I, Naghi P, Stefan L et al. (2023) Comparative Study of Sperm Selection Techniques for Pregnancy Rates in an Unselected IVF-ICSI Population. J Pers Med 13:619. ► https://doi.org/10.3390/jpm13040619. PMID: 37109005; PMCID: PMC10145657

9

Documentation and Quality Assurance in Reproductive Medicine

Contents

Supplementary Information The online version contains supplementary material available at
▶ https://doi.org/10.1007/978-3-662-73035-5_10.

Quality Management Measures

Errors in a fertility center can have serious consequences. In the event of mix-ups, for example, a couple could receive a child from another couple. It is therefore not surprising that, due to such mix-ups, many fertility centers introduced a **quality management system (QM system)** more than 30 years ago. To prevent errors, a QM system includes, among other things, active patient identity checks at all critical steps in the ART laboratory (for example, through the documented four-eyes principle or automated monitoring systems with alarm functions), functional monitoring with alarm forwarding for critical equipment (e.g., incubators), daily data backups, equipment maintenance, regular team meetings and training sessions, continuing education, internal quality controls and audits, as well as error documentation and management. **One should learn from mistakes**. The focus is not on who made a mistake, but why it happened. To prevent the error in the future, it is actively discussed within the practice and a strategy for avoiding the error is developed.

Legal Obligation and Certification

A QM system documents, analyzes, improves, and monitors processes. With the implementation of the European Tissue Directive 2007 into national law (GewebeG), a QM system is mandatory for fertility centers. Proof is provided by a certificate from an accredited and recognized certification body (e.g., DEKRA, TÜV Nord, and TÜV Süd). Oocytes, embryos, and sperm cells are considered tissues within the meaning of the GewebeG (Annex 1.2). This is not an independent law, but an **article law** (a collection of amendments to existing laws). It includes the AMG with the AMWHV, the TPG with the TPG-GewV, and the TFG (see ▶ Chap. 1, ◻ Table 10.1). This law also includes a

◻ **Table 10.1**   Legal and professional regulatory frameworks in assisted reproduction

Legal, regulatory, and professional regulatory frameworks	Explanation	Scope of application
Medicinal Products Act (AMG), associated Ordinance on the Manufacture of Medicinal Products and Active Substances (AMWHV)	Law on the circulation of medicinal products, reporting obligations Single European Code (SEC code)	PEI reporting in the event of serious reactions and incidents involving germ cells and germ cell tissue
Transfusion Act (TFG)	Law regulating transfusion services, regulates documentation obligations	Donor eligibility, traceability
Transplantation Act (TPG), associated TPG Tissue Ordinance (TPG-GewV)	Regulates legal requirements for the donation, removal, and transfer of tissues, documentation and reporting obligations	PEI annual report on treated germ cells and germ cell tissue
Civil Code (BGB)	regulates legal relationships between private individuals, keeping of patient records	Documentation of medical history, findings, treatments as well as consents, information, and medical letters
Guideline of the German Medical Association (BÄK)	Removal and transfer of human germ cells or germ cell tissue in the context of assisted reproduction	All procedures of assisted reproduction

general ban on trade in non-industrially produced tissue and tissue preparations such as oocytes, sperm cells, and embryos. The ISO 9001 quality management standard is internationally recognized. It defines requirements for the quality management system. Meeting these requirements is intended to ensure that the organization has appropriate processes in place to provide products and services of sufficient quality. Certification as proof of a functioning QM system is costly. The costs for the audit during initial certification according to ISO 9001 are high and depend on the number of employees. The certificate is valid for three years. In addition, there are costs for the annual surveillance audits. Besides the ISO 9001 quality management standard, there are other, more affordable QM procedures such as "Quality and Development in Practices®" (QEP) from the National and Regional Association of Statutory Health Insurance Physicians (KBV and KVs), the "KV Practice Quality Management" (KPQM) from the Association of Statutory Health Insurance Physicians of Westphalia-Lippe (KVWL), or the "Cooperation for Transparency and Quality" (KTQ) certification procedure.

Quality Management in the Fertility Center

The introduction of a QM system is intended to help improve the quality of services in a fertility center at all levels, beyond the ART laboratory. Optimization of **management processes** can not only better ensure quality, but also contribute to competitive advantage and economic success. The **core process** is the provision of reproductive medicine services. Through improved marketing, easier appointment scheduling, and professionally competent staff, for example, more patients can be attracted for initial consultations and treatments (Fig. 10.1). The "product" of a fertility center is the desired child. This means that the reproductive medicine service was successful and led to the birth of a child. With a high pregnancy rate and good freezing and thawing rates of cryopreserved material, as well as competent and empathetic counseling and treatment, the **requirements** of fertility and fertility preservation **patients** (**clients**) are met. This also increases client **satisfaction**, as well as that of interested internal and external stakeholders. These include employ-

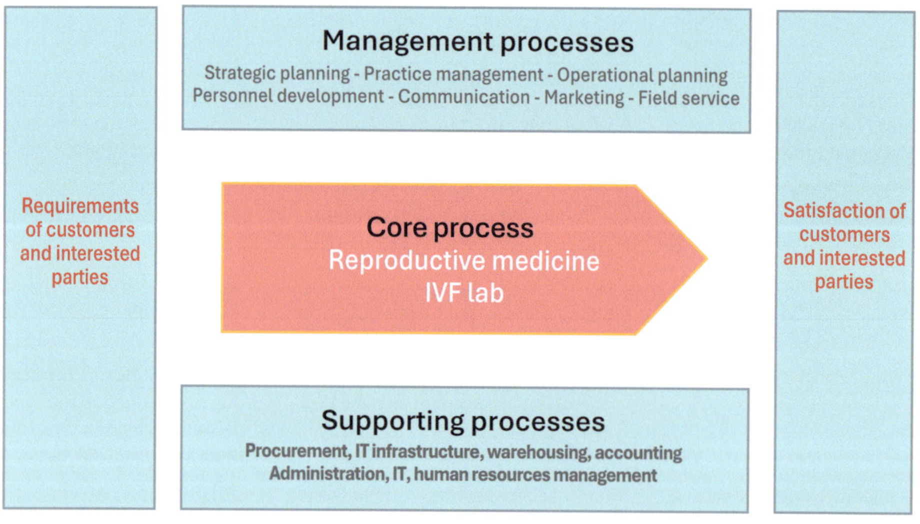

Abb. 10.1 Quality management in the fertility center. (According to Kazazi E [Specialization in Reproductive Medicine])

ees and shareholders, cooperation partners, suppliers, health insurance companies, higher-level organizations, and authorities. A patient- and client-friendly administration and accounting, as well as human resources, data processing, maintenance, and procurement, are **supporting processes**. Improved management processes can further enhance the reputation of a fertility center. Usually, all areas from gynecological endocrinology and reproductive medicine, including all laboratory services, to administration, practice and personnel management, and procurement are certified.

occupational health and safety (**ArbSchG**), occupational safety (**ASiG**), the Technical Rules for Workplaces (**ASR**), and the regulations of the German Statutory Accident Insurance (**DGUV**). The QMR also monitors the representatives for data protection and IT security (General Data protection Regulation **GDPR**) as well as the representative for equipment in accordance with the Medical Devices Law Enforcement Act (**MPDG**). There are now software programs suitable for regular use of the QM system in daily practice, which simplify the monitoring, updating, and further development of the QM system for the QMR.

Basic Structure of a QM System

◼ Figure 10.2 shows, by way of example, the basic structure of a QM system in a fertility center. The **quality management representative (QMR)** is responsible for ensuring that the requirements of the QM system are implemented and that process flows are regularly updated, as a QM system must adapt to the constant changes in practice operations. This includes the introduction of new methods in the ART laboratory, new legal and regulatory requirements, or personnel changes. The QMR monitors the assigned **qualified representatives** for hygiene and safety in the implementation of the Infection Protection Act (**IfSG**) and the laws for

Process Optimization

In quality management, the **Plan-Do-Check-Act (PDCA) cycle** has proven itself as an approach for the "continuous improvement process" (CIP). In the first step, goals and the resources required to achieve them are defined (**Plan**). This is followed by implementation of the project (**Do**). Next comes the review of whether the goals have been achieved (**Check**). If necessary, corrections to the procedure must be made (**Act**) and taken into account in the next PDCA cycle. If no problems have arisen and everything works as planned, we have achieved an improved state and will pro-

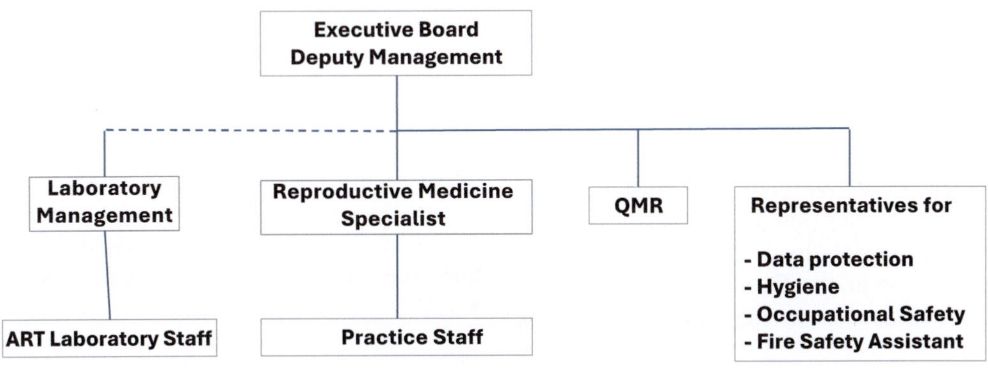

◼ **Abb. 10.2**   Organizational chart of quality management in a fertility center

ceed in the future according to the new insights gained.

Documentation

According to Section 630f of the Civil Code (BGB), the physician is fundamentally required to keep a **patient record**. All measures and their results that are essential for the current and future treatment from a professional point of view must be recorded. The patient record must also include consents, information, and medical letters. The retention period for the patient record after completion of treatment is 10 years. For the collection, processing, and handling of oocytes and sperm cells in the context of artificial fertilization, a separate **donor record** must be kept for both the woman and the man in accordance with Section 5 of the TPG Tissue Ordinance (GewV), which must be retained for 30 years (Section 15 TPG). The content of counseling and information, along with the consent form prior to donation, must also be documented. Here, "donation" also refers to the provision of oocytes and sperm for one's own fertility treatment. For sperm donations, the documentation must comply with the regulations of the **SaRegG**. The German Institute for Medical Documentation an Information (DIMDI) stores the data according to the maximum life expectancy of donor children for 110 years. The recipient should confirm in writing that she has consented to the treatment after being informed, including the associated reporting obligations (see ▶ Chap. 6).

A fertility center is considered a tissue establishment according to the GewebeG. **Every transferred germ cell** must be documented by the treating physician or under their responsibility in accordance with the provisions of the GewebeG (§ 13a TPG, § 7 TPG-GewV). In the case of donations, the Single European Code (**SEC code**) must also be documented (§ 4 paragraph 30a of the Medicinal Products Act). This enables **traceability** and risk assessment. Every tissue that is collected, processed, handled, stored, dispensed, or otherwise used, as well as imported and exported tissue, must be reported, specifying the type and quantity (§ 8d TPG). Based on this, the fertility center is required to prepare an annual **report** for the **PEI** as the responsible federal authority. The data are entered into the PEI database and published as annual **aggregate reports**. The **PEI** publishes annually not only a summary statistic on the germ cells and germ cell tissue collected and used, but also a vigilance report ("safety report") with suspected cases of **serious reactions** and **events**. This report can be accessed in the "Newsroom" on the PEI website (▶ www.pei.de). Serious reactions and events refer to complications and events during artificial fertilization, such as OHSS or the mix-up of embryos. Every **suspected case of a serious reaction**, such as hospitalization due to OHSS, and every **serious event**, such as events related to the collection, examination, processing, handling, preservation, storage, or dispensing, must be reported in accordance with the Tissue Act § 63i AMG (reporting forms in Appendices 6.3 and 6.4). In addition, the **laboratory tests** required for collection must be fully documented in the tissue donor laboratory (§ 33 para. 4 AMWHV) and recorded in the donor record. The responsible person must confirm by signature in the test protocol that the laboratory tests were carried out according to the work instructions and that the test results are correct. The QM system of a tissue establishment must ensure that the defined minimum requirements, such as appropriate **standard operating procedures**, are met (§ 32 para. 3 AMWHV).

Fee Schedules (EBM, GOÄ)

The key differences between the **private medical fee schedule (GOÄ)** and the **statutory fee schedule** according to the Uniform Value Scale **(EBM)** are summarized in ◻ Table 10.2. In the EBM, the fee item schedule (GOP codes) specify **individual services** or **basic flat rates**. In addition to a basic flat rate, **additional flat rates** can be billed in reproductive medicine. Billing to statutory health insurance (GKV) is done quarterly. The statutory physician's fee is settled several months later.

Authorization According to § 121 a SGB V

Most patients are insured under statutory health insurance, and most office-based physicians are accredited as contract physicians with the Association of Statutory Health Insurance Physicians (KV). This also applies to fertility centers, which are run in the outpatient sector by office-based physicians. In order to ensure that couples with statutory health insurance have adequate access to assisted reproduction within a reasonable distance, comprehensive coverage must be guaranteed. For this reason, official authorization for assisted 1 reproduction is granted as needed (e.g., planning areas with a radius of 80 km). In "oversupplied" planning areas, some fertility centers lack this additionally required official **authorization** to perform assisted reproduction according to § 121 a Social Code Book (SGB) Five (V) (see ▶ Chap. 1). These centers can therefore only offer assisted 1 reproduction methods as private services.

Guidelines on Assisted Reproductive Technology (ART) and § 27 a SGB V

Only fertility centers with authorization according to § 121 a SGB V can bill assisted reproduction as services covered by statutory health insurance (see ▶ Chap. 1). These are regulated in SGB V – Statutory Health Insurance – in **§ 27 a Assisted Reproduction**. Insured persons are entitled to adequate, needs-based medical treatment in accordance with the generally accepted state of medical science. In accordance with the **principle of cost-effectiveness**, treatments must be **adequate**, **appropriate**, and **economical**, and must not exceed what is

◻ **Table 10.2** Comparison of billing according to EBM and GOÄ

Fee schedule	GOÄ (private practice)	EBM (statutory practice)
Assignment of GOP code	each individual medical service	Assignment of individual medical services to billable GOP codes (flat rates, also individual services), basic and additional flat rates
GOP codes	Points, amount	Points, amount
Multipliers	depending on degree of difficulty and time required (1x to 2.3x, up to 3.5x with justification)	not applicable
Billing time	Possible at any time	quarterly
Remuneration	Patient pays doctor's bill, reimbursement by health insurance	Presentation of electronic Health Card (eGK), payment after quarterly billing Fee paid by the Association of Statutory Health Insurance Physicians (KV)

necessary. The details are set out by the **Federal Joint Committee (G-BA)** in binding "Guidelines of the Federal Committee of Physicians and Health Insurance Funds on Medical Measures for Artificial Insemination (**'Guidelines on Assisted Reproduction'**)" (Appendix 10.1). The ART methods, the number of treatments, and the catalog of indications for these procedures are summarized in ◘ Table 10.3. The method in 10.4 ("intratubal gamete transfer," abbreviated GIFT) is still listed in the G-BA guidelines, although it is no longer performed.

Methods and Counting of Cycles

Assisted Reproduction may only be performed at the expense of statutory health insurance if, according to the guidelines, there is a reasonable prospect of achieving pregnancy. By law, a **reasonable prospect of success** no longer exists if the **number of procedures** for the chosen treatment method has been exceeded (◘ Table 10.3). If, however, a clinical pregnancy is achieved for the chosen treatment method, the cycle counts as a successful attempt. It can be repeated in the event of a **miscarriage**. The number of successful attempts is not limited. If a **live** or **stillbirth** occurs within the maximum number of unsuccessful attempts, there is a **renewed entitlement** to assisted reproduction **including** the **maximum number** of **unsuccessful attempts**.

A treatment method is generally considered **fully performed** when insemination or embryo transfer has been carried out. However, in IVF and ICSI treatment, special considerations apply once the **oocyte culture has been initiated**, i.e., oocytes and sperm have been combined. If **no embryo transfer** can be performed, for example due to fertilization failure or developmental arrest of a fertilized oocyte, such a cycle is still considered fully performed under the guideline. Contrary to the stated maximum number of unsuccessful attempts, in **IVF** or **ICSI treatment** there is **no longer a reasonable prospect of success** if **fertilization has failed twice**. If fertilization failure occurs in the first IVF attempt, the ICSI method can subsequently be performed up to two times. If fertilization failure occurs again, there is no longer a reasonable prospect of success. However, a cycle is **not considered fully**

◘ **Table 10.3** Indications for ART and number of procedures according to G-BA guideline on artificial insemination

Treatment method	Number	Medical indications
10.1 Insemination in spontaneous cycle	8	11.1 somatic causes, impaired sperm-mucus interaction, male subfertility, immunologically induced infertility.
10.2 Insemination with gonadotropin stimulation	3	11.2 male subfertility, immunologically induced infertility
10.3 In vitro fertilization (IVF) with embryo transfer (ET)	3	11.3 tubal amputation, tubal occlusion not treatable by other means (including microsurgery), tubal functional loss not treatable by other means, also in endometriosis, – idiopathic (unexplained) infertility, male subfertility or immunologically induced infertility, if 10.2 is not promising or has failed
10.5 Intracytoplasmic sperm injection (ICSI)	3	11.5 a) Severe male fertility disorder, documented by two current semen analyses and prior examination by an andrologist; b) ICSI after cryopreservation in the presence of a proven fertility disorder in the female insured person

performed and can be repeated if, for example, after follicle puncture, no oocyte culture could be initiated because unexpectedly no oocytes or sperm were available. A gonadotropin-stimulated insemination cycle can also be repeated if, for example, it is canceled before the planned insemination due to the risk of multiple pregnancy.

Case Study
A 29-year-old patient with statutory health insurance gave birth to a child a year ago after her second IVF treatment for tubal occlusion. She now wishes to have a second child and, after the birth, is entitled to three IVF cycles. Surprisingly, fertilization fails in the first IVF cycle after the birth, so after a change of method, the second cycle is performed using ICSI. The patient becomes pregnant but suffers a miscarriage in the ninth week of pregnancy. After a treatment break, another ICSI cycle is performed, which does not result in pregnancy. The health insurance company approves another ICSI cycle on the follow-up cost plan, as the cycle with the miscarriage can be repeated.

Eligibility Requirements

An **entitlement** to assisted reproduction exists if the **requirements** according to ▣ Table 10.4 are met. In particular, the age limits of both partners at the time of treatment must be observed. Assisted reproduction procedures can only be accessed by **referral** from specialists. **Counseling** of the **couple** on the individual medical, psychological, and social aspects of assisted reproduction is provided by physicians authorized to use the specialty title "gynecologist" as well as by physicians with special expertise in reproductive medicine (e.g., specialists in urology or dermatology). Another requirement is authorization to participate in basic psychosomatic care (sample form in Appendix 10.2). Before **ICSI** is performed, a **documented andrological examination** of the man by a physician with additional training in andrology is also required (e.g., physician's letter). This also allows for the detection of testicular tumors, which peak in frequency during the reproductive phase of men and can be a cause of reduced semen quality. The **treatment plan** (sample treatment plan Appendix 10.3) is completed by the fertility center. The costs for medical services plus material costs and costs for of-

▣ **Table 10.4**   Eligibility requirements for artificial insemination

Eligibility requirement	Woman	Man
Marital status	married	
Homologous treatment	Egg and sperm cells from the spouses	
Age	at least 25 and at most 39 years	at least 25 and at most 49 years
Counseling on artificial insemination according to guideline	Submission of medical certificate of counseling for insemination, IVF, or IVF/ICSI treatment	
Specialist referral	by gynecologist	by andrologist, urologist
ICSI: Clinical-andrological examination according to guideline	not applicable	Submission of confirmation of examination by physician with additional training in andrology
Approved treatment plan	Woman's health insurance	Man's health insurance

fice supplies as well as the estimated medication costs are entered separately for the woman and the man. Before treatment begins, the treatment plan must be approved by both the woman's and the man's health insurance companies. The treatment costs for the woman and the man are covered by their respective health insurance companies. The couple's co-payment is 50 percent. The costs for insemination in a spontaneous cycle, including medication, are about €250, for insemination in a stimulated cycle about €1,000 (high-priced stimulation medications), for IVF treatment about €3,000, and for ICSI treatment about €3,500. **No entitlement** exists after sterilization of the woman or man, for same-sex couples, or for unmarried heterosexual couples.

Mixed Insurance Situation

If only one partner is insured with a statutory health insurance fund (GKV) and the other with a **private health insurance (PKV)**, billing in this **mixed insurance situation** becomes complicated and requires individual clarification, since in the GKV, remuneration is set in the Uniform Value Scale (EBM) (□ Table 10.2). A billing code (GOP) in the EBM can include several different services and service complexes as a flat rate. In the PKV, each individual service is billed according to the fee schedule for physicians (GOÄ). The two systems are different, and the GOPs cannot be reconciled. A PKV will cover the costs of fertility treatment if there is an organic cause (**principle of causation, polluter pays principle**) and the insurance tariff does not exclude fertility treatments. If a tubal occlusion is present as an organic cause and both partners are privately insured, the woman's private health insurance must cover the full IVF treatment costs according to the principle of causation. Courts have ruled that a **probability of success** of at least **15%** must be present as a prerequisite for benefits. The **number** of **treatment cycles** is **not limited** under this condition. If, on the other hand, ICSI treatment is necessary for the privately insured couple because of severely impaired semen quality, the man's private health insurance must cover all treatment costs. This includes all treatment costs such as cycle monitoring, follicle puncture, and embryo transfer, as well as the costs of stimulation medications. In principle, with a PKV, but also in mixed insurance situations with GKV and/or government aid, free medical care, or the armed forces, **individual cost clarifications** are necessary. An overview of the often complex billing situations is illustrated in □ Table 10.5 using three case examples.

□ **Table 10.5**   Billing examples for IVF treatment depending on marital status and health insurance provider (GKV and PKV)

	Case Example I	**Case Example II**	**Case Example III**
Medical indication	Non-treatable tubal occlusion	Non-treatable tubal occlusion	**Non-treatable tubal occlusion**
Age woman/man	33 years/35 years	33 years/35 years	33 years/35 years
Health insurance	Both statutorily insured	Both statutorily insured	Both privately insured
Marital status	Married	**Not married**	**Not married**
Entitlement	Yes	**No**	Yes
Billing method	EBM: Treatment plan approved: 50% GKV, 50% co-payment	According to GOÄ: 100% self-pay	According to GOÄ: principle of causation, 100% via woman's PKV

Statutory Benefits and Funding by State and Federal Government

To provide financial relief for their members, some statutory health insurance funds offer **statutory benefits**. Since 2012, the options for statutory benefits offered by health insurance funds have been expanded under the GKV Health Care Structure Act, including for assisted reproduction. The nationwide program "BKK Kinderwunsch" is a statutory benefit of the Bavarian State Association of Company Health Insurance Funds together with the Bavarian Association for Reproductive Medicine (BRB). About one third of centers in Germany now participate. Additional benefits in "BKK Kinderwunsch" include, among others, a **subsidy** for the **4th cycle,** for **blastocyst culture,** for a **frozen embryo transfer cycle**, and for **IVF** and **ICSI cycles** for **women up to 41 years** (Appendix 10.5).

To support couples seeking fertility treatment with IVF or ICSI, there is an additional government funding program. Most federal states participate in this program (▶ https://www.informationsportal-kinderwunsch.de). In this combined federal and state **"state funding"** program, a subsidy of 25% of treatment costs is paid up to the third attempt and a subsidy of 50% of treatment costs for the fourth attempt. Unmarried couples receive a half subsidy of 12.5% up to the third cycle and 25% for the fourth cycle. However, since the beginning of 2024, there has been a funding freeze, as federal funds for the financial support of involuntarily childless couples have been lacking since the 2024 federal budget.

Data Protection Measures

Data protection refers to the safeguarding of every individual (natural person) during the processing of personal data. Every data controller must ensure compliance with the legal principles listed in Article 5 of the **General Data Protection Regulation (GDPR)**, and, in principle, each individual has the right to determine how their personal data is used (■ Table 10.6). This includes ethnic and cultural origin, political, religious, and philosophical beliefs, health, or sexuality.

Data Protection in Practice Premises

The protection of personal data begins at the **reception** in the fertility center. Data collection should take place in a screened area. The privacy policy should be explained to patients before obtaining their

□ Table 10.6   Principles for the processing of personal data (GDPR Art. 5)

Principles	Explanation
Lawfulness, fair processing, transparency	Data must be processed lawfully, fairly, and in a manner that is transparent to the data subject
Purpose limitation	Data may only be collected for specified, explicit, and legitimate purposes and must not be further processed for other purposes
Data minimization	Limitation to what is necessary for the purposes of processing
Accuracy	Personal data must be accurate and, where necessary, kept up to date
Storage limitation	Data must be stored in a form that permits identification of data subjects only as long as necessary for the purposes for which they are processed
Integrity and confidentiality	Data must be processed using appropriate technical and organizational measures to ensure adequate security, including protection against unauthorized or unlawful processing, and against accidental loss, destruction, or damage

written consent. For patients with statutory insurance, master data is usually transferred from the electronic health card (eGK), and for privately insured patients, either from the insurance card or entered directly into the **practice software**. The practice software must be password-protected with individual access rights for staff to prevent unauthorized access. Screens must be shielded from third-party view, either spatially or with a privacy filter. When leaving the computer workstation, a password-protected screensaver must be activated. **Telephone calls** with patients must not be overheard by other patients. Whenever possible, phone conversations should be conducted in a back office. If this is not possible, calls at the reception must be handled discreetly and without mentioning names. Information about personal data may only be given over the phone if the caller's identity is verified (e.g., by calling back). In **treatment rooms**, it must be ensured that documents of other patients cannot be viewed. Patient data is sent encrypted by email or by **mail**. Information to third parties may only be provided if a **confidentiality waiver** is present.

Access, Maintenance, and Protection of IT Systems and Compliance Monitoring for the GDPR

Patient data and documents are recorded, generated, received, imported, processed, stored, or transmitted using a **hardware and software system**. Employees with a **home office workstation** must ensure that third parties cannot access data by implementing individualized measures. Depending on the requirements of their role, employees should be assigned different **viewing** and **editing rights** in the practice software. Every staff member should be provided with documented information about medical confidentiality and the requirements of the GDPR. **Access** to the central **data processing system** should remain **restricted** to a few individuals. Only this group should perform regular **data backups**. Antivirus programs and firewalls must be installed and kept up to date. If, despite all precautions, there is a **failure** of the **data processing systems**, for example due to malware, the availability of personal data must be quickly restored using existing backups. Professional

Table 10.7 Record of personal data processing according to GDPR Art. 30

Processing activity	Patients	Employees
Description	Use and operation of practice management software	Maintaining personnel files
Purpose	Medical documentation, billing, quality assurance, appointments	Conducting employment relationship
Category of persons	Patients	Employees
Data category	Health data, if applicable genetic data	Personnel data
Categories of recipients	Internal: practice staff External: other physicians/psychotherapists, Association of Statutory Health Insurance Physicians, health insurance, medical service, medical association, private billing agency	Internal: practice owner External: health insurance, tax offices, pension insurers
Retention period	10 years after completion of treatment/30 years for ART	10 years after end of employment

IT service providers can offer assistance here. A **data protection agreement** should be concluded with such a company for the **maintenance** and **servicing** of the **IT** systems. Maintenance, including updates or software installation, is usually performed via **remote maintenance**, which must be included in such a data protection agreement. A data protection agreement must be concluded with all cooperating software partners who require remote access for updates or troubleshooting. The practice premises should also be secured against **theft and burglary** to protect the data processing system. The **disposal of patient records** in paper form or on other data carriers must comply with the data protection regulations of the GDPR, e.g., according to DIN standard 66399.

A fertility center must appoint a company **data protection officer** (DPO) if at least 10 employees are regularly involved in the automated processing, use, or collection of personal data. The data protection officer is the point of contact for management, employees, as well as external parties and supervisory authorities. They are particularly responsible for **compliance with data protection policies**. This includes monitoring the record of processing activities for personal data of patients and employees (**Table 10.7**). A completed sample form "Record of Processing Activities" can be found in Appendix 10.4. If a **data breach** occurs, such as the loss of a data carrier, the data protection officer must report it to the supervisory authority within 72 hours.

Data Collection Programs

The **German IVF Registry** (D·I·R) was established as early as 1982 by the first five IVF working groups, all of which were university institutions. The data analysis formed the basis for clinical and **scientific exchange**. In addition, the registry data was intended to provide a high level of transparency, as at that time, public debate about the new possibilities of reproductive medicine was highly controversial.

D·I·R Annual Reports for Science and Public Relations

IVF treatment data has been systematically collected since 1985. The **registry analyses** are presented and discussed at the annual IVF meetings in the following year. **Annual reports** from 1991 onward are available on the website of the German IVF Registry (▶ https://www.deutsches-ivf-register.de). Since 2009, these reports have been published in the Journal für Reproduktionsmedizin und Endokrinologie (JRE) in both German and English. Special editions for couples, as a commented excerpt from the respective annual report, have been published since 2021. The association was founded as the German IVF Registry e.V. (D·I·R) in 2008. The association is a consortium of reproductive medicine specialists in medical institutions in Germany that practice assisted reproduction techniques. In 2024, the D·I·R had 142 members. Since 1997, data has been documented electronically. Various **data collection programs** are available. The software "DIRpro" was developed by the D·I·R. Not only cycle data but also the medical histories of both woman and man, including previous findings and the baseline semen analysis, are documented. The data is encrypted, assigned a treatment number, and transmitted electronically to the D·I·R office without identity data such as name or address. For the transmission **of these pseudonymized treatment data sets**, patient consent is required if the fertility center is located in Baden-Württemberg, Bavaria, Hamburg, Hesse, Rhineland-Palatinate, Saarland, Saxony, Saxony-Anhalt, or Thuringia. Consent can be withdrawn at any time. In other federal states, physicians are required to report due to state-specific medical professional laws. In these cases, informing the couples is sufficient. Deletion of this data cannot be requested, but data can be blocked, meaning it can only be processed in a limited way.

Nationally and internationally, the D·I·R enjoys a high reputation. It is the only registry worldwide that records cycles **prospectively**. A registry is of high quality if data is entered prospectively rather than retrospectively. Prospective data collection means in practice that a treatment cycle must be documented from the 7th day of stimulation, i.e., before the outcome of the treatment is known. Analyses of prospectively collected data yield more reliable results, as all initiated treatment cycles are included and analyses are not based on a selection of cycles with, for example, good outcomes.

Quality Assurance by AG QSReproMed

While the D·I·R focuses on scientific questions in its data analyses, the **state medical associations** use the treatment data for **quality assurance**. From 1995 to 2011, the D·I·R office was located at the Schleswig-Holstein Medical Association. To continue this function, with the founding of the D·I·R association in 2008 and the move of the office to Berlin in 2012, the state medical associations formed the Working Group for Quality Assurance in Reproductive Medicine (AG **QSReproMed**) in 2013, based at the Schleswig-Holstein Medical Association. Currently, only the medical associations of Berlin and North Rhine do not participate in this working group. Data is transferred from the fertility center to the QSReproMed receiving office via an interface. Only data required for quality assurance is exported. This data is **pseudonymized**, meaning that medical history and treatment data are assigned a treatment number without identity data such as name, first name, addresses, insurance numbers, or other contact information. It is no longer possible to link the data to personal information. A brief information sheet for patients about the export of a treatment data set can be found in Appendix 10.6. The analysis is based on 22 quality indicators. These include **plausibility** (traceability) and **prospectivity** of the data, as well as **multiple birth** and **birth rates**. A panel of representatives from the medical associations and reproductive medicine specialists defines the reference ranges. The QSReproMed analysis for a center shows **deviations** from the reference values. This allows results to be compared. If a center's results fall outside the reference range, the medical association initiates a **collegial dialogue**.

The Ideal Patient and Comparability of Center Data

To better compare treatment outcomes between centers, both the D·I·R and AG QS-ReproMed consider the **ideal patient** or the **ideal scenario**. The definitions have been revised several times in the past. Here are the current definitions:

Definitions

- **Definition of "ideal" patient in the D·I·R** (Annual Report 2023): Patient age $\leq$ 35 years, fresh cycle, 1st cycle, $\geq$ 8 oocytes retrieved, $\geq$ 5 2PN stages, sperm obtained orthogradely (ejaculation)
- **Definition of "ideal scenario" AG QS-ReproMed** (Center analysis 2023): Patient age 26 to 35 years, number of PN $\geq$ 4, SET = single embryo transfer.

Definition of "pregnancy": intrauterine chorionic cavity *or* cardiac activity *or* ectopic pregnancy *or* miscarriage

---

Data Collection Software

Currently, three **data collection programs** are available for documenting D·I·R and QSReproMed registry data, each with an interface for data export. This consists of hardware and software, the so-called "**ARTbox.**" This small device organizes the export to the D·I·R and to the QS-ReproMed receiving office at the Schleswig-Holstein Medical Association, with adjustable settings. Only the required data is sent. This ensures a uniform data set regardless of the data collection software used. The main program used for data export is MedITEX IVF (CRITEX GmbH). DIRproNOVA is the second program. It is a dedicated D·I·R data collection software from CRITEX GmbH without additional features such as automated physician letters with treatment data. The third program is QuinniPro from Austria (QuinniSoft).

Learning Objectives
- Retention periods for patient and donor records
- Know the tasks of the QMR
- Know the requirements for coverage of assisted reproduction costs by statutory and private health insurance (GKV and PKV)

Fertility centers voluntarily introduced a quality management system (QM system) decades ago. This is now legally required. The personnel structure is defined in an organizational chart. The quality management representative (QMR) is appointed by the management of the fertility center. In line with ongoing changes and challenges in the provision of reproductive medicine services, the QMR regularly updates and improves work processes. When handling oocytes, sperm, and germ cell tissue in the ART laboratory, additional documentation requirements and retention periods must be observed in accordance with the Tissue Act. Private health insurance (PKV) covers the costs of assisted reproduction if the insured person has an organic cause (causation principle). For statutory health insurance (GKV), the requirements, benefits, and billing for fertility treatment are regulated in the "Guidelines on Assisted Reproduction." Since the GKV only partially covers the costs of fertility treatment for a limited number of cycles, some statutory health insurers offer additional benefits in their statutes. When collecting and processing data, the principles for processing personal data according to the General Data Protection Regulation (GDPR) must be observed. Medical history and treatment data are documented using various data collection programs. Data export for quality assurance and scientific analysis is carried out via a combined hardware and software solution ("ARTbox") to ensure a uniform data set.

Below is the link to the electronic supplementary material.

10

Psychosocial Care and Support

Contents

Supplementary Information The online version contains supplementary material available at ▶ https://doi.org/10.1007/978-3-662-73035-5_11.

Psychosocial Stress in the Context of Fertility Desire

Patients seeking fertility treatment are often perceived as "difficult." This makes it all the more important to welcome and care for them in a friendly and empathetic manner from the outset. They wish to have children, but conception is not occurring. Previously, they used contraception, and now pregnancy—the "most natural thing in the world"—is not happening (Fig. 11.1). Affected women and couples are therefore emotionally tense and react very sensitively. One in six women experiences a period of unfulfilled desire for children (see ▶ Chap. 3). Fertility disorders are rarely psychosocial in origin. For a long time, an initially unexplained, so-called idiopathic infertility was mistakenly equated with psychogenic infertility. Naturally, there are also fertility patients with psychopathology. The prevalence in the general population is 15 to 20%. Symptoms of **psychosocially influenced infertility** include, despite education, behaviors that impair fertility (such as poor nutrition, competitive sports, substance abuse), no intercourse on fertile days, or not starting fertility treatment even though pregnancy is desired.

Support Services

Infertility is a taboo subject, even though it is common. In their circle of friends, there are usually already children or a friend has become pregnant again. An open conversation with friends is usually not possible. Friends probably would not be able to empathize with the situation either. This explains why unfulfilled desire for children can become a life crisis for some couples or lead to withdrawal and isolation. It is therefore important to offer **low-threshold professional support services** to fertility patients from the very beginning. The availability of such services can vary greatly by region and may range from an interdisciplinary network to a **competence network** for fertility. In such a competence network, various therapists can pool their counseling and seminar offerings. A concept for establishing local competence networks for fertility, supported by the Federal Ministry for Family Affairs, has already been developed (Mayer-Lewis 2024). Pregnancy counseling centers are also increasingly staffed with **qualified counseling professionals** for fertility counseling. The German Society for Fertility Counseling (BKiD) qualifies and certifies appropriate professionals. The society

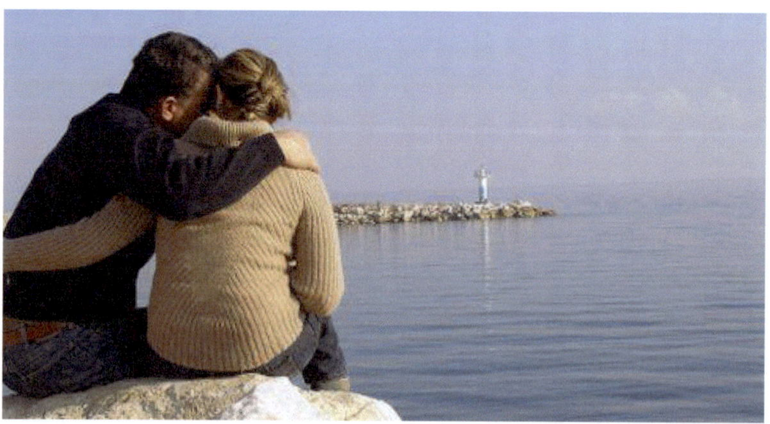

Fig. 11.1   Time of wanting a child

also offers continuing education for medical assistants. With a BKID checklist (Appendix 11.1), patients can assess whether they are likely to benefit from fertility counseling ("fertility coaching"). However, many affected individuals are not even aware that such support options exist.

Fertility Treatment

Fertility disorders can also lead to stress and relationship conflicts. Around 50% of all couples report changes in sexuality during counseling (see ▶ Chap. 5). The woman feels socially responsible for children and for the childlessness. She is repeatedly reminded of her desire for children by her recurring menstruation. Career planning is challenging. The man, on the other hand, often adopts a pragmatic and goal-oriented attitude and is less emotionally tense. When a couple seeks help at a fertility center, their expectations for **fertility treatment** are very high. However, the treatment is essentially carried out on the woman, so the man often feels "marginalized" or even helpless. The ability to absorb the large amount of information before and during treatment is usually limited. The woman undergoes invasive medical treatment and can thus transfer responsibility for the unfulfilled desire for children to the physician. However, this situation is sometimes also experienced as a loss of control. There is a strong desire for sufficient medical consultation time during ongoing treatment. Disappointment is great when this is not possible for organizational reasons. It is therefore understandable that women experience the treatment process as assembly-line work and feel hurt. If a fertility treatment ends unsuccessfully, depressive grief reactions occur. This is normal. Self-esteem decreases, and one in three women and one in five men feel a reduction in well-being. Grief reactions can last up to two years. In the long term, however, these couples are just as satisfied as couples with children. A favorable outcome after unsuccessful therapy is more likely if an alternative life plan ("Plan B") already exists during fertility treatment, since treatment success cannot be guaranteed. Such a "Plan B" should be actively addressed in psychosocial counseling before and during fertility treatment.

Support Work by Medical Support Staff

During the course of treatment, a qualified and competent medical assistant (MFA), nurse, or other medical support staff at the fertility center can provide valuable support. They can answer the **many questions** from patients before, during, and after a treatment cycle with assisted reproduction, **for which the physician often has little or no immediate time**. Questions about treatment contracts can be discussed and the organization of procedures explained. This helps patients feel safer and well cared for during treatment. Written **information material** is often not read by patients. However, it can be used as a valuable support tool in personal conversations. For example, during a treatment cycle, from the pre-cycle to the pregnancy test, a center-specific individualized "workbook" can be used to explain the therapy step by step.

If fertility treatment is successful and pregnancy occurs, there may be a further need for support or counseling. Pregnancy follows a timeline, so counseling appointments are required under some time pressure. Acute counseling needs often arise when miscarriages or multiple pregnancies are diagnosed (see ▶ Chap. 7).

Miscarriages

If the pregnancy test is positive after fertility treatment, there is great joy. A clinical pregnancy is documented after reproductive medical treatment when a gestational sac and/or fetal heartbeat can be detected. This is possible from the seventh week of pregnancy. After previous **miscarriages**, the fear is high that the pregnancy will not continue. If, unexpectedly, a few days after a positive pregnancy test, bleeding and a drop in the pregnancy hormone hCG occur, the disappointment is severe. Some women even experience this situation as the loss of a child. Therefore, affected women should be offered close psychosocial support as soon as a miscarriage is imminent. It is beneficial to continue such counseling after a miscarriage and to include the partner. Referrals to counseling centers and self-help groups (e.g., initiative-regenbogen.de) are often helpful for those affected. The miscarriage rate increases with maternal age. It is below 20% for women up to age 35 and rises to over 50% for women aged 43 and older. For a woman who is "older" from a reproductive medicine perspective, a miscarriage often also means the end of fertility treatment.

Multiple Pregnancies

The goal of fertility treatment is an ongoing singleton pregnancy resulting in the birth of a healthy child. **Multiple pregnancies** are not desired, as they increase health risks for both mothers and children. In any case, intensified obstetric and prenatal medical care

is indicated. Fortunately, the risk of multiples after ART has decreased significantly in recent years (Fig. 11.2), as more and more centers recommend transferring only one embryo to patients. As a result, from 1997 to 2022, **multiple birth rates** after fresh and frozen embryo transfer (FET) cycles have been **reduced** by about 35 to 40% (D·I·R Annual Report 2023). Dizygotic multiple pregnancies due to the transfer of two or three embryos are avoidable; monozygotic multiple pregnancies are not. The latter are rare but more often lead to the problematic twin-to-twin transfusion syndrome, or TTTS (see ▶ Chaps. 6 and 7). In this syndrome, the fetuses share a placenta. The main **maternal risks** of dizygotic multiple pregnancies are summarized in Table 11.1. For mothers, the main risk is preeclampsia, often associated with gestational diabetes and postpartum hemorrhage. Severe preeclampsia is life-threatening. For the **children**, the risk of prematurity is highest at 85 to 90%. Extremely premature infants with brain injury are more likely to develop movement disorders and muscle stiffness (cerebral palsy), seizures, blindness, and deafness. This requires long-term regular physical and speech therapy. Since the children are usually born underweight (microsomic), intrauterine gene reprogramming (**fetal programming**) increases the later

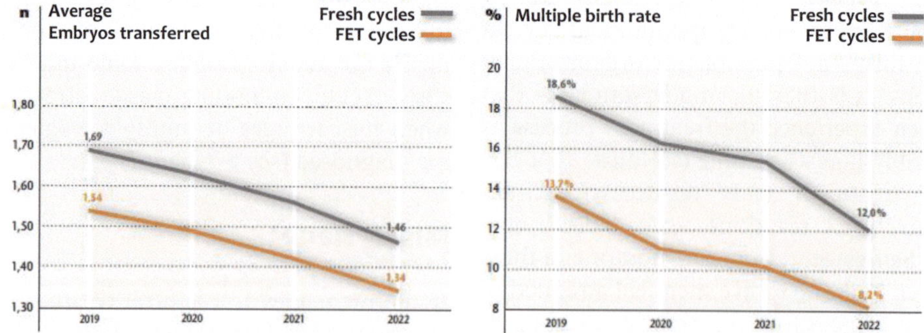

Fig. 11.2 Embryos per transfer and multiple birth rate 2019–2022; FET = frozen embryo transfer (With kind permission from D·I·R-(2024) Annual Report 2023)

▣ Table 11.1 Maternal and child health in multiples*

	Mothers	Children
Risks	Gestational diabetes	Prematurity (esp. respiratory distress, intestinal disease, brain injury)
	Preeclampsia	Malformations
	Anemia	Microsomia
	Postpartum hemorrhage	Behavioral disorders (esp. emotional and social)
	Risk of chronic exhaustion, depression, relationship conflicts	Delayed development (including motor and learning disorders)

*dizygotic only; esp. = especially; incl. = including

risk of insulin resistance. This also increases susceptibility to type 2 diabetes, hypertension, heart attack, and stroke in adulthood (see ▶ Chap. 9). Preterm infants also have an increased risk of behavioral problems and developmental disorders. Long-term consequences for the mother can include chronic exhaustion and depression. An increased separation rate among parents of multiples is known.

Gamete Donation

Family structures have changed significantly over the decades. Traditionally, mother and father are married and raise their children together. In 1996, this traditional family form was still present in over 80% of families, but by 2016 it had dropped to 66%. At the same time, the proportion of unmarried couples and single parents with children has risen to 10% and 25%, respectively (▣ Table 11.2). This situation has significantly changed the daily routine in psychosocial counseling, as the need for advice on family law and child support has increased. In addition, donor treatments with gametes are on the rise. The proportion of family forms, especially with children conceived via **sperm donation**, is increasing. Psychosocial counseling is recommended before any gamete donation (social parenthood, inform-

▣ Table 11.2 Change in family structures and children after donation and surrogacy 1996 to 2016 (According to P. Thorn (Specialization in Reproductive Medicine))

Family structures and children's parentage	1996	2016
Mother, father, biological child, married	81%	65.7%
Mother, father, biological child, not married	4%	9.7%
Single parent, biological child	14%	24.7%
Partnerships and single parents, child after sperm donation	approx. 1200	approx. 2000
Partnerships and single parents, child after egg cell donation	approx. 800	approx. 2000
Partnerships and single parents, child after embryo donation or surrogacy	isolated cases	

ing the child and the environment, child development, family handling of the conception story, contact between child and donor). Since 2018, the Sperm Donor Registry Act (SaRegG) applies to sperm donation, protecting the rights of the child and the donor. For married lesbian couples, the non-biological co-mother is not the legal second mother at the child's birth.

She must adopt the child. This process is called stepchild adoption. The law on parentage has not yet been amended. It determines who is legally recognized as the mother and father of a child. **Egg Cell donation** is prohibited in Germany. Couples therefore often seek treatment abroad (◘ Table 11.2). In many countries, donations are anonymous. Thus, donor-conceived children later have no right to information about the donor. **Embryo donation** is permitted in Germany. It is coordinated by the Network Embryo Donation Germany e.V. as a non-profit organization. The child's right to information about their biological parents is secured through a notary. Psychosocial counseling is recommended for both the donating and receiving parents (informing the child and the environment, child development, family handling of the conception story, significance of full siblings in a second family, contact between child and family). Due to the increase in gamete donations, about 50% of psychosocial counseling sessions for fertility now concern sperm, egg cell, and embryo donation. One fifth of these counseling sessions relate to treatments abroad. A newer counseling topic is the preparation, support, and follow-up of contacts between donor-conceived children and their donor and families.

🎓 **Learning Objectives**
- Know support services for couples with fertility desire and the relevance and frequency of psychopathologies
- Recognize and support psychosocial stress in miscarriages and multiple pregnancies, including maternal and child risks
- Understand the role of psychosocial counseling in gamete donation

For affected couples, the period of wanting a child is a life phase characterized by anxiety, optimism, hope, disappointment, and grief. Professional support is often helpful, as fertility treatment is not a guarantee for the birth of a child. Competent MFAs, nurses, and other medical support staff provide valuable assistance in daily practice, especially for female patients. Miscarriages and multiple pregnancies lead to particular stress situations after a desired pregnancy is achieved. Treatments involving donations are taking up an increasing share, now accounting for 50% of counseling time in psychosocial fertility counseling. In 20% of these sessions, the focus is on egg cell donation abroad. Recently, counseling has also included supporting donor-conceived children in meeting their donor.

Below is the link to the electronic supplementary material.

Reference

D·I·R-Jahrbuch 2023 (2024) J Reproduktionsmed Endokrinol 21 (Sonderheft 4), 1–64

Practical Knowledge, Experience, and Skills

Contents

Differences in the Daily Practice of Fertility Centers

All fertility centers perform assisted reproductive technology (ART) techniques in accordance with legal requirements and laboratory standards. However, they differ in their spatial facilities and the practical implementation of individual steps during planning as well as before, during, and after treatment. Fertility centers use different practice management software programs, each offering various advantages for the administration and processing of patient data. These are used for the appointment calendar and for reading the electronic Health Card (eHC). In addition, the practice management programs are indispensable for billing with statutory and private health insurance. One of the three approved **data collection programs** must be used for documenting reproductive medicine treatment data in the center (see ▶ Chap. 10). The MedITEX IVF program, which is predominantly used, can also serve as an electronic patient record, a word processor for automated medical letters, and for additional applications such as importing an online medical history. Furthermore, it offers interfaces for external programs such as electronic signatures for consent forms and treatment contracts. For **video consultations**, patients must sign an additional information and consent form. When using practice IT systems, compliance with data protection regulations is mandatory. For this reason, all visitors to a center, including observers, must sign a data protection declaration.

The workflow of consultations is handled very differently within each center. The duration of **appointment types** (such as initial consultation, follow-up, start of an ART cycle, and monitoring) also varies considerably. Some centers employ room assistants for organizational preparation and follow-up as well as documentation to support and relieve the physician. This also includes entering ultrasound measurements into the data collection program for export to the D·I·R and QSReproMed. This ensures that for **prospective data collection**, cycle data from the 7th day of stimulation are documented.

During patient contact, it is very helpful for patients if the attending MFAs, nurses, or other medical support staff are also familiar with the regional **support services** offered by counseling centers with qualified psychosocial counselors, as they are more intensively confronted with the patients' emotional burdens than the physicians. Fertility centers often train their staff in communication with fertility patients in difficult situations (e.g., cancellation of an embryo transfer or diagnosis of a miscarriage). The satisfaction of fertility patients largely depends on how well they feel cared for in a fertility center. As part of quality management, it is important to regularly measure **"customer satisfaction."** The proven but labor-intensive method is a questionnaire. To save paper and reduce workload, digital apps are also used. This allows the center to quickly and anonymously receive the results of patient surveys.

For hygiene reasons, the **ART laboratory** is accessible only to laboratory staff during oocyte treatments in many centers. Otherwise, the various workstations at the lab benches, the andrology workstation, and the cryostorage room can be visited in the ART laboratory. Preimplantation genetic diagnosis with trophectoderm biopsy can be explained and illustrated with case examples. With a time-lapse incubator, the development of an oocyte up to a blastocyst can be demonstrated.

To work competently in a fertility center, MFAs, nurses, and other medical support staff can be qualified according to the **model training curriculum** for medical assistants "Reproductive Medicine" of the German Medical Association (BÄK, 2022). It covers the entire spectrum of reproductive medicine.

Action Competencies

Medical assistants are expected to support and relieve reproductive medicine specialists by taking on delegable tasks based on their qualifications. These include:

1. Supporting the preparation, execution, and follow-up of diagnostic procedures (e.g., ultrasound in the stimulation cycle with documentation of findings)
2. Preparation, execution, and follow-up of reproductive medical procedures (e.g., follicular puncture with documentation)
3. Communication, counseling, and information for couples seeking fertility treatment
4. Knowledge of legal foundations and medical limitations of fertility therapy
5. Data collection, quality assurance, and billing in compliance with data protection (e.g., documentation of relevant fields in the data collection program for an ART treatment for data export to D·I·R and QSReproMed, billing of reproductive medical services for private and statutory health insurance)

Practical Training

In order to apply the specific knowledge in reproductive medicine with the above-mentioned **complex action competencies** 1 to 5, a supervised, structured internship in a fertility center is important. Such a "**practical day**" should begin with a tour of the facilities involving the center's MFAs. To train action competencies, small group work directly at the workstations is advisable. Hands-on exercises on simulators, laboratory equipment, and computer workstations are also possible (◘ Fig. 12.1).

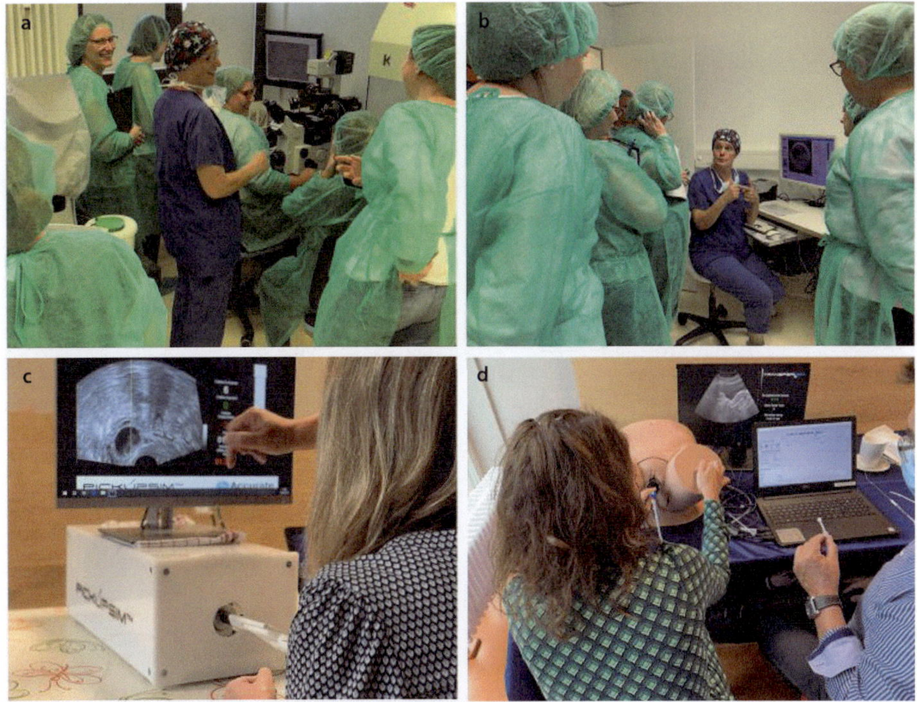

◘ **Fig. 12.1** Hands-on procedure room area and ART laboratory. **a**: ICSI microscope "catching" sperm, **b**: evaluation of time-lapse images (time-lapse incubator), **c**: follicular puncture on a phantom, **d**: embryo transfer on a phantom

The following **sample schedule for the practical day** is possible:

8:00–9:00 am:	Welcome
	Introduction round
	Participants' expectations
9:00–10:00 am:	Tour of the fertility center
10:00–1:00 pm:	Division into small groups
	Tour and explanation of work areas and processes
	Alternating discussion, practical exercises, and applications
	depending on availability - IVF laboratory, cryopreservation - Andrology laboratory - Hormone laboratory - Procedure room including follicular punctures, inseminations - Reception including appointment scheduling, telecommunications, IT - Examination and treatment room including hormone treatments
1:00–2:00 pm:	Lunch break with catering
2:00–4:15 pm:	Discussion of the following topics with practical examples - Documentation and quality assurance - MedITEX IVF - Billing - Topics requested by participants
4:15–4:30 pm:	Feedback
	Farewell

Duration: 10 teaching units (450 min)

Objectives of the practical day:

- Introduction to work areas and processes
- practical exercises and applications
- Discussion of different approaches
- Exchange of experiences ("best practice")

For this, the **presence is desirable** of

- Medical director or deputy
- Laboratory director or deputy
- Head MFA or deputy
- additional supervisors for the small groups as needed

Repeating the content of webinars and eLearning is not part of the practical day.

All fertility centers perform assisted reproductive technology (ART) techniques as their main service in accordance with legal requirements and laboratory standards. However, the centers differ in their spatial facilities and in the practical implementation of individual steps during planning and before, during, and after treatment. Therefore, MFAs, nursing staff, and other medical support staff are very curious to gain insight into another fertility center. There is also a desire for collegial exchange and to be able to ask: How do you do it? It is about patient care from scheduling the initial consultation to the final appointment after the end of fertility treatment. These wishes are fulfilled in the model training curriculum of the German Medical Association through internships ("practical day") in another fertility center. The internships take place after completion of the theoretical training. On the "practical days," practical exercises in small groups can also be conducted, for example at computer workstations with explanations of billing for reproductive medical services, or demonstrations of data entry and documentation in the software programs. Hands-on exercises on laboratory equipment in the ART laboratory (e.g., "catching" sperm with the ICSI microscope) and on simulators for follicle aspirations and embryo transfers are also possible.

Reference

BÄK. Musterfortbildungscurriculum für Medizinische Fachangestellte „Reproduktionsmedizin". Berlin, 2022. ▶ https://www.bundesaerztekammer.de/fileadmin/user_upload/BAEK/Gesundheitsfachberufe/MFA_Fortbildungscurricula/Musterfortbildungscurriculum_Reproduktionsmedizin_MFA.pdf. Zuletzt 10.6.2025

Supplementary Information

M. Bals-Pratsch et al., *Workplace: Fertility Clinic*, https://doi.org/10.1007/978-3-662-73035-5

Appendix

Appendix 1.1 Act for the Protection of Embryos (Embryo Protection Act—ESchG) of December 13, 1990

Law
on the Protection of Embryos
(Embryo Protection Act   - ESchG)

December 13, 1990

The Bundestag has passed the following law:

§ 1

Abusive use of reproductive technologies

(1) Anyone who

1. transfers a foreign unfertilized egg cell to a woman,

2. attempts to artificially fertilize an egg cell for any purpose other than to induce pregnancy in the woman from whom the egg cell originates,

3. attempts to transfer more than three embryos to a woman within one cycle,

4. attempts to fertilize more than three egg cells within one cycle by means of intratubal gamete transfer,

5. fertilizes more egg cells from a woman than are to be transferred to her within one cycle,

6. removes an embryo from a woman before it has completed implantation in the uterus in order to transfer it to another woman or to use it for a purpose other than its preservation, or

7. it undertakes to perform assisted reproduction on a woman who is prepared to give up her child to third parties on a permanent basis after birth (surrogate mother) or to transfer a human embryo to her.

(2) The same punishment shall apply to anyone who

1. artificially causes a human sperm cell to penetrate a human egg cell, or

2. artificially transfers a human sperm cell into a human egg cell

without the intention of causing pregnancy in the woman from whom the egg cell originates.

(3) The following shall not be punished

1. in the cases referred to in paragraph 1, nos. 1, 2, and 6, the woman from whom the egg cell or embryo originates, as well as the woman to whom the egg cell is transferred or to whom the embryo is to be transferred, and

2. in the cases referred to in paragraph 1, no. 7, the surrogate mother and the person who intends to take the child into their permanent care.

(4) In the cases referred to in paragraph 1, no. 6, and paragraph 2, the attempt shall be punishable.

§2

Abusive use of human embryos

(1) Anyone who sells or transfers a human embryo that has been created extracorporeally or removed from a woman before it has implanted in the uterus for a purpose other than its preservation shall be punished with imprisonment of up to three years or a fine.

(2) Anyone who causes a human embryo to develop extracorporeally for a purpose other than bringing about a pregnancy shall also be punished.

(3) Attempting to do so is punishable.

§ 3
Prohibition of sex selection

Anyone who attempts to artificially fertilize a human egg cell with a sperm cell selected on the basis of the sex chromosome it contains shall be punished with imprisonment for up to one year or a fine. This shall not apply if the selection of the sperm cell by a physician serves to protect the child from Duchenne muscular dystrophy or a similarly serious sex-linked hereditary disease, and the disease threatening the child has been recognized as correspondingly serious by the competent authority under state law.

§ 4
Unauthorized fertilization, unauthorized embryo transfer, and artificial insemination after death

(1) Anyone who

1. attempts to artificially fertilize an egg cell without the consent of the woman whose egg cell is being fertilized and the man whose sperm is being used for fertilization,
2. attempts to transfer an embryo to a woman without her consent, or
3. knowingly artificially fertilizes an egg cell with the sperm of a man after his death.

(2) In the case of paragraph 1, no. 3, the woman on whom the artificial fertilization is performed shall not be punished.

§ 5
Artificial modification of human germ cells

(1) Anyone who artificially modifies the genetic information of a human germ cell shall be punished with imprisonment of up to five years or a fine.

(2) Anyone who uses a human germ cell with artificially altered genetic information for fertilization shall also be punished.

(3) Attempting to do so is punishable.

(4) Paragraph 1 shall not apply to

1. artificial modification of the genetic information of a germ cell outside the body, if it is impossible for it to be used for fertilization,
2. artificial modification of the genetic information of any other germ cell from the body that has been taken from a dead fetus, a human being, or a deceased person, if it is impossible for

a) it is transferred to an embryo, fetus, or human being, or

b) a germ cell is created from it, and

3. vaccinations, radiation, chemotherapy, or other treatments that are not intended to alter the genetic information of germ cells.

§ 6
Cloning

(1) Anyone who artificially causes a human embryo to be created with the same genetic information as another embryo, fetus, human being, or deceased person shall be punished with imprisonment of up to five years or a fine.

(2) Anyone who transfers an embryo as described in paragraph 1 to a woman shall also be punished.

(3) Attempting to do so is punishable.

§ 7
Chimera and hybrid formation

(1) Anyone who attempts

1. to combine embryos with different genetic information into a cell cluster using at least one human embryo,
2. to combine a cell containing genetic information different from that of the cells of the embryo with a human embryo and to allow it to continue to differentiate with the embryo, or
3. to produce a differentiable embryo by fertilizing a human egg cell with the sperm of an animal or by fertilizing an animal egg cell with the sperm of a human,

shall be punished with imprisonment of up to five years or a fine.

(2) The same penalty shall apply to anyone who attempts

1. an embryo created by an act under paragraph 1

a) a woman or

b) an animal

or

2. a human embryo to an animal.

§ 8
Definition

(1) For the purposes of this Act, an embryo shall be deemed to be a fertilized human egg cell capable of development from the moment of nuclear fusion, as well as any totipotent cell removed from an embryo which, under the necessary conditions, is capable of dividing and developing into an individual.

(2) In the first twenty-four hours after nuclear fusion, the fertilized human egg cell is considered capable of development unless, even before

At the end of this period, it is determined that it is unable to develop beyond the single-cell stage.

(3) Germ line cells within the meaning of this Act are all cells that lead in a cell line from the fertilized egg cell to the egg and sperm cells of the human being that has developed from it, as well as the egg cell from the introduction or penetration of the sperm cell to the completion of fertilization with nuclear fusion.

§ 9
Medical reservation

Only a physician may perform:

1. assisted reproduction

2. the transfer of a human embryo to a woman,

3. the preservation of a human embryo or a human egg cell into which a human sperm cell has already penetrated or been artificially introduced.

§ 10
Voluntary participation

No one is obliged to carry out or cooperate in measures of the type specified in § 9.

§ 11
Violation of the physician's reservation

(1) Anyone who, without being a physician,

1. performs assisted reproduction contrary to § 9 No. 1, or

2. transfers a human embryo to a woman contrary to § 9 No. 2,

shall be punished with imprisonment for up to one year or a fine.

(2) In the case of § 9 No. 1, the woman who performs artificial insemination on herself and the man whose semen is used for artificial insemination shall not be punished.

Section 12
Provisions on fines

(1) Anyone who, without being a physician, preserves a human embryo or a human egg cell as described in § 9 No. 3 shall be guilty of an administrative offense.

(2) The administrative offense may be punished with a fine of up to five thousand German marks.

§ 13
Entry into force

This law shall enter into force on January 1, 1991.

––––––––

The constitutional rights of the Federal Council are preserved.

The above law is hereby enacted and will be published in the Federal Law Gazette.

Bonn, December 13, 1990

The Federal President
Weizsäcker

The Federal Chancellor
Dr. Helmut Kohl

The Federal Minister of Justice
Engelhard

The Federal Minister
for Youth, Family, Women, and Health
Ursula Lehr

The Federal Minister
for Research and Technology
Riesenhuber

Appendix 1.2 Act on the Quality and Safety of Human Tissues and Cells (Tissue Act) of 20.07.2007

Act

on the quality and safety of human tissues and cells
(Tissue Act)*)

July 20, 2007

The Bundestag has passed the following law:

Article 1
Amendment
of the Transplantation Act

The Transplantation Act of November 5, 1997 (Federal Law Gazette I, p. 2631), last amended by Article 42 of the Act of March 26, 2007 (Federal Law Gazette I, p. 378), is amended as follows:

1. The heading shall read as follows:

"Act
on the Donation, Removal, and Transfer of Organs and Tissues (Transplantation Act - TPG)."

2. The following table of contents shall be inserted before Section 1:

"Table of Contents

Section 1

General provisions

§ 1 Scope

§ 1a Definitions

§ 2 Public information, declaration on organ and tissue donation, organ and tissue donation register, organ and tissue donor cards

Section 2

Removal of organs

and tissues from deceased donors

§ 3 Removal with the consent of the donor

§ 4 Removal with the consent of other persons

§ 4a Removal from dead embryos and fetuses

§ 5 Verification procedure

§ 6 Respect for the dignity of organ and tissue donors

§ 7 Data collection and use; obligation to provide information

Section 3

Removal of organs and tissues from living donors

§ 8 Removal of organs and tissues

§ 8a Removal of bone marrow from minors

§ 8b Removal of organs and tissues in special cases

§ 8c Removal of organs and tissues for reimplantation

Section 3a

Tissue establishments, testing laboratories, registries

§ 8d Special obligations of tissue establishments

§ 8e Testing laboratories

§ 8f Register of tissue establishments

Section 4

Mediation and transfer of certain organs, transplant centers, cooperation in the removal of organs and tissues

§ 9 Admissibility of organ transfer, priority of organ donation

§ 10 Transplant centers

§ 11 Cooperation in the removal of organs and tissues, coordination center

§ 12 Organ allocation, allocation agency

Section 5

Notifications, documentation, traceability, data protection, deadlines

§ 13 Reports, accompanying documents for organs subject to allocation

§ 13a Documentation of tissues transferred by medical care facilities

§ 13b Reporting of serious incidents and serious adverse reactions involving tissues

§ 13c Traceability procedures for tissues

§ 14 Data protection

§ 15 Retention and deletion periods

---

*) This Act implements Directive 2004/23/EC of the European Parliament and of the Council of March 31, 2004, on setting standards of quality and safety for the donation, procurement, testing, processing, preservation, storage, and distribution of human tissues and cells (ABI. EU No. L 102 p. 48). The obligations arising from Directive 98/34/EC of the European Parliament and of the Council of June 22, 1998, laying down a procedure for the provision of information in the field of technical standards and regulations and of rules on Information Society services (OJ EC No. L 204 p. 37), as amended by Directive 98/48/EC of the European Parliament and of the Council of July 20, 1998 (OJ EC No. L 217 p. 18), have been complied with.

Section 5a

Guidelines on the state of medical science, regulatory authority

§ 16 Guidelines on the state of medical science for organs

§ 16a Prescription authorization

§ 16b Guidelines on the state of medical science regarding the removal of tissue and its transfer

Section 6

Prohibitions

Section 17 Prohibition of organ and tissue trafficking

Section 7

Penal and administrative fine provisions

§ 18 Trade in organs and tissues

§ 19 Further criminal provisions

§ 20 Administrative fine provisions

Section 8 Final provisions

§ 21 Competent federal authority

§ 22 Relationship to other areas of law

§ 23 Armed Forces

§ 24 Amendment to the Criminal Code

§ 25 Transitional provisions

§ 26 Entry into force, expiry".

3. The heading of Section 1 shall read as follows:

"Section 1

General provisions."

4. § 1 shall be worded as follows:

Section 1
Scope

(1) This Act applies to the donation and removal of human organs or tissues for the purpose of transplantation, as well as to the transplantation of organs or tissues, including the preparation of these measures. It also applies to the prohibition of trade in human organs or tissues.

(2) This Act shall not apply to

1. tissue removed from a person during the same surgical procedure for the purpose of being transplanted back to that person,

2. blood and blood components."

5. The following Section 1a is inserted after Section 1:

"Section 1a

Definitions

For the purposes of this Act

1. organs, with the exception of skin, are all parts of the human body consisting of different tissues which form a functional unit in terms of structure, blood supply, and ability to perform physiological functions, including parts of organs and individual tissues or cells

of an organ that can be used for the same purpose as the entire organ in the human body;

2. organs subject to mandatory allocation are the organs heart, lung, liver, kidney, pancreas, and intestine within the meaning of number 1, which have been removed in accordance with § 3 or § 4;

3. non-regenerative organs are all organs that cannot regenerate in the donor after removal;

4. Tissues are all components of the human body consisting of cells that are not organs as defined in number 1, including individual human cells.

5. Next of kin are, in order of priority

   a) the spouse or registered civil partner,

   b) the adult children,

   c) the parents or, if the potential organ or tissue donor was a minor at the time of death and only one parent, guardian, or caregiver was responsible for his or her care at that time, that caregiver,

   d) siblings of legal age,

   e) grandparents;

6. Removal means the extraction of organs or tissues;

7. transplantation means the use of organs or tissues in or on a human recipient, as well as their use in humans outside the body;

8. a tissue establishment is an establishment that procures, examines, processes, preserves, labels, packages, stores, or distributes tissue for the purpose of transplantation;

9. a medical care facility is a hospital or other facility providing direct patient care, which is under constant medical supervision and in which medical services are provided;

10. A serious incident is any undesirable event in connection with the collection, examination, preparation, processing, preservation, storage, or distribution of tissues that could result in the transmission of an infectious disease, death, or a life-threatening condition, disability, or loss of function in patients, or that could necessitate or prolong hospitalization, or that could lead to or prolong an illness; A serious incident is also defined as any incorrect identification or mix-up of germ cells or embryos in the context of medically assisted fertilization procedures.

11. A serious adverse reaction is an unintended reaction, including a communicable disease, in the donor or recipient in connection with the removal or transfer of tissue, which is fatal or life-threatening, results in disability or loss of ability, or requires or prolongs hospitalization, or leads to or prolongs illness.

6. Section 2 is amended as follows:

a) The heading is worded as follows:

§2

Informing the public, declaration on organ and tissue donation, organ and tissue donation register, organ and tissue donation cards."

b) Paragraph 1 is amended as follows:

aa) In sentence 1, the word "organ donation" is replaced by the words "organ and tissue donation," the word "organ removal" is replaced by the words "organ and tissue removal," and the word "organ transfer" is replaced by the words "organ and tissue transfer, including the possible medical use of medicinal products manufactured from tissues."

bb) In sentence 2, the word "organ donation" is replaced by the words "organ and tissue donation" and the word "organ donor cards" is replaced by the words "organ and tissue donor cards."

cc) In sentence 3, the word "organ donation" is replaced by the words "organ and tissue donation."

c) Paragraph 2 is amended as follows:

aa) In sentence 1, the words "organ donation" are replaced by the words "organ and tissue donation" and the word "organ removal" is replaced by the words "organ and tissue removal."

bb) In sentence 2, the words "or tissue" are inserted after the word "organs."

d) Paragraph 3 is amended as follows:

aa) In sentence 1, the words "and social security" are deleted, the word "organ donation" is replaced by the words "organ or tissue donation" and the word "organ donor register" is replaced by the words "organ and tissue donor register".

bb) In sentence 2, the word "organ removal" is replaced by the words "organ or tissue removal."

cc) Sentence 3 is amended as follows:

aaa) In number 1, the word "organ donation" is replaced by the words "organ or tissue donation."

bbb) In numbers 2 and 3, the word "organ donor registry" is replaced by the word "registry."

ccc) In number 4, the word "code numbers" is replaced by the words "user IDs and passwords."

ddd) In number 6, the word "organ donor registry" is replaced by the word "registry."

e) Paragraph 4 is amended as follows:

aa) In sentence 1, the word "organ donor register" is replaced by the word "register" and the word "organ donors" is replaced by the words "organ or tissue donors," and the words "or tissue" are inserted after the word "organs."

bb) In sentence 2, the reference to "§ 3 (1) No. 2" is replaced by the reference to "§ 3 (1) sentence 1 No. 2."

cc) In sentence 3, the word "organ removal" is replaced by the words "organ or tissue removal" and the words "or under whose responsibility the tissue removal is carried out in accordance with Section 3 (1) sentence 2" are inserted after the word "perform."

f) In paragraph 5, the words "The Federal Ministry of Health" are replaced by the words "The Federal Government" and the words "an organ donor card" are replaced by the words "the organ and tissue donor card."

7. The heading of Section 2 shall be worded as follows:

"Section 2

Removal of organs
and tissues from deceased donors."

8. Section 3 is amended as follows:

a) The heading shall read as follows:

"Section 3

Removal with

the consent of the donor."

b) Paragraph 1 is amended as follows:

aa) In the sentence before number 1, the words "or tissues" are inserted after the word "organs" and the words "or § 4a" are inserted after the reference to "§ 4".

bb) In number 1, the word "organ donor" is replaced by the words "organ or tissue donor."

cc) In number 2, the word "organ donor" is replaced by the words "organ or tissue donor."

dd) The following sentence is added:

"Notwithstanding sentence 1 no. 3, tissue may also be removed by other qualified persons under the responsibility and according to the professional instructions of a physician."

c) Paragraph 2 is amended as follows:

aa) In the part of the sentence before number 1, the words "or tissues" are inserted after the word "organs."

bb) In number 1, the word "organ removal" is replaced by the words "organ or tissue removal."

cc) In number 2, the word "organ donor" is replaced by the words "organ or tissue donor."

d) Paragraph 3 is amended as follows:

aa) In sentence 1, the word "organ donor" is replaced by the words "organ or tissue donor" and the word "organ removal" is replaced by the words "organ or tissue removal."

bb) In sentence 2, the words "He has" are replaced by the words "The person performing the removal has" and the word "organ removal" is replaced by the words "organ or tissue removal."

9. Section 4 is amended as follows:

a) The heading is worded as follows:

"Section 4

Removal with

the consent of other persons."

b) Paragraph 1 is amended as follows:

aa) In sentence 1, the words "perform organ removal" are replaced by the words "perform organ or tissue removal or under whose responsibility the tissue removal is performed in accordance with § 3 (1) sentence 2", the word "organ donor" is replaced by the words "organ or tissue donor" and the word "organ donation" is replaced by the words "organ or tissue donation."

bb) In sentence 2, the words "Section 3 (1) Nos. 2 and 3 and (2)" are replaced by the words "Section 3 (1) sentence 1 Nos. 2 and 3, sentence 2 and (2) No. 2" and the word "organ removal" is replaced by the words "organ or tissue removal," and the word "next" is inserted before the word "relatives" in each case.

cc) The following sentence is inserted after sentence 2: "If the removal of several organs or tissues is being considered, consent shall be obtained together."

dd) In the new sentence 4, the word "next" is inserted before the word "relatives" and the word "organ donor" is replaced by the words "organ or tissue donor."

ee) In the new sentence 5, the word "next" is inserted before the word "relatives."

ff) In the new sentence 6, the word "next" is inserted before the word "relatives" and the period is replaced by a semicolon

and the words "the agreement must be in writing" are added.

c) Paragraph 2 is amended as follows:

aa) Sentence 1 is deleted.

bb) In the new sentence 1, the word "organ donor" is replaced by the words "organ or tissue donor."

cc) In the new sentence 2, the word "next" is inserted before the word "relatives."

dd) In the new sentence 3, the word "next" is inserted before the word "relatives."

ee) In the new sentence 4, the word "next" is inserted before the word "relative" and the words "next available subordinate relatives" are replaced by the words "first available next of kin".

ff) In the new sentence 5, the word "organ donor" is replaced by the words "organ or tissue donor."

d) In paragraph 3, the word "organ donor" is replaced by the words "organ or tissue donor" and the word "organ removal" is replaced by the words "organ or tissue removal."

e) Paragraph 4 is worded as follows:

"(4) The physician shall record the course, content, and outcome of the involvement of the next of kin and the persons referred to in paragraph 2, sentence 5, and paragraph 3. The next of kin and the persons referred to in paragraph 2, sentence 5, and paragraph 3 have the right to inspect the records."

10. The following § 4a is inserted after § 4:

"Section 4a

Removal from

dead embryos and fetuses

(1) The removal of organs or tissues from a dead embryo or fetus is only permissible if

1. the death of the embryo or fetus has been determined in accordance with rules that correspond to the state of medical science,

2. the woman who was pregnant with the embryo or fetus has been informed by a physician about the possible removal of organs or tissue and has given her written consent to the removal of organs or tissue, and

3. the procedure is performed by a physician.

In the cases referred to in sentence 1 no. 3, § 3 (1) sentence 2 shall apply mutatis mutandis. The information must be provided and consent obtained only after death has been determined.

(2) The physician shall record the course, content, and result of the explanation and consent pursuant to paragraph 1, sentence 1, no. 2. The person performing the removal shall record the course and extent of the organ or tissue removal.

The woman who was pregnant with the embryo or fetus has the right to inspect the records. She may consult a person she trusts. Consent may be revoked in writing or orally.

(3) In the cases referred to in paragraph 1, the woman who was pregnant with the embryo or fetus shall be considered the donor only for the purposes of documentation, traceability, and data protection.

11. Section 5 is amended as follows:

a) Paragraph 1 is amended as follows:

aa) In sentence 1, the word "organ donor" is replaced by the words "organ or tissue donor" and the words "sentence 1" are inserted after "paragraph 1".

bb) In sentence 2, the words "sentence 1" are inserted after the words "para. 1".

b) Paragraph 2 is amended as follows:

aa) In sentence 1, the words "organs of the organ donor" are replaced by the words "organs or tissues of the donor."

bb) In sentence 3, the word "immediately" is inserted after the word "examination findings."

cc) In sentence 4, the words "sentence 6" are replaced by the words "sentence 5."

c) The following paragraph 3 is added:

"(3) The determination pursuant to Section 4a (1) sentence 1 no. 1 shall be made by a physician who may not be involved in the removal or transfer of the organs or tissues of the embryo or fetus. Nor may he be subject to the instructions of a physician who is involved in these measures. The examination results and the time of their determination shall be recorded and signed by the physicians without delay in a separate document, stating the underlying examination findings. The woman who was pregnant with the embryo or fetus shall be given the opportunity to inspect the document. She may consult a person she trusts."

12. Section 6 is amended as follows:

a) The heading is worded as follows:

"Section 6

Respect for the dignity

of the organ and tissue donor."

b) In paragraph 1, the word "organ removal" is replaced by the words "organ or tissue removal from deceased persons" and the word "organ donor" is replaced by the words "organ or tissue donor."

c) In paragraph 2, sentence 1, the word "organ donor" is replaced by the words "organ or tissue donor."

d) The following paragraph 3 is added:

"(3) Paragraphs 1 and 2 shall apply mutatis mutandis to dead embryos and fetuses."

13. Section 7 shall be worded as follows:

„§ 7

Data collection

and use; duty to provide information

(1) The collection and use of personal data of a potential organ or tissue donor, a next of kin, or a person pursuant to Section 4 (2) sentence 5 or (3) and the transmission of this data to the persons entitled to information pursuant to paragraph 3 sentence 1 is permissible insofar as this is necessary to clarify whether organ or tissue removal is permissible pursuant to Section 3 (1) and (2), § 4 (1) to (3) and § 9 (2) sentence 2, and whether there are medical reasons preventing it, as well as for informing the next of kin pursuant to § 3 (3) sentence 1.

(2) The following persons are obliged to provide immediate information on the data required under paragraph 1: 1. Physicians who treated the potential organ or tissue donor for an illness preceding death,

2. Physicians who have received information about the potential organ or tissue donor from the organ and tissue donor registry pursuant to Section 2 (4),

3. the medical care facility in which the death of the potential organ or tissue donor was determined in accordance with Section 3 (1) sentence 1 no. 2,

4. Physicians who performed the postmortem examination on the potential organ or tissue donor,

5. the authorities in whose custody or joint custody the body of the potential organ or tissue donor is or has been, and

6. the person commissioned by the coordination center (§11) or a tissue procurement organization, insofar as they have received information about the data required under paragraph 1.

The obligation to provide information without delay shall only apply after the death of the potential organ or tissue donor has been determined in accordance with § 3 (1) sentence 1 no. 2.

(3) The following persons have a right to information about the data required under paragraph 1

1. Physicians who intend to remove organs pursuant to § 3 or § 4 and who work in a hospital that is licensed to transplant such organs pursuant to § 108 of the Fifth Book of the Social Code or other legal provisions, or who cooperate with such a hospital for the purpose of removing such organs,

2. Physicians who intend to remove tissue in accordance with

§ 3 or § 4 or under whose responsibility tissue is to be removed in accordance with § 3 (1) sentence 2 and who work in a medical care facility that removes such tissue or cooperate with such a facility for the purpose of removal

643255_1_En_BookBackmatter_Figh

3. the person appointed by the coordinating body.

The information shall be obtained for all organs or tissues intended for removal. It may only be obtained after the death of the potential organ or tissue donor has been determined in accordance with Section 3 (1) sentence 1 no. 2.

14. The heading of Section 3 shall be worded as follows:

"Section 3

Removal of organs

and tissues from living donors."

15. Section 8 is amended as follows:

a) The heading shall read as follows:

"Section 8

Removal of

organs and tissues."

b) Paragraph 1 is amended as follows:

aa) Sentence 1 is amended as follows:

aaa) In the part of the sentence before number 1, the words "from a living person" are replaced by the words "or tissues for the purpose of transfer to others is from a living person, unless otherwise specified in § 8a."

bbb) In number 1 letter b, the words "and 2" are inserted after the words "sentence 1".

ccc) In number 2, the words "or tissue" are inserted after the word "organ."

ddd) In number 3, the words "in the case of organ removal" are inserted before the word "one."

bb) In sentence 2, the words "of organs that cannot regenerate" shall be replaced by the words "of a kidney, part of a liver, or other non-regenerative organs" and the word "registered" shall be inserted before the word "partner."

c) Paragraph 2 is amended as follows:

aa) Sentence 1 is replaced by the following sentences: "The donor must be informed by a physician in an understandable manner about

1. the purpose and nature of the procedure,

2. the examinations and the right to be informed of the results of the examinations,

3. the measures taken to protect the donor, as well as the extent and possible, including indirect, consequences and long-term effects of the intended organ or tissue removal on his or her health,

4. medical confidentiality,

5. the expected chances of success of the organ or tissue transplant and other circumstances that the donor recognises as being of significance for the donation, and

6. the collection and use of personal data.

The donor must be informed that his or her consent is a prerequisite for organ or tissue removal."

bb) In the new sentence 4, the word "organ donor" is replaced by the word "donor."

cc) The following sentence is added:

"Sentence 3 shall not apply in the case of the intended removal of bone marrow."

d) Paragraph 3 is amended as follows:

aa) Sentence 1 is worded as follows:

"In the case of a living person, organs may only be removed after the donor and the recipient have agreed to the removal, and tissue may only be removed after the donor has agreed to participate in medically recommended follow-up care."

bb) In sentence 2, the words "for the removal of organs from a living person" are inserted after the word "requirement."

16. The following Sections 8a to 8c are inserted after Section 8:

"Section 8a

Removal of

bone marrow from minors

The removal of bone marrow from a minor for the purpose of transplantation is permissible, notwithstanding Section 8(1) sentence 1 no. 1 letters a and b and no. 2, subject to the following condition:

1. The bone marrow is intended for use by first-degree relatives or siblings of the minor.

2. According to medical assessment, the transfer of the bone marrow to the intended recipient is suitable for curing a life-threatening disease in that recipient.

3. A suitable donor in accordance with Section 8 (1) sentence 1 no. 1 is not available at the time of bone marrow extraction.

4. The legal representative has been informed in accordance with Section 8 (2) and has consented to the removal and use of the bone marrow. Section 1627 of the Civil Code shall apply. The minor must be informed by a physician in accordance with Section 8 (2), insofar as this is possible in view of their age and mental maturity. If the minor refuses the intended collection or use, or

expresses this in any other way, this must be taken into account.

5. If the minor is capable of understanding the nature, significance, and implications of the removal and of expressing their will accordingly, their consent is also required.

If the bone marrow of the minor is to be used for first-degree relatives, the legal representative must notify the family court immediately in order to obtain a decision in accordance with Section 1629 (2) sentence 3 in conjunction with Section 1796 of the Civil Code.

§ 8b

Removal of organs and tissues in special cases

(1) If organs or tissues have been removed from a living person as part of medical treatment of that person, their transfer is only permissible if the person is capable of giving consent and has been informed in accordance with Section 8 (2) sentences 1 and 2 and has consented to the transfer of the organs or tissues. Section 8 (2) sentence 4 shall apply mutatis mutandis to the recording of the information and consent.

(2) Paragraph 1 shall apply mutatis mutandis to the procurement of human sperm cells intended for medically assisted fertilization.

(3) Section 8 (2) sentence 6 shall apply mutatis mutandis to the revocation of consent.

Section 8c

Removal of organs and tissues for re-transfer

(1) The removal of organs or tissues for the purpose of reimplantation is only permissible in the case of a living person if

1. the person

    a) is capable of giving consent,

    b) has been informed in accordance with Section 8 (2) sentences 1 and 2 and has consented to the removal and reimplantation of the organ or tissue,

2. the removal and reimplantation of the organ or tissue are carried out as part of medical treatment and are necessary for this treatment according to the generally accepted state of medical science, and

3. the removal and reimplantation are carried out by a physician.

(2) Notwithstanding paragraph 1, no. 1, the removal of organs or tissues for the purpose of reimplantation in a person who is unable to understand the nature, significance, and implications of the intended removal and to express their will accordingly is only permissible if the legal representative or an authorized representative

has been informed in accordance with Section 8 (2) sentences 1 and 2 and has consented to the removal and reimplantation of the organ or tissue. Sections 1627, 1901 (2) and (3) and Section 1904 of the Civil Code shall apply.

(3) The removal of organs or tissues for the purpose of reimplantation in a living embryo or fetus is only permissible under the conditions of paragraph 1, nos. 2 and 3, if the woman who is pregnant with the embryo or fetus has been informed in accordance with § 8 (2) sentences 1 and 2 and has consented to the removal and reimplantation of the organ or tissue. If this woman is not in a position to understand the nature, significance, and implications of the planned removal and to express her will accordingly, paragraph 2 shall apply mutatis mutandis.

(4) Section 8 (2) sentence 4 shall apply mutatis mutandis to the recording of the information and consent.

(5) Section 8 (2) sentence 6 shall apply mutatis mutandis to the revocation of consent."

17. The following Section 3a shall be inserted before Section 4:

"Section 3a

Tissue establishments,
testing laboratories, registries

Section 8d

Special obligations of tissue establishments

(1) Notwithstanding the provisions of pharmaceutical law, a tissue establishment that procures or tests tissue may only operate if it has appointed a physician who possesses the necessary expertise in accordance with the state of medical science. The tissue establishment is obliged to

1. comply with the requirements for the procurement of tissues in accordance with the state of medical science and technology, in particular with regard to donor identification, the procurement procedure, and donor documentation,

2. ensure that tissue is only collected from donors who have been medically assessed in accordance with the state of the art in medical science and technology and found to be medically suitable for donation,

3. ensure that the laboratory tests required for tissue donors in accordance with the state of medical science and technology are carried out in a testing laboratory in accordance with Section 8e,

4. ensure that tissues are only released for preparation, processing, preservation, or storage if the medical assessment pursuant to number 2 and the laboratory tests pursuant to

Number 3 have determined that the tissue is suitable for these purposes,

5. to ensure that the necessary medical care is provided to living donors before and after tissue removal, and

6. ensure quality assurance for the measures referred to in numbers 2 to 5.

Further details are regulated by a statutory order pursuant to Section 16a.

(2) Notwithstanding medical documentation requirements, a tissue establishment shall document every tissue collection and donation and the associated measures, as well as information on products and materials that come into contact with the collected or donated tissues, for the purposes regulated in this Act, for traceability purposes, for the purposes of medical care for the donor, and for the purposes of risk assessment and monitoring in accordance with the provisions of the German Medicines Act or other legal provisions in accordance with a statutory order pursuant to Section 16a.

(3) Each tissue establishment shall keep records of its activities, including details of the type and quantity of tissue collected, examined, processed, treated, preserved, stored, distributed, or otherwise used, imported, and exported, as well as the origin and destination of the tissue, and shall make a description of its activities publicly available. It shall submit an annual report to the competent federal authority containing information on the type and quantity of tissue collected, processed, preserved, stored, distributed or otherwise used, imported and exported. The report shall be submitted on a form issued by the federal authority and published in the Federal Gazette. The form may also be made available and used electronically. The report shall be submitted after the end of the calendar year, by March 1 of the following year at the latest. The competent federal authority shall compile the information submitted by the tissue establishments in an anonymized form in a comprehensive report and make it publicly available. If a tissue establishment's report is incomplete or is not available by the deadline specified in sentence 5, the competent federal authority shall inform the authority responsible for monitoring. Tissue establishments shall send the competent authority a list of the medical care facilities to which they supply tissue at least every two years or upon request.

§8e

Testing laboratories

The laboratory tests prescribed for tissue donors in accordance with Section 8d (1) sentence 2 no. 3 may only be carried out by a testing laboratory for which a license has been granted in accordance with the provisions of the German Medicines Act. The testing laboratory is obliged to ensure quality assurance for the laboratory tests prescribed in § 8d (1) sentence 2 no. 3.

§8f

Register of tissue establishments

(1) The German Institute for Medical Documentation and Information shall maintain a publicly accessible register of tissue establishments operating within the scope of this Act and shall ensure its ongoing operation. The register contains information on the tissue establishments and their accessibility, as well as on the activities for which the manufacturing license, the license for processing, preservation, storage, or marketing, or the import license has been granted in accordance with the provisions of the German Medicines Act. The competent authorities of the federal states shall transmit the information referred to in sentence 2 to the German Institute for Medical Documentation and Information. The German Institute for Medical Documentation and Information may charge fees for the use of the register. The fee schedule requires the approval of the Federal Ministry of Health in consultation with the Federal Ministry of Finance. The competent authorities of the federal states and the European Commission are exempt from paying fees.

(2) The Federal Ministry of Health may, by statutory order with the consent of the Bundesrat, specify in detail the information to be included in the register pursuant to paragraph 1, sentence 2, and regulate the details of its transmission by the competent authorities of the federal states and the use of the register. The statutory order may also provide for the transmission of information to institutions and authorities within and outside the scope of this Act."

18. The heading of Section 4 shall be worded as follows:

"Section 4

Mediation and transfer of certain organs, transplant centers, cooperation in the removal of organs and tissues."

19. Section 9 is amended as follows:

a) The heading shall be worded as follows:

"Section 9

Admissibility of

organ transplantation, priority of organ donation."

b) The previous wording becomes paragraph 1 and sentence 2 is worded as follows:

"The transfer of organs subject to mandatory allocation is only permissible if the organs have been allocated by the allocation agency in accordance with the provisions of § 12."

c) The following paragraph 2 is added:

"(2) The possible removal and transfer of an organ subject to mandatory allocation takes precedence over the removal of tissue; it must not be impaired by tissue removal. The removal of tissues from a potential donor of organs subject to allocation pursuant to Section 11 (4) sentence 2 is only permissible if a person commissioned by the coordination center has documented that the removal or transfer of organs subject to allocation is not possible or is not impaired by the tissue removal."

20. Section 10 is amended as follows:

a) In paragraph 1, sentence 1, the reference to "Section 9, sentence 1" is replaced by the reference to "Section 9 (1), sentence 1."

b) Paragraph 2 is amended as follows:

aa) In number 1, the word "transplantation" is replaced by the word "organ transfer."

bb) In number 4, the word "immediately" is inserted after the word "organ transfer."

c) Paragraph 3 is repealed.

21. Section 11 is amended as follows:

a) In the heading, the word "organ removal" is replaced by the words "removal of organs and tissues."

b) In paragraph 3, sentence 1, the words "and social security" are deleted.

c) Paragraph 4 is amended as follows:

aa) In sentence 1, the words "for the removal of organs subject to mediation and for the removal of tissues from potential donors of organs subject to mediation" are inserted after the word "coordination center."

bb) The following sentence is inserted after sentence 2:

"If these patients are also eligible as tissue donors, this must be communicated at the same time."

cc) In the new sentence 4, the word "organ removal" is replaced by the words "organ or tissue removal."

dd) In the new sentence 5, the words "or tissue removal" are inserted after the words "organ removal and allocation."

d) Paragraph 6 is repealed.

22. Section 12 is amended as follows:

a) In paragraph 4, sentence 2, no. 1, the words "processing and use" are replaced by the word "use."

b) In paragraph 5, sentence 1, the words "and social security" are deleted.

c) Paragraph 6 is repealed.

23. The heading of Section 5 is worded as follows:

"Section 5

Notifications, documentation, traceability, data protection, deadlines."

24. Section 13 is amended as follows:

a) The heading is amended to read as follows:

"Section 13

Notifications, accompanying documents of bodies subject to mediation."

b) In paragraph 2, the words "process and use" are replaced by the word "use."

25. The following Sections 13a to 13c are inserted after Section 13:

"§ 13a

Documentation of transferred tissue by medical care facilities

Medical care facilities must ensure that, for the purposes of traceability or risk assessment in accordance with the provisions of the German Medicines Act or other legal provisions, every tissue transferred is documented by the attending physician or under his or her responsibility in accordance with a statutory order pursuant to Section 16a.

Section 13b

Reporting of serious incidents and serious adverse reactions involving tissues

Healthcare facilities must

1. any serious incident that can be attributed to the procurement, testing, preparation, treatment or processing, preservation, storage or distribution, including transport, of the tissues used, and

2. any serious adverse reaction observed during or after the transfer of the tissues and which may be related to the quality and safety of the tissues,

immediately after their discovery and report them to the tissue establishment from which they received the tissue immediately in accordance with sentence 2. In doing so, they shall provide all information necessary for traceability and for quality and safety control in accordance with a statutory order pursuant to § 16a.

Section 13c

Traceability procedure for tissues

(1) Each tissue establishment shall establish a procedure for immediately identifying any tissue that may be affected by a serious incident or serious adverse reaction, excluding it from distribution, and notifying the establishments to which it has been supplied.

(2) The state health insurance funds shall be informed of any changes in medical care.

(2) If a tissue establishment or a medical care facility has reasonable grounds to suspect that tissue may cause a serious disease, it shall immediately investigate the cause and trace the tissue from the donor to the recipient or vice versa. It shall also identify, examine, and block any previous tissue donations from the donor if the suspicion is confirmed."

26. Section 14 is amended as follows:

a) Paragraph 1 is amended as follows:

aa) Sentence 1 shall be worded as follows:

"If the coordinating body, the intermediary body, or the tissue establishment is a non-public body within the scope of this Act, Section 38 of the Federal Data Protection Act shall apply with the proviso that the supervisory authority shall also monitor compliance with the provisions on data protection insofar as their scope of application is broader than that provided for in Section 38 (1) sentence 1 of the Federal Data Protection Act."

bb) In sentence 2, the words "processing and use" are replaced by the word "use" and the word "organ donor register" is replaced by the words "organ and tissue donor register."

b) Paragraph 2 is amended as follows:

aa) In sentence 1, the words "organ removal, allocation, or transfer" are replaced by the words "organ or tissue removal, organ allocation or transfer, or tissue donation or transfer" and the words "organ donor and organ recipient" are replaced by the words "donor and recipient."

bb) In sentence 2, the words "or § 4a" are inserted after the reference to "§ 4" and the word "organ removal" is replaced by the words "organ or tissue removal."

cc) In sentence 3, the words "processed or used" shall be replaced by the word "used."

dd) In sentence 4, the words "processed and used" are replaced by the word "used."

ee) The following sentence is added:

"The bodies referred to in paragraph 1, sentence 1, shall take technical and organizational measures to ensure that the data is protected against unauthorized addition, deletion, or alteration and that no unauthorized disclosure takes place."

c) The following paragraph 3 is added:

"(3) In the case of sperm donation, these provisions shall not affect the right of the child

of the recipient. In the case of bone marrow donation, notwithstanding paragraph 2, the identity of the tissue donor and the tissue recipient may be disclosed to each other or to their respective relatives if the tissue donor and the tissue recipient or their legal representatives have expressly consented to this.

27. § 15 is worded as follows:

"Section 15

Retention and deletion periods

(1) The records of participation pursuant to Section 4 (4), of the explanation pursuant to Section 4a (2), for the determination of the test results pursuant to Section 5 (2) sentence 3 and (3) sentence 3, for the explanation pursuant to Section 8 (2) sentence 4, also in conjunction with Section 8a sentence 1 no. 4, § 8b (1) and (2), § 8c (1) No. 1 letter b and (2) and (3), and for expert opinions pursuant to § 8 (3) sentence 2, as well as documentation of organ removal, allocation, and transplantation, shall be retained for at least ten years. The personal data contained in these records and documentation shall be deleted at the latest by the end of a further year. Sentence 2 shall not apply if the data referred to therein are stored together with the information referred to in paragraph 2; these data shall be deleted or anonymized at the latest after 30 years.

(2) Notwithstanding paragraph 1, for the purposes of traceability, the information to be documented in accordance with Section 8d (2) must be retained for at least 30 years after the expiry date of the tissue and the data to be documented in accordance with Section 13a must be retained for at least 30 years after the transfer of the tissue and must be available immediately. After the retention period has expired, the information must be deleted or anonymized."

28. The following heading is inserted before Section 16:

"Section 5a

Guidelines on the state of medical science, regulatory authority."

29. Section 16 is amended as follows:

a1) The heading is worded as follows:

"Section 16

Guidelines on the state of medical science with regard to organs."

a) Paragraph 1, sentence 1 is amended as follows:

aa) In number 1, the words "sentence 1" are inserted after the words "Section 3 (1)".

bb) The following number 1a is inserted after number 1:

"1a. the rules for determining death pursuant to § 4a (1) sentence 1 no. 1,".

b) In paragraph 2, the words " , 1a" are inserted after the words "No. 1".

30. The following § 16a is inserted after § 16:

"Section 16a

Regulatory authority

The Federal Ministry of Health may, by statutory order with the consent of the Bundesrat and after consulting the German Medical Association and other experts, regulate the requirements for the quality and safety of tissue procurement and transplantation, insofar as this is necessary to avert dangers to human health or to prevent risks. The statutory order may, in particular, specify the details of the requirements for

1. the removal and transfer of tissues, including their documentation and the protection of the documented data,

2. the medical assessment of medical suitability as a tissue donor,

3. the examination of tissue donors,

4. the reporting of quality and safety deficiencies and serious adverse reactions by medical care facilities, and

5. the provision of information to and obtaining of the consent of tissue donors or the consent to tissue procurement

are regulated. The Federal Ministry of Health may transfer the authorization pursuant to sentence 1 to the competent higher federal authority by statutory order without the consent of the Bundesrat."

30a. The following Section 16b is inserted after Section 16a:

"Section 16b

Guidelines on the state of medical science regarding the removal of tissue and its transfer

(1) In addition to the provisions of the statutory order pursuant to Section 16a, the German Medical Association may, in agreement with the competent higher federal authority, establish guidelines on the generally accepted state of medical science regarding the removal of tissues and their transfer, in particular with regard to the requirements for

1. the medical assessment of medical suitability as a tissue donor,

2. the examination of tissue donors, and

3. the removal, transfer, and use of human tissue.

When developing the guidelines, the appropriate participation of experts from the relevant professional and trade circles, including the competent federal and state authorities, shall be ensured. The guidelines shall be published by the competent federal authority in the Federal Gazette.

(2) Compliance with the state of the art in medical science is presumed

if the guidelines of the German Medical Association pursuant to paragraph 1 have been observed."

31. The heading of Section 6 shall be worded as follows:

"Section 6

Prohibitions."

32. Section 17 is amended as follows:

a) In the heading, the word "organ trade" is replaced by the words "organ and tissue trade."

b) Paragraph 1 is amended as follows:

aa) In sentence 1, the words "or tissues" are inserted after the word "organs" and the words "of another" are inserted after the word "medical treatment."

bb) Sentence 2 is amended as follows:

aaa) In number 1, the words "or tissue" are inserted after the word "organs."

bbb) Number 2 is worded as follows:

"2. Medicinal products manufactured from or using organs or tissues and subject to the provisions on authorization pursuant to Section 21 of the Medicinal Products Act, also in conjunction with Section 37 of the Medicinal Products Act, or registration pursuant to Section 38 or Section 39a of the German Medicinal Products Act, or are exempt from authorization by statutory order pursuant to Section 36 of the German Medicinal Products Act or from registration pursuant to Section 39 (3) of the German Medicinal Products Act, or active substances within the meaning of Section 4 (19) of the German Medicinal Products Act that are manufactured from or using cells."

c) In paragraph 2, the words "or tissue" are inserted after the word "organs."

33. The heading of Section 7 shall be worded as follows:

"Section 7

Penal and administrative fine provisions."

34. Section 18 is amended as follows:

a) In the heading, the word "organ trade" is replaced by the words "organ and tissue trade."

b) In paragraph 1, the words "or tissue" are inserted after the word "organ."

c) In paragraph 4, the words "organ donors" are replaced by the words "organ or tissue donors," the word "organs" is replaced by the words "organs or tissues," and the word "organ recipients" is replaced by the words "organ or tissue recipients."

35. Section 19 is amended as follows:

a) Paragraphs 1 to 3 are worded as follows:

"(1) Anyone who

1. contrary to Section 8 (1) sentence 1 no. 1 letter a or letter b or no. 4 or Section 8c (1) no. 1 or no. 3, (2) sentence 1, also in conjunction with (3) sentence 2, or Section 8c (3) sentence 1, removes an organ or tissue,

2. removes an organ contrary to § 8 (1) sentence 2, or

3. contrary to § 8b (1) sentence 1, also in conjunction with (2), uses an organ or tissue for transfer to another person or obtains human sperm cells,

shall be punished with imprisonment of up to five years or a fine.

(2) Anyone who, contrary to § 3 (1) sentence 1 or (2), § 4 (1) sentence 2 or § 4a (1) sentence 1, removes an organ or tissue shall be punished with imprisonment of up to three years or a fine.

(3) Anyone who

1. provides or passes on information contrary to § 2 (4) sentence 1 or sentence 3,

2. uses information contrary to § 13 (2), or

3. discloses or uses personal data contrary to § 14 (2) sentence 1, also in conjunction with sentence 2, or sentence 3,

shall be punished with imprisonment of up to one year or a fine."

b) In paragraph 5, the reference to "paragraph 1" is replaced by a reference to "paragraph 2."

36. Section 20 shall be worded as follows:

"Section 20

Provisions on fines

(1) Anyone who intentionally or negligently

1. contrary to Section 5 (2) sentence 3 or (3) sentence 3, fails to make a record, or makes an incorrect, incomplete, or untimely record,

2. contrary to § 8d (1) sentence 2 no. 3 in conjunction with a statutory order pursuant to § 16a sentence 2 no. 3, fails to ensure that a laboratory test is carried out,

3. contrary to Section 8d (2) in conjunction with a statutory order pursuant to Section 16a sentence 2 no. 1, fails to document a tissue sample, a tissue donation, an associated measure or a statement specified therein, or does so incorrectly, incompletely or untimely,

4. contrary to Section 9 (1), transfers an organ,

5. contrary to Section 10 (2) No. 4, fails to document the organ transfer, or does so incorrectly, incompletely, or untimely,

6. contrary to Section 13a in conjunction with a statutory order pursuant to Section 16a sentence 2 no. 1, fails to ensure that a transferred tissue is documented,

7. contrary to § 13b sentence 1 in conjunction with a statutory order pursuant to § 16a sentence 2 no. 4, fails to document a quality or safety defect or a serious adverse reaction, or documents it incorrectly, incompletely, or late, or fails to report it, or reports it incorrectly, incompletely, or late,

8. contravenes a statutory order pursuant to Section 16a sentence 1 or an enforceable order based on such a statutory order, insofar as the statutory order refers to this provision on fines for a specific offense.

(2) The administrative offense may be punished with a fine of up to thirty thousand euros."

37. The heading of Section 8 shall be worded as follows:

"Section 8

Final provisions."

38. Sections 21 to 23 shall be worded as follows:

"Section 21

Competent federal authority

The competent federal authority within the meaning of this Act is the Paul Ehrlich Institute.

Section 22

Relationship to
other areas of law

The provisions of the Embryo Protection Act and the Stem Cell Act remain unaffected.

§23

German Armed Forces

Within the remit of the Federal Ministry of Defense, the competent authorities and experts of the German Armed Forces are responsible for monitoring the implementation of this Act.

Article 2
Amendment
to the Medicinal Products Act

The Medicinal Products Act, as published on December 12, 2005 (Federal Law Gazette I, p. 3394), last amended by Article 2 of the Act of June 14, 2007 (Federal Law Gazette I, p. 1066), is amended as follows:

1. The table of contents is amended as follows:

a) The following information is inserted after the information on Section 20a:

"Section 20b Permit for the procurement of tissue and laboratory testing

Section 20c Permit for the processing, preservation, storage, or marketing of tissue or tissue preparations."

b) The following information is inserted after the information on § 21:

"Section 21a Approval of tissue preparations."

c) The following information is inserted after the information on Section 63b:

"Section 63c Special documentation and reporting requirements for blood and tissue preparations."

d) The following information is inserted after the information on Section 72a:

"§ 72b Import license and certificates for tissues and certain tissue preparations."

e) The following information is added:

"Fourteenth subsection

§ 142 Transitional provisions arising from the Tissue Act."

2. Section 2 (3) No. 8 is worded as follows:

"8. Organs within the meaning of Section 1a No. 1 of the Transplantation Act, if they are intended for transfer to human recipients."

3. Section 4 is amended as follows:

a) In paragraph 20, the words "biotechnology" are inserted after the word "procedures."

b) The following paragraph 30 is added:

"(30) Tissue preparations are medicinal products that are tissues within the meaning of Section 1a No. 4 of the Transplantation Act or have been produced from such tissues. Human sperm and egg cells, including impregnated egg cells (germ cells), and embryos are neither medicinal products nor tissue preparations."

4. Section 4a is amended as follows:

a) Sentence 1 is amended as follows:

aa) No. 2 is worded as follows:

"2. the procurement and marketing of germ cells for artificial insemination in animals,".

bb) Number 4 is worded as follows:

"4. tissue removed from a person during a treatment procedure for the purpose of being transferred back to that person."

b) Sentence 3 is deleted.

5. The following sentences are added to Section 10(8):
"In the case of tissue preparations, at least the information specified in paragraph 1, sentence 1, nos. 1 and 2, without specifying the strength, dosage form, and group of persons, Nos. 3, 4, 6, and 9, as well as the indication "Biological hazard" in the case of confirmed infectivity. In the case of autologous tissue preparations, the indication "For autologous use only" must also be provided, and in the case of autologous and directed tissue preparations, additional information on the recipient must also be provided."

6. Section 13 is amended as follows:

a) The following sentence is added to paragraph 1:
"Sentence 1 does not apply to tissue within the meaning of Section 1a No. 4 of the Transplantation Act or to tissue preparations for which a permit is granted in accordance with Section 20c."

b) In paragraph 4, sentence 2, a comma and the word "tissue preparations" are inserted after the word "blood preparations."

7. Section 14 is amended as follows:

a) Paragraph 1 is amended as follows:

aa) No. 5c is worded as follows:

"5c. contrary to Section 4, sentence 1, No. 2 of the Transfusion Act, no senior medical officer has been appointed or this person does not have the necessary expertise according to the state of medical science, or contrary to Section 4, sentence 1, No. 3 of the Transfusion Act, no medical officer is present when the donation is taken from a human being."

bb) In number 6a, the words "and, in the case of the collection of blood and blood components, additionally in accordance with the provisions of the second section of the Transfusion Act" are inserted after the word "technology."

b) In paragraph 2b, the word "transplants" is replaced by the word "tissue preparations."

c) Paragraph 4 is amended as follows:

aa) Number 4 is worded as follows:

"4. the collection or testing, including laboratory testing of donor samples, of substances of human origin intended for the manufacture of medicinal products, with the exception of tissue, in other establishments or facilities,".

bb) The clause after number 4 is worded as follows:

"which do not require a separate permit, provided that suitable premises and facilities are available for this purpose and that it is ensured that the manufacture and testing are carried out in accordance with the state of the art and that the head of manufacturing and the head of quality control are able to fulfill their responsibilities."

8. Section 15 is amended as follows:

a) In paragraph 3, sentence 3, no. 2, the comma after the word "fresh plasma" is deleted and the words "as well as for active substances and blood components for the manufacture of blood preparations" are inserted.

b) Paragraph 3a is amended as follows:

aa) In sentence 1, the word "transplants" is replaced by the word "tissue preparations."

bb) In sentence 2, the word "may" is replaced by the word "must" and the words "for transplants, at least three years of experience in the field of tissue transplantation" are replaced by the words "for tissue preparations, at least two years of experience in the field of manufacturing and testing such medicinal products in establishments or facilities that require a manufacturing authorization under this Act or hold a license under Community law."

9. In Section 16, the words "or the other" shall be inserted after the word "appointed."

10. (deleted)

11. (deleted)

11a. The following Section 20b is inserted after Section 20a:

"Section 20b
Permission for the extraction
of tissue and laboratory testing

(1) An institution that wishes to harvest tissue intended for use in humans within the meaning of Section 1a No. 4 of the Transplantation Act (harvesting institution) or to carry out the laboratory tests necessary for harvesting requires a permit from the competent authority. Procurement within the meaning of sentence 1 is the direct or extracorporeal removal of tissue, including all measures intended to preserve the tissue in a condition suitable for processing or treatment, to clearly identify it, and to transport it. The permit may only be refused if

1. there is no suitably trained person with the necessary professional experience who, in the case of a collection facility, can also be the medical professional within the meaning of Section 8d (1) sentence 1 of the Transplantation Act,

2. other participating personnel are not sufficiently qualified,

3. there are no suitable rooms for the respective tissue procurement or for laboratory tests, or

4. it cannot be guaranteed that the tissue procurement or laboratory tests will be carried out in accordance with the state of the art in medical science and technology and in accordance with the provisions of Sections 2, 3, and 3a of the Transplantation Act.

The competent authority may refrain from conducting an inspection within the meaning of Section 64 (3) sentence 2 before granting permission in accordance with this provision. The competent authority shall grant permission to the procurement facility for a specific establishment and for specific tissue, and to the laboratory for a specific establishment and for specific activities. In doing so, the competent authority may involve the competent higher federal authority.

(2) A separate permit pursuant to paragraph 1 is not required for anyone who carries out these activities on a contractual basis under contract with a processor or processor who holds a permit pursuant to § 13 or § 20c for the processing of tissue or tissue preparations. In this case, the manufacturer or processor shall notify the extraction facility or laboratory to the locally competent authority and attach the information and documents referred to in paragraph 1, sentence 3, to the notification. One month after the notification pursuant to sentence 2, the manufacturer or processor shall notify the competent authority of the procurement facility or laboratory, unless the competent authority for the procurement facility or laboratory has objected. In exceptional cases, the period specified in sentence 3 shall be extended by a further two months. The manufacturer or processor shall be notified of this before the expiry of the deadline, stating the reasons. If the competent authority has objected, the time limits in sentences 3 and 4 shall be suspended until the reason for the objection has been removed. Paragraph 1, sentences 3 to 6 shall apply mutatis mutandis, with the proviso that the permit pursuant to paragraph 1, sentence 5 shall be granted to the manufacturer or processor.

(3) The permit shall be withdrawn if it subsequently becomes known that one of the grounds for refusal under paragraph 1, sentence 3, existed at the time of issuance. If one of these grounds for refusal subsequently arises, the permit shall be revoked; instead of revocation, the permit may also be suspended. The competent authority may temporarily prohibit the procurement of tissue or laboratory testing if the procurement facility, laboratory, manufacturer, or processor fails to provide the evidence required for tissue procurement or laboratory testing."

11b. The following Section 20c is inserted after Section 20b:

"Section 20c
Permit for the processing, preservation, storage, or marketing of tissues or tissue preparations

(1) Notwithstanding Section 13(1), an establishment that wishes to process, preserve, store, or place on the market tissues or tissue preparations that are not processed using industrial methods and whose essential processing methods are sufficiently well known in the European Union requires a license from the competent authority in accordance with the following provisions. This also applies to tissues or tissue preparations whose processing methods are new but comparable to a known method. The decision on whether to grant the authorization shall be taken by the competent authority of the state in which the establishment is or is to be located, in consultation with the competent federal authority.

(2) The permit may only be refused if 1. there is no person with the necessary expertise and experience in accordance with paragraph 3 (responsible person in accordance with § 20c) who is responsible for ensuring that the tissue preparations and tissues are processed, preserved, stored, or placed on the market in accordance with the applicable legal provisions,

2. other personnel involved are not sufficiently qualified,

3. suitable premises and facilities for the intended activities are not available,

4. there is no guarantee that the processing, including labeling, preservation, and storage, as well as testing, is carried out in accordance with the state of the art in science and technology, or

5. a quality management system based on the principles of good professional practice has not been established or is not kept up to date.

(3) Proof of the necessary expertise of the responsible person pursuant to § 20c shall be provided by a certificate of an examination taken after completion of a university degree in human medicine, biology, biochemistry, or a degree recognized as equivalent, as well as at least two years of practical experience in the field of processing or treatment of tissues or tissue preparations.

(4) If there are objections to the documents submitted, the applicant shall be given the opportunity to remedy the deficiencies within a reasonable period of time. If the deficiencies are not remedied, the permit shall be refused. The permit shall be granted for a specific establishment and for specific tissues or tissue preparations.

(5) The competent authority shall take a decision on the application for a permit within a period of three months. If a permit holder applies for a change to the permit, the authority shall take a decision within a period of one month. In exceptional cases, the period shall be extended by a further two months. The applicant shall be notified of this before the expiry of the period, stating the reasons. If the authority gives the applicant the opportunity to remedy deficiencies in accordance with paragraph 4, sentence 1, the time limits shall be suspended until the deficiencies have been remedied or until the expiry of the time limit set in accordance with paragraph 4, sentence 1. The suspension shall commence on the day on which the request to remedy the deficiencies is delivered to the applicant.

(6) The holder of the permit shall notify the competent authority in advance of any change to the information specified in paragraph 2, submitting supporting evidence, and may only make the change once the competent authority has issued written permission. In the event of an unforeseen change of the responsible person pursuant to Section 20c, the notification must be made immediately.

(7) The permit shall be withdrawn if it subsequently becomes known that one of the grounds for refusal under paragraph 2 existed at the time of issuance. If one of these grounds for refusal subsequently arises, the permit shall be revoked; instead of revocation, the permit may also be suspended. Paragraph 1, sentence 3 shall apply mutatis mutandis. The competent authority may provisionally order the suspension of the processing of tissues or tissue preparations if the processor fails to provide the evidence required for processing. If the processing of tissues or tissue preparations is suspended, the processor shall ensure that tissue preparations and tissues still in storage continue to be stored in a manner that ensures quality and are transferred to other manufacturers, processors, or distributors with a permit in accordance with paragraph 1 or Section 13 (1). This also applies to the data and information on processing or treatment required for the traceability of these tissue preparations and tissues."

12. The following number 1d is inserted after Section 21 (2) No. 1c:

"1d. Tissue preparations that are subject to the approval requirement under the provisions of § 21a (1),".

12a. The following Section 21a is inserted after Section 21:

"Section 21a

Approval of tissue preparations

(1) Tissue preparations that are not processed or treated using industrial methods and whose essential processing or treatment methods are sufficiently well known in the European Union and whose effects and side effects are evident from scientific knowledge may only be placed on the market within the scope of this Act if, by way of derogation from the authorization requirement under Section 21(1), they have been approved by the competent federal authority. This also applies to tissue preparations whose processing methods are new but comparable to a known method. Sentence 1 applies accordingly to blood stem cell preparations intended for autologous or directed use for a specific person. The approval covers the procedures for collection, processing, and testing, donor selection, and documentation for each step of the process, as well as the quantitative and qualitative criteria for tissue preparations. In particular, critical processing procedures must be evaluated to ensure that the procedures do not render the tissues clinically ineffective or harmful to patients.

(2) The applicant shall enclose the following information and documents with the application for approval:

1. the name or company name and address of the processor,

2. the name of the tissue preparation,

3. the areas of application and the type of application and, in the case of tissue preparations that are only to be used for a limited period of time, the duration of use,

4. information on the processing of the tissue preparation and on the procurement, donor testing, preservation, and storage of the tissue preparation,

5. the method of preservation, the shelf life, and the method of storage,

6. a description of the functionality and risks of the tissue preparation,

7. documentation on the results of microbiological, chemical, and physical tests and the methods used to determine them, insofar as this documentation is necessary, and

8. all information and documentation relevant to the evaluation of the medicinal product.

(3) For the information referred to in paragraph 2, No. 3, scientific evidence may be submitted, which may also consist of medical experience data prepared using scientific methods. Studies by the manufacturer of the tissue preparation, data from publications, or subsequent evaluations of the clinical results of the manufactured tissue preparations may be considered for this purpose.

(4) The competent federal authority shall decide on the application for approval within a period of five months. If the applicant is given the opportunity to remedy deficiencies, the time limits shall be suspended until the deficiencies have been remedied or until the expiry of the time limit set for remedying them. The suspension shall commence on the day on which the request to remedy the deficiencies is served on the applicant.

(5) The competent authority may attach conditions to the approval. Section 28 shall apply mutatis mutandis.

(6) The competent authority may only refuse the approval if

1. the documents submitted are incomplete,

2. the tissue preparation does not correspond to the state of scientific knowledge, or

3. the tissue preparation does not fulfill its intended function or the risk-benefit ratio is unfavorable.

(7) The applicant or, after approval, the holder of the approval shall immediately notify the competent federal authority, enclosing the relevant documents, if there are changes in the information provided in the application.

and documents pursuant to paragraphs 2 and 3. In the event of a change in the documents pursuant to paragraph 3, the change may only be implemented once the competent federal authority has given its approval.

(8) The approval shall be withdrawn if it subsequently becomes known that one of the grounds for refusal under paragraph 6 nos. 2 and 3 existed. It shall be revoked if one of these grounds for refusal subsequently arises. In both cases, the suspension of the approval may also be ordered for a limited period. Before a decision is made in accordance with sentences 1 to 3, the holder of the approval shall be heard, unless there is imminent danger. If the approval has been withdrawn or revoked or if the approval is suspended, the tissue preparation may not be placed on the market or brought within the scope of this Act.

(9) Notwithstanding paragraph 1, tissue preparations that may be placed on the market in a Member State of the European Union or in another State party to the Agreement on the European Economic Area require a certificate from the competent federal authority when they are first brought into the scope of this Act. Before issuing the certificate, the competent federal authority shall verify whether the processing or treatment of the tissue preparations complies with the requirements for collection and processing procedures, including donor selection procedures and laboratory tests, as well as the quantitative and qualitative criteria for tissue preparations in accordance with this Act and its regulations. The competent federal authority shall issue the certificate if the equivalence of the requirements under sentence 2 is evident from the approval certificate or another certificate issued by the competent authority of the country of origin and proof of approval in the Member State of the European Union or the other signatory state to the Agreement on the European Economic Area is provided. Any change in the requirements under sentence 2 must be notified to the competent federal authority in good time before further transfer into the scope of this Act. The certificate must be withdrawn if one of the conditions under sentence 2 has not been met; it must be revoked if one of the conditions under sentence 2 has subsequently ceased to apply."

13. (deleted)

14. In Section 25(8), sentence 1, the words "tissue preparations" shall be inserted after the words "blood preparations".

14a. Section 33 is amended as follows:

   a) In paragraph 1, the words "on the approval of tissue preparations" shall be inserted after the word "authorization."

b) In paragraph 2, sentence 2, the words "on the approval of tissue preparations" shall be inserted after the word "approval".

15. In Section 54 (1) sentence 1, the words "and for tissues" are inserted after the word "substances."

16. Section 63b is amended as follows:

a) In paragraph 1, the word "blood preparations" is replaced by the words "blood and tissue preparations, with the exception of blood preparations within the meaning of paragraph 2, sentence 3, and tissue preparations within the meaning of Section 21a."

b) In paragraph 5, sentence 7, the word "blood preparations" is replaced by the words "blood and tissue preparations, with the exception of blood preparations within the meaning of paragraph 2, sentence 3, and tissue preparations within the meaning of Section 21a."

17. The following Section 63c is inserted after

Section 63b:

"Section 63c
Special documentation
and reporting requirements for
blood and tissue preparations

(1) The holder of a license or authorization for blood preparations within the meaning of Section 63b (2) sentence 3 or for tissue preparations within the meaning of Section 21a shall keep detailed records of suspected serious adverse events or reactions that have occurred in the Member States of the European Union or in the signatory states to the Agreement on the European Economic Area or in a third country and that affect or can be attributed to the quality and safety of blood or tissue preparations, as well as on the number of recalls.

(2) The holder of a license or authorization for blood or tissue preparations within the meaning of paragraph 1 shall also document any suspected serious incident that may affect the quality or safety of the blood or tissue preparations, and any suspected serious adverse reaction that may affect the quality or safety of the blood or tissue preparations or be attributed to them, and report them to the competent federal authority without delay, at the latest within 15 days of becoming aware of them. The report must contain all the necessary information, in particular the name or company name and address of the pharmaceutical company, the name and number or identification code of the blood or tissue preparation, the date and documentation of the occurrence of the suspected serious incident or serious adverse reaction, the date and place of blood component or tissue collection, the establishments or institutions supplied, and information on the donor. The incidents or reactions reported in accordance with sentence 1 shall be investigated and evaluated in terms of their cause and effect, and the results shall be communicated immediately to the competent federal authority, as shall the measures taken to trace and protect donors and recipients.

supervisory authority without delay, as well as the measures taken to trace and protect donors and recipients.

(3) Blood and plasma donation establishments or tissue establishments shall, in the case of blood or tissue preparations not subject to authorization or approval, as well as in the case of blood and blood components and tissues, report to the competent authority without delay any suspected serious adverse event that may affect the quality or safety of the blood or tissue preparations, and any suspected serious adverse reaction that may affect or be attributed to the quality or safety of blood or tissue preparations to the competent authority without delay. The report must contain all necessary information, such as the name or company name and address of the donation or tissue establishment, the name and number or identification code of the blood or tissue preparation, the date and documentation of the occurrence of the suspected serious incident or serious adverse reaction, the date of manufacture of the blood or tissue preparation, and information about the donor. Paragraph 2, sentence 3 shall apply mutatis mutandis. The competent authority shall forward the reports referred to in sentences 1 and 2 and the notifications referred to in sentence 3 to the competent federal authority.

(4) The holder of a marketing authorization or approval for blood or tissue preparations within the meaning of paragraph 1 shall, on the basis of the obligations referred to in paragraph 1, submit an updated report on the safety of the medicinal products to the competent federal authority immediately upon request or, in the case of recalls or cases or suspected cases of serious incidents or serious adverse reactions, at least once a year.

(5) The provisions of Section 63b (5a) shall apply to blood and plasma donation establishments or tissue establishments, and the provisions of Section 63b (5b) shall apply mutatis mutandis to the holders of a license for blood or tissue preparations.

(6) A serious incident within the meaning of the above provisions is any adverse event related to the procurement, testing, preparation, treatment, processing, preservation, storage, or distribution of tissues or blood preparations that could result in the transmission of an infectious disease, death, or a life-threatening condition, disability, or loss of function in patients, or that could require or prolong hospitalization, or that could lead to or prolong illness.

(7) A serious adverse reaction within the meaning of the above provisions is an unintended reaction, including a communicable disease, in the donor or

recipient in connection with the procurement of tissue or blood or the transfer of tissue or blood preparations, which is fatal or life-threatening, results in disability or loss of capacity, or requires or prolongs hospitalization, or leads to or prolongs illness."

18. Section 64 is amended as follows:

a) Paragraph 1 is amended as follows:

aa) In sentence 2, the words "and tissue" are inserted after the words "certain substances" and a comma and the words "pursuant to Section 54" are inserted after the reference to "Section 54."

bb) The following sentence is inserted after sentence 2: "In the case of Section 20b (2), the collection facilities and laboratories are subject to monitoring by the locally competent authority."

b) In paragraph 2, sentence 3, a comma and the words "tissues and tissue preparations" shall be inserted after the word "blood preparations."

c) In paragraph 3, sentence 1, after the word "health care," a comma and the words "of Section 2 of the Transfusion Act, Sections 2, 3, and 3a of the Transplantation Act" shall be inserted.

19. In Section 65 (1), sentence 1, after the word "health care," a comma and the words "of the second section of the Transfusion Act, sections 2, 3, and 3a of the Transplantation Act" shall be inserted.

19a. The following paragraph 3 is added to Section 72:

"(3) Paragraph 1 shall not apply to tissue within the meaning of Section 1a No. 4 of the Transplantation Act and to tissue preparations within the meaning of Section 20c."

19b. The following paragraph 4 is added to Section 72a:

"(4) Paragraph 1 shall not apply to tissue within the meaning of Section 1a No. 4 of the Transplantation Act and to tissue preparations within the meaning of Section 20c."

19c. The following Section 72b is inserted after Section 72a:

"Section 72b

Import license and certificates
for tissue and certain tissue preparations

(1) Anyone who wishes to import tissue within the meaning of Section 1a No. 4 of the Transplantation Act or tissue preparations within the meaning of Section 20c on a commercial or professional basis for the purpose of supplying them to others or for processing or treatment from countries that are not Member States of the European Union or other signatory states to the Agreement on the European Economic Area into the scope of this Act requires a permit from the competent authority. Section 20c (1) sentence 3 and (2) to (7) shall apply mutatis mutandis.

(2) The importer referred to in paragraph 1 may only import the tissues or tissue preparations into the scope of this Act if

1. the authority of the country of origin has confirmed by means of a certificate that the procurement or processing and the laboratory tests have been carried out in accordance with standards that are at least equivalent to the standards of good professional practice laid down by the Community, and such certificates are mutually recognized, or

2. the authority responsible for the importer has certified that the aforementioned basic rules have been complied with during the procurement or processing and laboratory testing, after it or a competent authority of another Member State of the European Union or another contracting state to the Agreement on the European Economic Area has verified in the country of origin that the standards of good professional practice are being complied with during harvesting or processing, or

3. the competent authority responsible for the importer has certified that the import is in the public interest if a certificate in accordance with number 1 is not available and a certificate in accordance with number 2 is not possible.

Notwithstanding sentence 1 no. 2, the competent authority may refrain from inspecting the procurement facilities in the country of origin if the documents submitted by the importer do not give rise to any objections or if it is already familiar with the facilities or operating sites and the quality assurance system of the party procuring the tissue in the country of origin.

(3) The Federal Ministry is authorized to determine, by statutory order with the consent of the Bundesrat, the further requirements for the import of tissues or tissue preparations in accordance with paragraph 2 in order to ensure the proper quality of the tissues or tissue preparations. In particular, it may lay down rules on the tests to be carried out by the responsible person pursuant to Section 20c and on the monitoring to be carried out in the country of origin by the competent authority.

(4) Paragraph 2, sentence 1 shall apply to the import of tissues and tissue preparations within the meaning of paragraph 1, insofar as their monitoring is regulated by a statutory order pursuant to § 54, § 12 of the Transfusion Act, or § 16a of the Transplantation Act."

19d. Section 96 is amended as follows:

a) The following number 4a is inserted after number 4:

"4a. obtains tissue or carries out laboratory tests without a permit pursuant to Section 20b (1) sentence 1 or (2) sentence 7, or without a permit pursuant to Section 20c (1) sentence 1 tissues or tissue preparations, or processes, preserves, stores, or markets them."

b) The following number 5a is inserted after number 5:

"5a. places tissue preparations on the market without authorization pursuant to Section 21a (1) sentence 1,".

c) The following numbers 18a and 18b are inserted after number 18:

"18a. imports tissue or tissue preparations without a permit pursuant to Section 72b (1) sentence 1,

18b. imports tissue or tissue preparations contrary to Section 72b (2) sentence 1,".

20. Section 97(2) is amended as follows:

a) In number 7, after the reference to "Section 20," a comma and the reference to "Section 20c (6), also in conjunction with Section 72b (1) sentence 2, § 21a (7) and (9) sentence 4" is inserted after the reference to "§ 63b (7) sentence 1 or 2," and the reference to "§ 63b (7) sentence 1 or sentence 2, § 63c (2) sentence 1," is replaced by the reference to "§ 63b (7) sentence 1 or sentence 2, § 63c (2) sentence 1,"

b) The following numbers 24e and 24f are inserted after number 24d:

"24e. fails to submit a report or fails to submit it on time, contrary to Section 63c (3) sentence 1,

24f. fails to submit a report or fails to submit it on time, contrary to § 63c (4),".

21. The following fourteenth subsection is added:

"Fourteenth Subsection

§ 142 Transitional provisions on the occasion of the Tissue Act

(1) A person who, on August 1, 2007, possesses the expertise pursuant to Section 15 (3a) in the version applicable at that time as a competent person may continue to perform the activity as a competent person.

(2) Anyone who, by October 1, 2007, has applied for a license pursuant to Section 20b (1) or (2) or Section 20c (1) or a manufacturing license pursuant to Section 13 (1), or by February 1, 2008, has applied for a license pursuant to Section 21a (1), or by September 30, 2008, has applied for a license pursuant to Section 21a (1), may continue to procure these tissues or tissue preparations, examine them in the laboratory, treat or process them, and preserve them. September 2008, may continue to procure, examine in the laboratory, process, preserve, store, or place on the market these tissues or tissue preparations until a decision has been made on the application.

(3) Anyone who, on August 1, 2007, holds a manufacturing license pursuant to Section 13 (1) for tissues or tissue preparations within the meaning of Section 20b (1) or Section 20c (1) or an authorization pursuant to Section 21 (1) for tissue preparations within the meaning of Section 21a (1) shall not be required to submit a new application pursuant to Section 20b (1), Section 20c (1) or Section 21a (1) "

Article 3

Amendment

of the Transfusion Act

The Transfusion Act of July 1, 1998 (Federal Law Gazette I p. 1752), last amended by Article 36 of the Ordinance of October 31, 2006 (Federal Law Gazette I p. 2407), is amended as follows:

1. Section 4, sentence 1 is amended as follows:

a) In number 2, the words "is a licensed physician (licensed medical professional) and" are deleted.

b) In number 3, the words "from a human being" are inserted after the word "donations" and the word "licensed" is deleted.

2. Section 5 is amended as follows:

a) In paragraph 1, sentence 1, the words "licensed" and "licensed" are deleted.

b) In paragraph 3, the words "The person designated in accordance with Section 2 (2) sentence 1 of the Operating Regulations for Pharmaceutical Companies" are replaced by the words "The person responsible for managing quality control in accordance with Section 14 (1) No. 2 of the German Medicines Act."

2a. In Section 7 (2), the word "licensed" is deleted.

2b. Section 8 (2) sentence 1 is amended as follows:

a) In number 2, the word "licensed" is deleted.

b) In number 3, the word "licensed" is deleted.

2c. In Section 9 (3) sentence 1, a comma and the words "including exemptions from payment" are inserted after the words "paragraph 2 sentence 2".

3. In Section 11a, the words "Section 1a, sentence 1, Section 2(1), sentences 1 and 2, Section 8(1), (2) and (4) and Section 15(1a) of the Operating Regulations for Pharmaceutical Companies" are replaced by the words "Section 3(1), sentences 1, 3 and 4, § 4 (1) sentences 1 and 2, § 7 (1) sentence 1, (2) and (4) and § 20 (2) of the Medicinal Products and Active Ingredients Manufacturing Ordinance."

4. Section 12 shall be worded as follows:

"Section 12

Regulatory authority

The Federal Ministry of Health may, by statutory order with the consent of the Bundesrat and after consulting the German Medical Association and other experts, regulate the technical requirements under this section, provided that this is necessary to avert dangers to human health or to prevent risks. The statutory order may, in particular, specify the details of the requirements for

1. the donation facilities,

2. the selection and examination of donors,

3. the information and consent of donors,

4. the procurement of donations,

5. donor immunization and pre-treatment for blood stem cell collection, and

6. the documentation of the donation collection and the protection of the documented data

The Federal Ministry of Health may transfer the authorization pursuant to sentence 1 to the competent higher federal authority by means of a statutory order without the consent of the Bundesrat.

4a. The following Section 12a is inserted after Section 12:

"Section 12a

Guidelines on the state
the state of medical science and technology for the collection of blood and blood components

(1) The German Medical Association may, in agreement with the competent higher federal authority, lay down guidelines on the generally accepted state of knowledge of medical science and technology for the collection of blood and blood components, supplementing the provisions of the statutory order pursuant to Section 12. When developing the guidelines, the appropriate participation of experts from the relevant professional and trade circles and the competent federal and state authorities shall be ensured. The guidelines shall be published by the competent federal authority in the Federal Gazette.

(2) Compliance with the state of the art in medical science and technology shall be presumed if the guidelines of the German Medical Association pursuant to paragraph 1 have been observed."

4b. Section 15 (1) is amended as follows:

a) In sentence 2, the word "licensed" is deleted.

b) In sentence 3, the word "licensed" is deleted.

5. Section 16 (2) is amended as follows:

a) In sentence 1, the word "side effect" is replaced by the words "adverse reaction."

b) In sentence 3, the word "side effects" is replaced by the words "adverse reactions."

6. The following sentence is added to Section 28:

"Sentence 1 shall also apply to blood intended for the preparation or multiplication of autologous body cells in the context of tissue cultivation for tissue regeneration."

7. In Section 32 (2), in number 1, the word "or" is replaced by a comma and in number 2, the full stop at the end is replaced by the word "or" and the following number 3 is added:

"3. contravenes a statutory order pursuant to Section 12 sentence 1 or an enforceable order based on such a statutory order, insofar as the statutory order refers to this provision on fines for a specific offense."

Article 4

Amendment to the Pharmacy Operating Regulations

In Section 17 (6a) of the Pharmacy Operating Regulations in the version published on September 26, 1995 (Federal Law Gazette I p. 1195), last amended by Article 35 of the Act of March 26, 2007 (Federal Law Gazette I p. 378), the words "preparations from other substances of human origin as well as" shall be inserted after the words "serums from human blood and".

Article 5

Amendment to the Operating Regulations for Pharmaceutical Wholesalers

The Operating Regulations for Pharmaceutical Wholesalers of November 10, 1987 (Federal Law Gazette I p. 2370), last amended by Article 3 of the Ordinance of November 3, 2006 (Federal Law Gazette I p. 2523), shall be amended as follows:

1. In Section 6(2) sentence 4 no. 2, the words "preparations from other substances of human origin as well as" shall be inserted after the words "sera from human blood and".

2. In Section 7 (3) sentence 2, the words "preparations from other substances of human origin as well as" shall be inserted after the words "sera from human blood and".

Article 6

Amendment of other legal provisions

(1) The Infection Protection Act of July 20, 2000 (Federal Law Gazette I p. 1045), last amended by Article 57 of the Ordinance of October 31, 2006 (Federal Law Gazette I p. 2407), is amended as follows:

1. In the table of contents, the reference to Section 25 is worded as follows:

"Section 25 Investigations, duty of the health authority to provide information on blood, organ, tissue, or cell donors."

2. In Section 9 (1) sentence 1 no. 13, the words "blood, organ, or tissue donation" are replaced by the words "blood, organ, tissue, or cell donation."

3. Section 25 is amended as follows:

a) The heading is worded as follows:

"Section 25

Investigations, duty of the health authority to provide information in the case of blood, organ, tissue, or cell donors."

b) Paragraph 2 is amended as follows:

aa) In sentence 1, the words "blood, organ, or tissue donors" are replaced by the words "blood, organ, tissue, or cell donors" and the words "tissue or organs" are replaced by the words "organs, tissue, or cells."

bb) Sentence 3 shall be worded as follows:

"In accordance with sentences 1 and 2, it shall also inform the coordination center established or designated in accordance with Section 11 of the Transplantation Act in the case of donors of organs subject to mandatory mediation (Section 1a No. 2 of the Transplantation Act) in the case of other organ, tissue, or cell donors, in accordance with the provisions of the Transplantation Act, the medical care facility where the organ, tissue, or cell was or is to be transplanted and the tissue establishment that removed the tissue or cell."

(2) In Section 5 No. 15 of the Criminal Code in the version published on November 13, 1998 (Federal Law Gazette I p. 3322), last amended by Article 1 of the Act of July 16, 2007 (Federal Law Gazette I p. 1327), the words "organ trafficking (Section 18 of the Transplantation Act)" are replaced by the words "organ and tissue trafficking (Section 18 of the Transplantation Act)".

(3) In Section 115a (2) sentences 2 and 4 of Book V of the Social Code – Statutory Health Insurance – (Article 1 of the Act of December 20, 1988, Federal Law Gazette I p. 2477, 2482), last amended by Article 6 of Act of June 14, 2007 (Federal Law Gazette I p. 1066), the words "paragraph 1" shall be inserted after the words "§ 9".

Article 7
Permission to publish

The Federal Ministry of Health may publish the text of the Transplantation Act and the Transfusion Act in the version applicable from August 1, 2007, in the Federal Law Gazette.

Article 7a
Experience report of the Federal Government

The Federal Government shall inform the legislative bodies of the Federation every four years, for the first time by August 1, 2010, about the situation regarding the supply of tissue and tissue preparations to the population.

Article 8
Entry into force

This Act shall enter into force on the first day of the month following its promulgation.

The constitutional rights of the Federal Council are preserved.

The above law is hereby enacted. It shall be published in the Federal Law Gazette.

Berlin, July 20, 2007

The Federal President
Horst Köhler

The Federal Chancellor
Dr. Angela Merkel

The Federal Minister of Health

Ulla Schmidt

Appendix 6.1 Information on the Prescription of Medications for Off-Label Use

As part of your fertility treatment, medications are used that are not directly approved for fertility treatment and use during pregnancy. These include, for example, the following medications:

Medication	Actual area of application	Function in fertility treatment
Brevactid® 1500	Restoration of fertility in men with certain conditions	Support of the luteal phase in an assisted reproduction cycle
Clomiphene	Induction of ovulation in women with infertility due to lack of ovulation.	Ovarian stimulation treatment in women with ovulation
Decapeptyl IVF® Or Triptofem®	Downregulation of the pituitary gland (no more FSH and LH are released) and prevention of premature LH surge	Triggering ovulation during fertility treatment.
Letrozole	Treatment of postmenopausal women with hormone receptor-positive primary breast cancer	Ovarian stimulation treatment in women with ovulation
Gynokadin® Dosage gel 0.6 mg/g gel	Hormone therapy during menopause	Proliferation of the uterine lining in artificial cycles, increased bleeding safety during artificial fertilization
Heparin (e.g., Fragmin P®)	Prevention of thrombosis (blood clots) after surgery and treatment of thromboembolism	In cases of known tendency to clot (thrombophilic diathesis): improvement of placenta formation and prevention of miscarriages
Metformin (e.g., Siofor®) or Metfoliquid	Diabetes mellitus	Improvement of pregnancy success in cases of risk for gestational diabetes (e.g., insulin resistance) **Goal:** optimal conditions for a successful pregnancy, as slight disturbances in Sugar metabolism before conception can lead to failure and pregnancy complications
Progynova®	Hormone therapy during menopause	Building up the uterine lining in an artificial cycle, increasing the reliability of bleeding during artificial fertilization

Prolutex®	Support of the luteal phase in ART when vaginal preparations are not possible	Support of the luteal phase

The medications mentioned have proven themselves internationally over decades, so their use is considered safe.

The drug manufacturer is only liable for the efficacy and safety of a drug when used within the scope of the indications specified in the marketing authorization. The manufacturer is exempt from liability for any damage to health if drugs are administered on medical prescription outside their approved scope of application under pharmaceutical law. However, the approval does not indicate whether the drug in question is also tolerable and appropriately effective for other indications. On the other hand, it cannot be ruled out with certainty that the drug will have side effects beyond what is considered acceptable according to medical science when used outside the approved scope of application. In certain areas of care and for individual clinical pictures, it is not possible to completely avoid the use of drugs beyond the limits of their approval if patients are not to be denied treatment in line with the latest medical findings. As a rule, these are clinical pictures that cannot be treated effectively in any other way due to a lack of therapeutic alternatives.

Typical risks of drug treatment include, in particular, undesirable harmful side effects and interactions, as well as possible long-term effects. For more information, please refer to the respective package inserts.

You must be aware that the prescription of drugs outside the area for which they are legally approved may entail particular risks, as their tolerability and efficacy have not been verified by the manufacturer in the approval process. It is also important to note that off-label drugs cannot be prescribed at the expense of statutory health insurance.

I confirm that detailed information about the above-listed prescribed drugs has been provided. In particular, it has been pointed out that the prescription is for a use not intended by the manufacturer.

Place, date   Signature of patient

Signature of physician

(c) Bals-Pratsch, et al. (2025). Workplace Fertility Center. Springer, Berlin, Heidelberg.
https://doi.org/10.1007/978-3-662-71659-5_6

Appendix 6.2 Information for the Recipient on the Legal Basis of Sperm Donation under the Sperm Donor Registry Act (SaRegG)

I was informed about the legal basis for sperm donation under the SaRegG at the fertility clinic (medical care facility). In particular, I was given a copy of the wording of the law.

1. It was explained to me that a child born through artificial reproduction using donated sperm has the right to information about the donor. The importance of knowing one's own ancestry for a person's development was explained to me. The possibility of external counseling on the consequences of artificial reproduction with sperm from an unknown donor was discussed.
2. After receiving this information, I understand that the fertility clinic must collect and store the following data before using the sperm donation:
   - Name
   - First name
   - Date and place of birth and country
   - Street and house number, postal code, and city

   This data will later, i.e., after successful treatment, be sent to the German Institute for Medical Documentation and Information (DIMDI) together with information about the date of sperm use, the facility where the sperm was obtained (collection facility/sperm bank), the donor number assigned there, and the expected date of birth or date of birth, as well as the number of children born, and stored there. The data will be deleted from the fertility clinic no later than six months after it has been transmitted. No report is made to the DIMDI if the fertility clinic is aware that no pregnancy has occurred.
3. I have been informed that I am legally obliged to notify the fertility clinic immediately after the birth, stating the date of birth, which child or how many children were born as a result of artificial reproduction. If I do not report this, the fertility clinic will contact me based on the calculated expected date of delivery. If I cannot be reached and the fertility clinic has no information about the birth, the aforementioned data will still be reported to DIMDI, with the expected delivery date being transmitted instead of the date of birth. DIMDI will store this data in the sperm donor registry and retain it for 110 years. Earlier deletion will only take place if pregnancy has not occurred as a result of treatment with the donor's sperm sample and this was not known beforehand.
4. I have been informed that, upon request, DIMDI will provide an eligible person (the child born or their legal representative) with information about the sperm donor's personal data. The right to information exists for the entire storage period. Once the child conceived through the sperm donation has reached the age of 16, only the child is entitled to obtain information.
5. When the child submits the request, a copy of their identity card and birth certificate must be provided. If the parents, as legal representatives, assert the right to information on behalf of their child who has not yet reached the age of 16, they must provide the child's birth certificate and copies of their identity cards. If the request is made by a legal representative, a legal

Power of representation required. Before providing information, DIMDI recommends that the person requesting information seek specific advice and refers them to existing counseling services.

6. I am aware that I only have a right to information and correction from DIMDI with regard to my data stored there. If my treatment with donor sperm has not resulted in the birth of a child, I have a right to have my stored data deleted by DIMDI.

7. I understand that, according to § 1600d paragraph 4 of the German Civil Code (BGB), it is not possible to establish the legal paternity of the sperm donor.

After receiving the information and sufficient time for consideration, I confirm

surname, first name, born on date, residing at street number, postal code, city, that I have understood the information provided.

Furthermore, I declare that I have been informed of my obligation to notify the fertility clinic of the birth of the child or children, stating the date of birth, no later than three months after the birth. I assure you that I will fulfill this obligation.

____

Place, date   Signature of patient

I have informed the above signatory and explained the content of this declaration to her.

____

Place, date   Signature of informing physician

(c) Bals-Pratsch, et al. (2025). Workplace Fertility Center. Springer, Berlin, Heidelberg.
https://doi.org/10.1007/978-3-662-71659-5_6

Appendix 6.3 Reporting of Suspected Serious Adverse Reaction in Donors of Tissues, Tissue Preparations, or Stem Cells in Accordance with § 63i AMG (Form G1b)

Speichern		Formular zurücksetzen

Reporting suspected serious adverse reactions in donors of tissue, tissue preparations, or stem cells in accordance with Section 63i of the German Medicines Act (AMG)

Form G1b

to the Paul Ehrlich Institute, Department SBD 2, Paul-Ehrlich-Straße 51-59, 63225 Langen

For further information, see: www.pei.de: Vigilance/Tissue Vigilance

Email biovigilance@pei.de

Tel.: (06103) 77-3117

Please do not fill in this field
PEI No.:

Fax: (06103) 77-1268

Reporting institution:

Street:

Postal code: City

Tel.   Fax

Internal case number

Donor details

Initials: _ _ _ _ _ Date of birth: _ _ _ _ _ _ _ _ _   ☐ Female   ☐ Male   ☐ Diverse

Tissue or tissue preparation (GWZ)

Type of tissue /TPP

☐ Oocytes (autologous)   ☐ Hematopoietic stem cells (bone marrow)   ☐ Autologous donation   ☐ Allogeneic donation

☐ Other: _

Single European Code/SEC (40 characters) or identification code	Date of collection	Transfer date

Tissue establishment

Name: _

EU tissue establishment code (TE code): _

Donation-related medication (e.g., stimulation protocol in the context of assisted reproduction):

_   _ _ _ _ _ _

_ _ _ _ _ _ _ _ _ _   _   _ _ _ _ _ _

_   _ _ _ _ _ _ _ _ _ _

Type of tissue/GWZ application: _ _ _ _ _ _ _ _ _ _ _ _ _

Information on serious adverse reactions in the donor

_   _ _ _ _ _ _

_   _ _ _ _ _ _

☐ Local reaction   ☐ Systemic reaction

☐ Ovarian hyperstimulation syndrome (OHSS) Severity: ☐ III ☐ IV   ☐ V (according to Golan) or

Severity: ☐ III (according to WHO)

☐ Other reaction: _   _ _ _ _ _ _

Hospitalization: ☐ no ☐ yes, duration: _ _ _ _ _

Outcome of the reaction: ☐ Recovered   ☐ Restored with consequential damage   ☐ Death

Time of occurrence of the reaction: Duration of the adverse reaction:

Causality assessment: ☐ certain   ☐ probable ☐ possible   ☐ unlikely   ☐ excluded

☐ Final report to follow

Measures implemented:

_   _ _ _ _ _ _

_   _ _ _ _ _ _

Additional organizations notified (e.g., BfArM): _

Impairment of the quality and safety of the harvested tissue/GWZ:

☐ No   ☐ Yes, which: _

Details of the reporting person:

Last name: First name: Tel. no.:

Zip code: City: Fax number:

Email

Signature: Date:

Version G-2023-01

Appendix 6.4 Reporting of a Serious Adverse Event (Incident) Related to the Manufacture or Application of Tissues, Tissue Preparations, or Stem Cells in Accordance with § 63i AMG

<table>
<tr><td>Form G1c</td><td colspan="2">**Reporting a serious incident (accident)**
in connection with the manufacture or use of tissues,
tissue preparations, or stem cells in accordance with Section 63i AMG
to the Paul Ehrlich Institute, Department SBD 2, Paul-Ehrlich-Straße 51-59, 63225 Langen
For further information, see: www.pei.de: Vigilance/ Tissue Vigilance
Email: biovigilance@pei.de</td></tr>
</table>

Tel.: (06103) 77-3117	Please do not fill in this field **PEI No.:**	Fax: (06103) 77-1268

Reporting   institution:

Street:

Postal code: City:

Tel.   Fax

Internal   case number

Tissues or tissue preparations affected   by the incident   (GWZ)

Type of tissue/GWZ   Single European Code/SEC (40 characters) / Identification code   Collection   Date of Transfer   Date of Incident

Date of Collection

Tissue establishment

Name: _ _ _ __ _____ _ ___ _ _ ______ _ __ ___ __ ____ _ _ __ ____ _ _____ __ __ _ ___ ____ EU

tissue establishment code (TE code): __ ____

Approval of the   tissue/GWZ   :

☐ Permission pursuant to Sections 20b and 20c of the German Medicines Act (AMG)☐ Approval pursuant to Section 21a (1) AMG☐ Authorization pursuant to Section 25 (1) AMG

Characterization of   the event

Defect detected outside the tissue establishment:	Yes ☐
Release of the affected tissue/GWZ:	yes ☐
Event occurred repeatedly:	yes ☐
Internal risk analysis assessed the event as serious:	Yes ☐

A report to the PEI is only required if at least one of the above criteria is met.

Serious incident affecting the quality or safety of tissues/tissue   -engineered products due to a deviation in the following processes:

☐ Collection	☐ Processing	☐ Preservation
☐ Examination	☐ Process ing	☐ Storage
☐ Delivery	☐ Transport	
☐ Other:		

Detailed description of the incident   (if necessary, attach an informal document as a report)

Rating

Measures   impl emented

Details of   the reporting person:

Name:	Telephone number:
Postal code:	Fax no.:
City:	Email:
Date:	Signature:

Version G-2023-01

Appendix 8.1 Directive of the Federal Joint Committee Kryo-RL from November 15, 2022

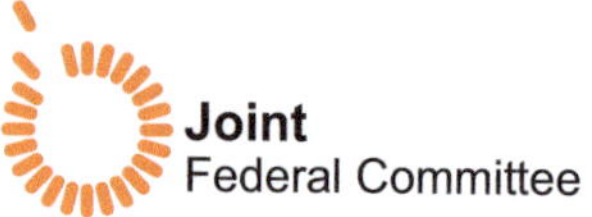

Directive

of the Joint Federal Committee on the cryopreservation of egg or sperm cells or germ cell tissue and corresponding medical measures due to germ cell-damaging therapy (Cryo-RL)

in the version dated July 16, 2020
published in the Federal Gazette (BAnz AT 19.02.2021 B7)

last amended on August 18, 2022
published in the Federal Gazette AT 14.11.2022 B2
entered into force on November 15, 2022

Contents

§ 1   Subject matter

This guideline specifies the conditions, nature, and scope of the insured persons' entitlement to cryopreservation of female and male germ cells and germ cell tissue due to germ cell-damaging therapy, as well as to the associated medical measures, as regulated in Section 27a (4) Social Code Book V (SGB V).

§ 2   Eligibility requirements

(1)   Insured persons are entitled to cryopreservation of egg or sperm cells or germ cell tissue and to the associated medical measures under the conditions specified below.

(2)   The prerequisite for entitlement under paragraph 1 is that

1. cryopreservation appears medically necessary for the insured person due to an illness (underlying illness) and its treatment with germ cell-damaging therapy within the meaning of § 3 in order to be able to carry out subsequent medical measures to bring about pregnancy in accordance with the guidelines on assisted reproduction

2. the specialist who diagnosed or treated the underlying disease provided medical advice in accordance with § 4 (2) No. 1 and a certificate in accordance with § 4 (2) No. 1 has been issued by this specialist for submission to a specialist qualified in reproductive medicine or andrology,

3. after submission of the medical certificate in accordance with Section 4 (2) No. 1, the patient received reproductive medicine and, where necessary, andrology counseling and information in accordance with Section 4 (2) No. 2, and

4. the requirements of the Transplantation Act (TPG) for consent have been observed. In accordance with the provisions set out therein, the patient must be capable of giving consent at the time of the removal of germ cells or germ cell tissue and must have consented to the performance of these measures. In the case of female insured persons, a legal representative or authorized representative may give consent if the patient is incapable of giving consent.

(3)   The entitlement under paragraph 1 does not exist or no longer exists

1. for male insured persons from the age of 50 and for female insured persons from the age of 40,

2. upon the death of the insured person.

§ 3   Medical indications

(1)   For the medical indication for cryopreservation and for the associated medical measures in accordance with this guideline, in addition to the general requirements for performing cryopreservation in relation to a disease, treatments must be planned which, according to the current state of scientific knowledge, may damage germ cells; these include in particular:

- surgical removal of the gonads,
- radiotherapy with expected damage to the gonads, or
- medication that may potentially damage fertility.

The specialist who diagnoses or treats the underlying disease shall determine whether this requirement is met.

(2)   The indication for cryopreservation of egg or sperm cells or germ cell tissue due to germ cell-damaging therapy and for the associated medical measures is made by specialists who are qualified to provide counseling in accordance with Section 4 (2) No. 2.

§ 4   Counseling

Close cooperation between the specialist disciplines involved must be ensured in order to provide comprehensive counseling to those affected and to integrate cryopreservation and the associated medical measures into the treatment of the underlying disease, taking into account the individual disease situation.

In order to be able to take advantage of the cryopreservation of egg or sperm cells or germ cell tissue and the associated medical measures in accordance with Section 5, the following must be done in advance:

1. Consultation with the specialist who diagnosed or is treating the underlying disease, taking into account the individual prognosis regarding the risks of germ cell damage associated with the treatment of the underlying disease and initial information about the possibility of reproductive medical treatment. This consultation also includes a medical assessment and certificate with the following information:

   a) Specification of the underlying disease for which a therapy that is potentially damaging to germ cells according to the current state of scientific knowledge is planned

   b) any previous treatment of the underlying disease,

   c) planned germ cell damaging therapy,

   d) known comorbidities,

   e) for female insured persons, information on whether a hormone-dependent tumor is present,

   f) Recommendation for counseling according to number 2,

g) a recommendation regarding the available time window for cryopreservation measures,

h) for female insured persons, information on whether menarche has already occurred and

j) that the consultation under number 1 has taken place.

As part of the consultation under number 1, a recommendation is made for a reproductive medicine consultation and, if necessary, an andrology consultation on cryopreservation and the associated medical measures under number 2.

2. reproductive medicine and, if necessary, andrology consultation and information on cryopreservation and the associated medical measures after presentation of the medical certificate in accordance with number 1. The following are authorized to carry out this consultation:

a) Specialists in gynecology and obstetrics with a focus on gynecological endocrinology and reproductive medicine in a practice or institution that meets the requirements of § 6 (1) and (2)

and

b) in the case of male insured persons, specialists who offer the necessary measures in accordance with Section 5 in connection with the collection of sperm cells and the removal of germ cell tissue and who meet the relevant requirements in accordance with Section 6.

The consultation referred to in number 2 shall be conducted taking into account the underlying disease itself, the age of the patient, and the prognosis. The consultation shall consider the advantages and disadvantages of the available options for fertility preservation, discuss the prospects of success and risks of the possible measures, and any associated psychosocial stress.

At the end of the consultation regarding germ cell-damaging therapy, the specialist shall conclusively examine the existence of the medical indication for cryopreservation in accordance with Section 3 (2), including the associated medical measures, taking all relevant aspects into account. If the indication is present, the insured person or their legal representative or authorized person shall determine together with the specialist whether egg cells, sperm cells, or germ cell tissue should be removed and cryopreserved.

§ 5 Scope of medical measures

(1) The medical measures associated with cryopreservation are the preparation, collection, processing, transport, freezing, storage, and subsequent thawing of egg or sperm cells and germ cell tissue.

(2)   The following medical procedures are covered by the preparation for cryopreservation:

1. Required laboratory tests in accordance with Section 6 (1) sentence 2 in conjunction with Annex 4 Nos. 1 and 3 of the TPG Tissue Ordinance (anti-HIV-1,2, HBsAg, anti-HBc, anti-HCV-Ab; in individual cases, where necessary, further tests in accordance with Annex 4, No. 1, letters d and e of the TPG Tissue Regulation) within three months prior to germ cell collection.

   The results of the tests must be available during the collection, processing, use, and storage of the germ cells or germ cell tissue. Otherwise, storage under quarantine conditions is required until the infection parameters are received.

2. Measures in connection with the collection of oocytes:

   Hormonal stimulation treatment in accordance with the limits of the drug approval (e.g., ovarian stimulation for egg cell retrieval), laboratory medical determinations of luteinizing hormone, estradiol, and progesterone; sonographic examinations and transvaginal or laparoscopic egg cell retrieval (follicular puncture).

3. Measures related to the retrieval of ovarian tissue for female children and adolescents from puberty onwards, at the earliest after menarche, and women up to the age of 40:

   a)   Surgical removal (laparoscopy, in exceptional cases laparotomy) of ovarian tissue, as well as preparation of the ovarian tissue prior to cryopreservation, in accordance with the German Medical Association's "Guideline on the Removal and Transfer of Human Germ Cells and Germ Cell Tissue in the Context of Assisted Reproduction" dated January 14, 2022.

   b)   The service requires comprehensive consultation of the insured person by the treating specialist in gynecology and obstetrics with a focus on "gynecological endocrinology and reproductive medicine" in accordance with Section 4 (2), No. 2 a).

4. Measures related to the collection, examination, and preparation of sperm cells in males from puberty onwards, including a semen analysis and, if necessary, testicular sperm extraction (TESE).

(3)   The cryopreservation procedure suitable for the insured person, including the associated measures, shall be selected in accordance with the provisions of the German Medical Association's guidelines on assisted reproduction pursuant to Section 16b TPG by the service providers authorized pursuant to Section 6.

§ 6   Authorized service providers

(1)   Measures pursuant to Section 5 may only be carried out by service providers who, in addition to the relevant requirements of paragraphs 2, 3, or 4 for the insured person, also meet the relevant requirements of the German Medical Association's guidelines on the removal and transfer of human germ cells or germ cell tissue in the context of assisted reproduction for the respective measures required pursuant to Section 5.

When providing the service components of transport, preparation, cryopreservation, and storage, service providers may also ensure compliance with the requirements set out in sentence 1 by means of cooperation agreements with institutions that meet the relevant requirements of the German Medical Association's guideline referred to in sentence 1 for the respective measures required and have the necessary approval in accordance with Section 20b or Section 20c of the German Medicinal Products Act (AMG)

(2)   Measures for germ cell procurement pursuant to Section 5 may only be performed by:

1. licensed physicians, authorized physicians, or authorized medically directed institutions that meet the following requirements:

   a)) The head of the practice or facility must be a specialist in gynecology and obstetrics and have a specialization in "gynecological endocrinology and reproductive medicine."

   b)) The practice or facility must have the following knowledge and experience:
   - Reproductive endocrinology
   - Gynecological sonography
   - Operative gynecology
   - Reproductive biology
   - and, in the treatment of male patients, andrology.

   Only two of these areas may be managed simultaneously by a physician or scientist at the practice or institution. Regular cooperation with a human geneticist and a psychotherapist must be ensured.

2. Hospitals that meet the requirements under number 1 letter b.

(3)   The surgical removal of ovarian tissue in accordance with Section 5 (2) No. 3 may be performed

1. in female children and adolescents from puberty onwards at the earliest after menarche, depending on physical development, either by specialists in gynecology and obstetrics or by specialists in pediatric surgery and

2. in women up to the age of 40 by specialists in gynecology and obstetrics.

(4)   In the case of male insured persons, measures pursuant to Section 5 in connection with the extraction of sperm cells and the removal of germ cell tissue may also be performed by specialists with additional training in andrology who offer all of the measures specified in Section 5 (2) No. 4. This applies accordingly to hospitals.

(5)   The specialist, focus, and additional designations used in the guideline are based on the (model) further training regulations of the German Medical Association and include physicians who hold a corresponding designation under the old law.

(6)   The relevant requirements for the measures in accordance with the German Medical Association's guideline on assisted reproduction pursuant to Section 16b TPG must be observed.

§ 7   Transitional cases

In cases where insured persons have already had their egg or sperm cells or germ cell tissue cryopreserved due to an illness and its treatment with germ cell-damaging therapy, or have already begun cryopreservation measures within the meaning of these guidelines, they are entitled to cryopreservation and the associated medical measures in accordance with these guidelines from the date of entry into force of the implementation of these guidelines in the Uniform Assessment Standard to the extent required in the specific individual case from that date. Corresponding benefits are granted at the request of the insured persons. The application must be accompanied by a medical certificate in accordance with Section 4, sentence 2, number 1.

§ 8   Review

The Joint Federal Committee shall review the scientific data on the cryopreservation of germ cell tissue, in particular in prepubertal children and adolescents, two years after the entry into force of this amendment to the guidelines and, on the basis of the results, shall discuss the need to adapt the regulations.

Appendix 8.2 Certificate of Existing Entitlement to Benefits for Insured Persons for Cryopreservation of Germ Cells Due to Germ Cell-Damaging Therapy

<table>
<tr><td>

Krankenkasse bzw. Kostenträger

Name, Vorname des Versicherten

geb. am

Kostenträgerkennung   Versicherten-Nr.   Status

Betriebsstätten-Nr.   Arzt-Nr.   Datum

</td><td>

Certificate confirming the insured person's entitlement to cryopreservation of germ cells due to germ cell-damaging therapy

</td></tr>
</table>

Entries by the specialist who diagnoses or treats the underlying disease

The above-named person is entitled to cryopreservation of egg or sperm cells or germ cell tissue and to the associated medical measures, as a disease and its treatment with germ cell-damaging therapy appear to be medically necessary in order to be able to carry out subsequent medical measures to bring about pregnancy in accordance with the guidelines on artificial insemination.

Diagnosis:________________________________ ICD-10________________________________

Any **previous treatment** of the underlying disease: ________________________________

Planned germ cell-damaging **therapy** (please tick):

      Surgical removal of the gonads **O**, Radiotherapy **O**, Fertility-damaging medication O

Known comorbidities: ________________________________

For female insured persons: Is there a **hormone-dependent tumor**? Yes **O** No **O**

Type: ________________________________

Recommendation regarding the available **time window** for cryopreservation measures:

____

A **consultation** has **been held**, taking into account the individual prognosis, the risks of germ cell damage associated with the treatment of the underlying disease, and initial information about the possibility of reproductive medicine treatment.

The underlying disease has been diagnosed.
and the indication for reproductive medicine/andrology counseling determined **by**:

Doctor's stamp/signature

Entries by the reproductive medicine specialist/andrologist

The consultation was conducted taking into account the underlying disease itself, the patient's age, and the prognosis. The chances of success, risks of possible measures, and potential psychosocial stress were discussed.

Doctor's stamp/signature

Appendix 9.1 Preimplantation Genetic Diagnosis Act—PreimpG of November 21, 2011

Law
regulating preimplantation genetic diagnosis
(Preimplantation Genetic Diagnosis Act - PräimpG)
of November 21, 2011

The Bundestag has passed the following law:

Article 1

Amendment to the

Embryo Protection Act

The Embryo Protection Act of December 13, 1990 (Federal Law Gazette I, p. 2746), which was amended by Article 22 of the Act of October 23, 2001 (Federal Law Gazette I, p. 2702), is amended as follows:

1. The following new Section 3a is inserted after Section 3:

"Section 3a

Preimplantation diagnosis;

Regulatory authority

(1) Anyone who genetically tests the cells of an embryo in vitro prior to its intrauterine transfer (preimplantation diagnosis) shall be punished with imprisonment of up to one year or a fine.

(2) If, due to the genetic disposition of the woman from whom the egg cell originates, or the man from whom the sperm cell originates, or both, there is a high risk of a serious hereditary disease for their offspring, it is not unlawful to genetically test the cells of the embryo in vitro prior to intrauterine transfer for the risk of this disease, with the written consent of the woman from whom the egg cell originates, in accordance with the generally accepted state of medical science and technology, in order to bring about a pregnancy. Nor shall anyone be acting unlawfully who, with the written consent of the woman from whom the egg cell originates, carries out preimplantation diagnosis to determine whether the embryo has a serious defect that is highly likely to result in stillbirth or miscarriage.

(3) Preimplantation diagnosis pursuant to paragraph 2 may only be performed

1. after providing information and counseling on the medical, psychological, and social consequences of the genetic testing of embryo cells requested by the woman, whereby the information must be provided before consent is obtained,

2. after an interdisciplinary ethics committee at the approved centers for preimplantation genetic diagnosis has checked that the requirements of paragraph 2 are met and given an approving assessment, and

3. by a physician qualified for this purpose in centers approved for preimplantation diagnosis that have the necessary equipment for performing preimplantation diagnosis measures.

The measures carried out as part of preimplantation diagnostics, including cases rejected by the ethics committees, shall be reported by the approved centers to a central office in anonymized form.

The measures carried out within the framework of preimplantation diagnosis, including cases rejected by the ethics committees, shall be reported by the approved centers to a central office in anonymized form and documented there. The Federal Government shall determine the details by statutory order with the consent of the Bundesrat

1. the number and requirements for the approval of centers in which preimplantation diagnostics may be performed, including the qualifications of the physicians working there and the duration of the approval,

2. on the establishment, composition, procedures, and financing of the ethics committees for preimplantation genetic diagnosis,

3. on the establishment and organization of the central office responsible for documenting measures carried out in the context of preimplantation diagnosis,

4. the requirements for reporting measures carried out within the framework of preimplantation genetic diagnosis to the central office and the requirements for documentation.

(4) Anyone who performs preimplantation genetic diagnosis contrary to paragraph 3, sentence 1, is guilty of an administrative offense. The administrative offense may be punished with a fine of up to fifty thousand euros.

(5) No physician is obliged to perform or participate in a measure pursuant to paragraph 2. Non-participation shall not result in any disadvantage for the person concerned.

(6) Every four years, the federal government shall prepare a report on experience with preimplantation genetic diagnosis. Based on the central documentation and anonymized data, the report shall contain the number of procedures performed annually and a scientific evaluation."

2. Section 9 is amended as follows:

a) The following new number 2 is inserted after number 1:

"2. preimplantation genetic diagnosis,"

b) The previous numbers 2 and 3 shall become numbers 3 and 4.

3. Section 11 (1) is amended as follows:

a) In number 1, the word "or" is replaced by a comma.

b) The following number 2 is inserted after number 1:
   "2. performs preimplantation genetic diagnosis
   contrary to Section 9, number 2, or".

c) The previous number 2 becomes number 3 and the reference to "No. 2" is replaced by the reference to "number 3."

4. In Section 12(1), the reference to "Section 9 No. 3" shall be replaced by the reference to "Section 9 No. 4."

Article 2

Entry into force*)

This Act shall enter into force on ...

The constitutional rights of the Federal Council are preserved.
The above law is hereby enacted. It shall be published in the Federal Law Gazette.

Berlin, November 21, 2011

The Federal President
Christian Wulff

The Federal Chancellor
Dr. Angela Merkel

The Federal Minister of Health
D. Bahr

*) Note from the editorial team: In accordance with Article 82, paragraph 2, sentence 2 of the Basic Law, this Act shall enter into force on the fourteenth day after the end of the day on which the Federal Law Gazette was published.

Appendix 9.2 Preimplantation Genetic Diagnosis Ordinance—PIDV of February 21, 2013

Regulation
regulating preimplantation genetic diagnosis
(Preimplantation Genetic Diagnosis Regulation - PIDV)

From February 21, 2013

On the basis of Section 3a (3) sentence 3 of the Embryo Protection Act, which was inserted by Article 1 number 1 of the Act of November 21, 2011 (Federal Law Gazette I p. 2228), the Federal Government decrees:

Section 1
General provisions

§1
Scope

This ordinance regulates the requirements for

1. the conditions for the approval of centers in which preimplantation genetic diagnosis may be carried out, and the duration of approval pursuant to Section 3a (3) sentence 3 number 1 of the Embryo Protection Act,

2. the qualifications of physicians working in approved centers pursuant to Section 3a (3) sentence 3 number 1 of the Embryo Protection Act,

3. the establishment, composition, procedures, and financing of the ethics committees for preimplantation genetic diagnosis pursuant to Section 3a (3) sentence 3 number 2 of the Embryo Protection Act,

4. the establishment and organization of the central office pursuant to Section 3a (3) sentence 3 no. 3 of the Embryo Protection Act, which is responsible for documenting measures carried out in the context of preimplantation diagnosis,

5. the reporting of measures carried out within the framework of preimplantation diagnostics pursuant to Section 3a (3) sentence 3 number 4 of the Embryo Protection Act, and

6. documentation pursuant to Section 3a (3) sentence 3 no. 4 of the Embryo Protection Act.

§2
Definitions

For the purposes of this Regulation

1. preimplantation diagnosis is the genetic examination of cells of an embryo in vitro prior to its intrauterine transfer (Section 3a (1) of the Embryo Protection Act),

2. a reproductive medicine procedure is artificial fertilization followed by the collection and preparation of cells,

3. cells within the meaning of numbers 1 and 2 are stem cells that

   a) have been removed from an embryo produced in vitro and have the ability to reproduce themselves through cell division in a suitable environment, and

   b) are capable of developing themselves or their daughter cells under suitable conditions into cells of different specializations, but not into an individual.

Section 2
Requirements for centers and ethics committees

§3
Requirements for the approval of centers

(1) Preimplantation diagnosis may only be carried out in a center that

1. has the necessary diagnostic, medical, and technical capabilities in accordance with the current state of scientific knowledge, both for the reproductive medicine procedure and for the genetic testing, and

2. is approved by the competent authority for the performance of preimplantation genetic diagnosis.

Reproductive medicine and human genetics facilities may also be approved as centers if a cooperation agreement ensures that the requirements specified in sentence 1 are met.

(2) Approval may only be granted upon application if

1. the center has an internal quality assurance system and participates in appropriate external quality assurance measures,

2. the center ensures that all measures associated with preimplantation genetic diagnosis

be carried out by qualified personnel,

3. the center ensures that the necessary counseling on the medical, psychological, and social consequences of the measures associated with preimplantation genetic diagnosis is provided by a physician who does not perform the measures themselves,

4. for the area of reproductive medicine measures

a) the person who heads the reproductive medicine facility is a specialist in gynecology and obstetrics and has a specialization in "gynecological endocrinology and reproductive medicine,"

b) the reproductive medicine facility has knowledge and experience in the fields of reproductive endocrinology, gynecological sonography, operative gynecology, reproductive biology with a focus on in vitro culture, andrology, and basic psychosomatic care,

c) the reproductive medicine facility has sufficient practical experience, in particular with in vitro fertilization, intracytoplasmic sperm injection or comparable procedures, with embryo transfer and with techniques for obtaining and processing cells,

d) the reproductive medicine facility has a cell biology laboratory with the necessary expertise in cell processing, and

5. for the genetic testing procedure

a) the person who heads the human genetics facility is a specialist in human genetics,

b) the human genetics facility has the following:

aa) accreditation by the German Accreditation Body for

aaa) comparative genome hybridization or molecular cytogenetic testing, and

bbb) molecular genetic testing, and

bb) sufficient practical experience in the application of these examination methods to individual cells.

There is no entitlement to approval. If it is necessary to choose between several suitable centers or institutions applying for approval, the competent authority shall decide taking into account the public interest, the diversity of applicants, and the need for centers for preimplantation genetic diagnosis.

(2a) The federal states may regulate by means of a state treaty that the centers in the participating federal states are approved by a joint body.

(3) The application for approval must be made in writing and must contain the following information and documents:

1. the name and address of the applicant; in the cases referred to in paragraph 1, sentence 2, the applicant shall be the person who heads the human genetics facility,

2. evidence demonstrating that the requirements set out in paragraph 2, sentence 1, numbers 1 to 5 are met; in the cases referred to in paragraph 1, sentence 2, also a copy of the cooperation agreement.

(4) The competent authority must issue the license for a center in writing. It shall be limited to five years. The license may be extended upon application in accordance with paragraph 2.

(5) The applicant is obliged to notify the competent authority immediately if there are any changes to the documents and information referred to in paragraph 3.

(6) The competent authority shall notify the central office pursuant to § 9 of the approval as a center for preimplantation diagnosis and its extension; notification shall also be given in the event of the withdrawal or revocation of the approval.

§4

Ethics committees for preimplantation genetic diagnosis

(1) The federal states shall establish independent interdisciplinary ethics committees for preimplantation genetic diagnosis (ethics committees) for the centers approved to perform preimplantation genetic diagnosis. The federal states may also establish joint ethics committees. The ethics committees shall be composed of four experts in the field of medicine, one expert each in the fields of ethics and law, and one representative each from the organizations responsible for representing the interests of patients and self-help groups for disabled persons at the state level. When composing the ethics committee, the appointing body shall take into account women and men with the aim of ensuring their equal participation.

(2) The members of the ethics committees shall be independent in their opinions and decisions and shall not be bound by any instructions. They shall be bound to confidentiality and discretion.

(3) The ethics committees shall charge fees and expenses for their activities as specified in Section 3a (3) sentence 1 number 2 of the Embryo Protection Act.

(4) Details regarding the composition, internal procedural rules, appointment of members of the ethics committees, and financing of the ethics committees shall be determined by state law. The term of appointment of the members of the ethics committees shall be limited.

Application for preimplantation genetic diagnosis

(1) The ethics committee shall only act for the purpose of examination and evaluation pursuant to Section 3a (3) sentence 1 number 2 of the Embryo Protection Act upon written application by the woman from whom the egg cell originates (applicant).

(2) The application must contain all information and documents required by the Ethics Committee to examine whether the conditions specified in Section 3a (2) of the Embryo Protection Act are met. The following must be submitted:

1. in the cases referred to in Section 3a (2) sentence 1 of the Embryo Protection Act, a medical-genetic report on the genetic disposition of the woman from whom the egg cell originates, or of the man from whom the sperm cell originates, or of both, including the name of the resulting hereditary disease, information on the probability of the offspring developing the disease and on the expected severity of the disease,

2. proof of the written consent of the persons entitled to apply pursuant to Section 8 (1) to the collection, processing, and use of their personal data by the ethics committee,

3. Proof of the written consent of the man from whom the sperm cell originates to the collection, processing, and use of his personal data by the ethics committee, insofar as his personal data is the subject of the application.

4. in the cases referred to in Section 3a (2) sentence 2 of the Embryo Protection Act, a medical assessment of the assumption that serious damage to the embryo is to be expected, which will most likely lead to a stillbirth or miscarriage,

5. the name of the center where the preimplantation genetic diagnosis is to be performed, including confirmation that it will be performed there in the event of an affirmative assessment,

6. information on whether another ethics committee for preimplantation genetic diagnosis has already made a decision on the facts submitted for assessment and, if so, a copy of that decision.

§6
Review of the application for preimplantation genetic diagnosis

(1) The ethics committee shall notify the applicant of its written decision on the application for preimplantation genetic diagnosis within three months of receiving the information and complete documentation required under § 5 (2).

(2) The ethics committees may, for the purpose of reviewing an application for preimplantation genetic diagnosis and the documents submitted for this purpose

1. utilize their own scientific findings,

2. consult experts who have experience with the health damage that is the subject of the application under review,

3. request expert opinions, or

4. hear the applicant orally.

In the cases referred to in sentence 1, numbers 2 and 3, the ethics committees are obliged to anonymize the personal data or, if anonymization is not yet possible in order to obtain the necessary findings, to pseudonymize it.

(3) Physicians are excluded from reviewing an application for preimplantation genetic diagnosis if, in the event of a favorable assessment of the application, they will perform the preimplantation genetic diagnosis, be involved in artificial insemination, or work at the center where the preimplantation genetic diagnosis or artificial fertilization is to be performed.

(4) The ethics committees shall approve the application for preimplantation genetic diagnosis if, after reviewing the information and documents referred to in § 5 (2) and taking into account the psychological, social, and ethical aspects relevant to the specific case, they conclude that the conditions set out in § 3a (2) of the Embryo Protection Act are met. They shall make their decision by a two-thirds majority of the members entitled to vote.

§7
Handling of data by ethics committees

(1) With the consent of the persons entitled to apply and, insofar as personal data relating to the man from whom the sperm cell originates is the subject of the application, also with his consent in accordance with Section 8 (1), the ethics committees may collect, process, and use the personal data referred to in Section 5 (2) for the purpose specified therein.

(2) The ethics committees are obliged to transmit the data referred to in § 8 (2) nos. 1, 3, and 4 to the centers in anonymized form.

(3) The ethics committees shall take the necessary technical and organizational measures to prevent the unauthorized use of the data.

(4) The ethics committees shall ensure that the information and documents referred to in Section 5 (2) and all documents relevant to the ethics committee's decision are retained for 30 years after the decision on the application. After expiry of the period specified in sentence 1, the information and documents shall be deleted without delay. The information and documents shall be deleted without delay before expiry of the period specified in sentence 1 if the application is withdrawn in accordance with Section 5 (1).

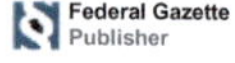

Section 8
Data collection, processing, and use

(1) The approved center for preimplantation genetic diagnosis shall obtain the written consent of the persons entitled to apply for the collection, processing, and use of personal data required for the performance of preimplantation genetic diagnosis and for the proceedings before the ethics committee. Prior to this, the approved center for preimplantation diagnosis shall provide the applicant with comprehensive information about the collection, processing, and use of personal data as provided for in sentence 1, both by the approved centers for preimplantation diagnosis themselves and by the ethics committees. Sentences 1 and 2 shall also apply to the consent of the man from whom the sperm cell originates, insofar as his personal data is required for the performance of preimplantation genetic diagnosis and in the proceedings before the ethics committee.

(2) Approved centers for preimplantation genetic diagnosis are required to submit the following data in anonymized form to the central office pursuant to § 9:
1. the number of applications for approval
   for the performance of preimplantation genetic diagnosis,
2. the number of preimplantation genetic diagnoses performed after approval,
3. the number of rejected applications for approval to perform preimplantation genetic diagnosis, and
4. the number of each type of justification for the indication pursuant to Section 3a (2) of the Embryo Protection Act, broken down by chromosomal disorders and autosomal dominant, autosomal recessive, and sex-linked hereditary diseases, including the respective genetic testing methods used in performing

whether the criteria for preimplantation genetic diagnosis were applied or should be applied.

(3) The information referred to in paragraph 2 must be reported by the approved centers for preimplantation genetic diagnosis to the central office pursuant to § 9 annually after the end of the calendar year, at the latest by March 1 of the following year.

(4) A form created by the central office shall be used for the data transmission pursuant to paragraph 2. The form may also be made available and used electronically.

Section 3
Central Office

Section 9
Central Office

(1) A central office shall be established at the Paul Ehrlich Institute, which shall be responsible for documenting the data reported in accordance with § 8 paragraph 2.

(2) The central office shall ensure that the information reported to it is documented and stored for ten years.

(3) The central office shall be obliged to forward the information reported to it and documented to the Federal Ministry of Health upon request so that it can prepare the Federal Government's report on experience with preimplantation genetic diagnosis.

Section 4
Final provisions

Section 10
Entry into force

This regulation shall enter into force on February 1, 2014.

The Federal Council has given its approval.

Berlin, February 21, 2013

The Federal Chancellor
Dr. Angela Merkel

The Federal Minister of Health
Daniel Bahr

**Appendix 10.1 Directives of the Federal Joint Committee
of Physicians and Health Insurance Funds on Medical Procedures
for Assisted Reproduction ("Directives on Assisted Reproduction")
of February 9, 2022**

Directives

of the Federal Committee of Physicians and Health Insurance Funds

on medical measures for assisted reproduction ("Directives on Assisted Reproductiondelines")

in the version dated August 14, 1990
published in the Federal Labor Gazette 1990, No. 12

last amended on December 16, 2021
published in the Federal Gazette (BAnz AT 08.02.2022 B3)
entered into force on February 9, 2022

The guidelines adopted by the Federal Committee of Physicians and Health Insurance Funds in accordance with Section 27a (5) in conjunction with Section 92 (1) sentence 2 no. 10 of the Fifth Book of the Social Code (SGB V) determine the medical details regarding the requirements, the type and scope of medical measures for achieving pregnancy through assisted reproduction in accordance with the legal requirements of Section 27a (1) SGB V in conjunction with Section 27a (4) SGB V.

Eligibility requirements

1. Medical measures in accordance with these guidelines may only be carried out if the measures to restore fertility in accordance with Section 27 SGB V (e.g., fertilization surgery, hormone stimulation alone), which are not covered by these guidelines, do not offer sufficient prospects of success, are not feasible, or are unreasonable.

2. Assisted reproduction services in accordance with these guidelines are only granted if they are performed in a homologous system, i.e., if the persons who wish to make use of these measures are married to each other. Only the egg cells and sperm of the spouses may be used. After sterilization, there is generally no entitlement to assisted reproduction services. Exceptions require the approval of the health insurance fund.

3. The health insurance fund is only responsible for services provided to its insured persons. This does not include any services that may be necessary for the spouse of the insured person in the context of assisted reproduction measures if the spouse is not insured with the same health insurance fund. The husband's health insurance fund is responsible for services related to the collection, examination, and preparation of male sperm, including capacitation if necessary, as well as for the laboratory tests on the husband mentioned in 12.1. The wife's health insurance fund is responsible for counseling the couple in accordance with No. 14 and for extracorporeal measures in connection with the combination of egg cells and sperm cells. The husband's health insurance fund is responsible for counseling the couple in accordance with No. 16 and for any human genetic counseling that may be required in this context.

4. Measures in accordance with these guidelines do not include services that go beyond assisted reproduction, such as the cryopreservation of sperm, impregnated egg cells, or embryos that have not yet been transferred.

5.   These guidelines apply exclusively to outpatient medical procedures performed by licensed physicians, authorized physicians, or authorized medically supervised facilities that have been granted approval by the competent authority in accordance with Section 121a of the German Social Code, Book V (SGB V) to perform the procedures in question. Medical procedures for assisted reproduction should, as far as possible, be performed on an outpatient basis. If medical procedures for assisted reproduction are performed as part of hospital treatment, the provisions of Section 112 (2) sentence 1 no. 6 SGB V apply.

6.   A prerequisite for the performance of assisted reproduction measures is that the HIV status of both spouses is known. Before treatment begins, the consultations specified in Section B, Number 5 of the Guideline on Contraception and Termination of Pregnancy (ESA-RL) should have taken place. For infectious samples, the conditions specified in the TPG Tissue Regulation (TPG-GewV) must be observed, which are only available in appropriately equipped facilities.

7.   Assisted reproduction procedures in accordance with sections 10.2, 10.3, 10.4, and 10.5 may only be performed if the spouses have first been advised by a physician who is not performing the procedures themselves on the medical, psychological, and social aspects of assisted reproduction (No. 14) and have been referred to one of the physicians or institutions authorized to perform these procedures (No. 17). Assisted reproduction procedures can therefore only be performed on referral.

8.   Assisted reproduction procedures may only be performed if there is a reasonable prospect that the chosen treatment method will result in pregnancy. There is no reasonable prospect of success for the respective treatment measures if they

-    up to eight times in the case of insemination in the spontaneous cycle (No. 10.1),

-    up to three times for insemination after hormonal stimulation (No. 10.2),

-    up to three times for in vitro fertilization (No. 10.3),

-    up to two times in the case of intratubal gamete transfer (No. 10.4),

-    up to three times in the case of intracytoplasmic sperm injection (No. 10.5) without a clinically confirmed pregnancy. If a clinically confirmed pregnancy has occurred without the subsequent birth of a child, this treatment attempt is not counted towards the above number. After the birth of a child, provided that the other requirements under these guidelines are met, there is a renewed entitlement to these measures within the respective maximum number of unsuccessful attempts. In this case, the treatment attempts preceding the birth are not counted towards the above number of attempts. If there is an indication both under No. 11.3 for in vitro fertilization measures and under No. 11.4 for intratubal gamete transfer measures the measures in question may, in principle, only be carried out alternatively, i.e. either the measures for in vitro fertilization or the measures for intratubal gamete transfer.

In vitro fertilization and intracytoplasmic sperm injection may also only be used alternatively due to the differentiated indications. The only exception is the case of total fertilization failure after the first attempt at in vitro fertilization. In this case, intracytoplasmic sperm injection (number 10.5) may be used in a maximum of two subsequent cycles, even if the requirements under number 11.5 are not met. A change of method within an IVF cycle (so-called rescue ICSI) is excluded. A change of method must be requested in a follow-up treatment plan. In the case of in vitro fertilization according to No. 10.3, the measures are considered to have been completed when the egg culture has been set up. In the case of in vitro fertilization, contrary to the above-mentioned number, there is no reasonable prospect of success after two complete cycles of treatment if fertilization has not occurred in either case and analysis of the relevant causes indicates that in vitro fertilization is not possible.

In the case of intracytoplasmic sperm injection according to No. 10.5, the procedure is considered to have been completed once the sperm has been injected into the egg(s). In the case of intracytoplasmic sperm injection, contrary to the aforementioned figure, there is no reasonable prospect of success after two complete procedures if fertilization has not occurred in either case.

If the method is changed to intracytoplasmic sperm injection after the first IVF treatment cycle with total fertilization failure, there is no reasonable prospect of success if fertilization has not occurred in both cycles (IVF and ICSI).

9.1 Only insured persons who have reached the age of 25 are entitled to assisted reproduction benefits. Female insured persons who have reached the age of 40 and male insured persons who have reached the age of 50 are not entitled to these benefits. For the indications listed in sections 11.1 to 11.5(a), the following applies: The specified age limits must be met for both partners in each treatment cycle (cycle case) on the first day of the spontaneous cycle, the first day of stimulation in the stimulated cycle, or the first day of downregulation. For the indication under number 11.5 letter b, the following applies: The specified age limits must be met for both partners in each attempt at the time of the first day of induction of hormonal preparation of the endometrium in accordance with number 12.3 letter b.

9.2 Before starting treatment, a treatment plan must be submitted to the health insurance fund for approval (see Appendix I for a sample).

The treatment plan must contain the following information:
- Date of birth of the spouses
- Indication(s) in accordance with sections 11.1 to 11.5(a) or (b)
- Treatment method in accordance with sections 10.1 to 10.5
- Type and number of assisted reproduction procedures performed to date
- Estimated treatment costs, including all medication costs per treatment cycle (cycle case).

The treatment plan covers a maximum of three consecutive cycles. Health insurance funds will only grant approval for the third IVF or ICSI cycle if fertilization has occurred in one of two treatment cycles (see section 8). For inseminations in the spontaneous cycle (in accordance with number 10.1), approval is granted for up to 8 consecutive cycles. If further cycles are eligible for approval, a follow-up treatment plan (see Appendix II for a sample) must be issued.

The follow-up treatment plan must contain the above information with the exception of the information on the type and number of assisted reproduction procedures performed to date. This information is replaced by the following
- type and number of assisted reproduction procedures performed to date without clinically proven pregnancy.

In the event of a change in the treatment method in accordance with numbers 10.1 to 10.5 or a change in method in accordance with number 8, paragraph 3, and at the latest one year after approval, a follow-up treatment plan (see Appendix II for a sample) must be submitted.

9.3 The Family Planning Subcommittee of the Joint Federal Committee is authorized to make changes to the templates for the treatment plan (Appendix I) and the follow-up treatment plan (Appendix II) that are necessary for practical application, provided that this does not alter the essential content of the treatment plan or follow-up treatment plan.

Methods

10. Medical measures for assisted reproduction in accordance with Section 27a of the German Social Code, Book V (SGB V) are used in the following procedures:

10.1 intracervical, intrauterine, or intratubal insemination in the spontaneous cycle, if necessary after triggering ovulation by administering HCG, if necessary after stimulation with antiestrogens,

10.2 intracervical, intrauterine, or intratubal insemination after hormonal stimulation with gonadotropins,

10.3 In vitro fertilization (IVF) with embryo transfer (ET), if necessary as zygote transfer or as intratubal embryo transfer (EIFT = embryo intrafallopian transfer),

10.4   intratubal gamete transfer (GIFT),

10.5   intracytoplasmic sperm injection (ICSI),

Medical indications

11.   The following are considered medical indications for performing medical procedures for artificial insemination:

11.1   For insemination according to No. 10.1:
-       somatic causes (e.g., impotentia coeundi, retrograde

         ejaculation, hypospadias, cervical canal stenosis, dyspareunia),
-       impaired sperm-mucus interaction,
-       male subfertility,

-       immunologically induced sterility.

11.2   For insemination according to No. 10.2:
-       male subfertility,

-       immunologically induced sterility.

Homologous insemination according to No. 10.2 should – apart from medically justified exceptional cases (e.g. certain forms of male subfertility) – only be performed if no more than three follicles have matured, due to the risk of high-order multiple pregnancies.

11.3 For in vitro fertilization (IVF) with embryo transfer (ET or EIFT), which may be intratubal:
-       Condition following tubal ligation,

-       tubal obstruction that cannot be treated in any other way (including microsurgery),

-       tubal dysfunction that cannot be treated in any other way, including in cases of endometriosis,
-       Idiopathic (unexplained) infertility, provided that all diagnostic and other therapeutic options for infertility treatment, including psychological evaluation, have been exhausted,
-       male subfertility, provided that treatment attempts in accordance with No. 10.2 are unlikely to be successful or have been unsuccessful,
-       immunologically induced infertility, provided that treatment attempts in accordance with No. 10.2 are unlikely to be successful or have been unsuccessful.

11.4   For intratubal gamete transfer (GIFT):
-       tubal dysfunction that cannot be treated in any other way, including in cases of endometriosis,
-       Idiopathic (unexplained) sterility, provided that all diagnostic and other

therapeutic options for infertility treatment have been exhausted,
- male subfertility, provided that treatment attempts in accordance with No. 10.2 are unlikely to be successful or have been unsuccessful.

11.5 For intracytoplasmic sperm injection (ICSI) with - intratubal embryo transfer (ET or EIFT), if applicable:

a) Severe male fertility disorder, documented by two recent semen analyses prepared on the basis of the WHO manual on "Examination and processing of human semen." The examination of the man as part of the assessment of the eligibility requirements under No. 1 by physicians with the additional designation "andrology" must precede the indication.

b) ICSI after cryopreservation in accordance with Section 27a (4) SGB V in cases of proven fertility problems in female insured persons, regardless of male fertility problems

The provision under number 8, sentence 15 remains unaffected.

Scope of measures

12. In detail, the following services may be considered in connection with the implementation of the measures under Nos. 10.1 to 10.5, depending on the method chosen:

12.1 Necessary laboratory tests in accordance with Section 6 (1) sentence 2 in conjunction with Annex 4 Nos. 1 and 3 TPG Tissue Ordinance for both spouses (anti-HIV-1,2, HBsAg, anti-HBc, anti-HCV-Ab; in individual cases, further tests in accordance with Annex 4, No. 1, letters d and e of the TPG Tissue Ordinance) within 3 months prior to the first germ cell collection and for subsequent germ cell collections, provided that these take place within the same partnership at a time that is 24 months after the first or a repeat laboratory test in accordance with the first half of the sentence. The results of the tests must be available during the collection, processing, use, or storage of the cells. In the case of sperm that is processed for intrauterine insemination and not stored, and provided that the tissue establishment can demonstrate that the risk of cross-contamination and exposure of staff has been addressed through the use of validated procedures, the physician responsible for the collection may refrain from performing the tests specified in Annex 4 of the TPG Tissue Ordinance.

12.2 Measures relating to the testing and processing – including capacitation, where applicable – of male semen,

12.3 implementation of measures
   a) hormonal stimulation treatment (only for measures under Nos. 10.2, 10.3, 10.4, and
       10.5
       or
   b) hormonal preparation of the endometrium according to 10.5 in the case of the medical
       indication in No. 11.5 letter b

12.4 Laboratory medical determinations of luteinizing hormone, estradiol, and progesterone,

12.5 Sonographic examinations,

12.6 Ultrasound-guided or laparoscopic egg cell retrieval (only for procedures under Nos. 10.3,
       10.4, and 10.5),

12.7 Measures relating to the combination of egg cells and sperm cells, including microscopic
       assessment of the maturity stages of egg cells (for measures under No. 10.4) or egg
       cell culture (for measures under Nos. 10.3 and 10.5),

12.8 . Insemination (for procedures under Nos. 10.1 and 10.2), embryo transfer (for
       procedures under Nos. 10.3, 10.5, including No. 10.5 in the case of the medical
       indication under No. 11.5(b), and intratubal gamete transfer (for procedures under No.
       10.4),

12.9 Counseling in accordance with Nos. 13-16.

Counseling of the married couple and referral for the implementation of the measures

13. Counseling of the married couple should – provided that the other legal requirements for
     benefits are met – only be carried out once the existence of one of the medical indications
     listed in No. 11 has been confirmed using appropriate diagnostic and, if necessary,
     therapeutic measures. If the doctor who made the indication is not the same as the
     consulting doctor, the counseling according to No. 7 should only be used on the basis of a
     corresponding referral from the doctor who made the indication.

14. The consultation pursuant to No. 7 should focus specifically on the individual medical,
     psychological, and social aspects of assisted reproduction. In addition to addressing the
     health risks and success rates of the treatment procedures, the physical and emotional
     stress involved, especially for the woman, as well as possible alternatives to having a
     child of their own (e.g., adoption) should also be discussed in detail. The couple should
     be informed that increased rates of malformation have been observed in children
     conceived through in vitro fertilization and intracytoplasmic sperm injection. An increased
     risk cannot be ruled out for other procedures either. The causes for this may lie in the
     procedures used as well as in the infertility itself.

15. A certificate must be issued confirming that the consultation has taken place. This certificate must be presented together with the referral to the doctor performing the artificial insemination.

16. Before performing intracytoplasmic sperm injection on the basis of the indication specified in section 11.5(a), the physician performing the procedure must inform the couple about the specific risks, including genetic risks, and possible malformations of the child. In doing so, the physician must also inform the couple about their right to human genetic counseling and, if necessary, testing prior to intracytoplasmic sperm injection.

    This counseling is particularly recommended for the couple in the case of certain findings (e.g., family history with indications of genetic malformations, bilateral congenital obstruction of the vas deferens in men). The conversation must be documented in an appropriate manner. If the couple refuses human genetic counseling, this must also be documented.

Authorized physicians

17. Assisted reproduction measures in accordance with these guidelines may only be performed by licensed physicians, authorized physicians, or authorized medically supervised facilities that have been granted approval to perform these measures by the competent authority in accordance with Section 121a of the German Social Code, Book V (SGB V). In the case of insemination, this only applies if it is carried out after stimulation procedures that increase the risk of pregnancies with 3 or more embryos.

18. Homologous inseminations without prior stimulation treatment (No. 10.1) may only be performed by physicians who are authorized to use the title "gynecologist."

19. Regulations in medical professional codes of conduct regarding the performance of assisted reproduction procedures remain unaffected.

20. Consultations pursuant to No. 14 may only be carried out by physicians who are authorized to use the title "gynecologist" and by other physicians who have special knowledge in the field of reproductive medicine (e.g., specialists in urology or dermatology). A further prerequisite for the provision of counseling in accordance with No. 14 is proof of authorization to participate in basic psychosomatic care.

21. In the case of assisted reproduction measures in accordance with this guideline, which involve stimulation treatment of the woman to obtain egg cells, this stimulation treatment should be carried out by the physician who performs the measure itself.

Recommendations for quality assurance

22. The following recommendations for quality assurance are made for the performance of assisted reproduction procedures:

22.1 Assisted reproduction services can only be performed and billed under statutory health insurance if certain quality requirements are met and verified in advance.
These include:

- The head of the practice or facility must be a specialist in gynecology and obstetrics and have completed the optional further training in "gynecological endocrinology and reproductive medicine."

- The practice or facility must have the following knowledge and experience:
    - Reproductive endocrinology
    - Gynecological sonography
    - Operative gynecology
    - Reproductive biology with a focus on in vitro culture
    - Andrology

Of these five areas, only two may be managed simultaneously by a physician or scientist at the practice or facility. In principle, physicians qualified in andrology (urologists, dermatologists, internists specializing in endocrinology) must be integrated into diagnostics and therapy in the context of assisted reproduction. Regular cooperation with a human geneticist and a medical psychotherapist must be ensured.

> The practice or facility must have the diagnostic and therapeutic capabilities necessary to perform assisted reproduction. The necessary technical equipment must be available, in particular for ultrasound diagnostics, hormone diagnostics, sperm diagnostics and preparation, egg cell retrieval, in vitro cultivation of egg cells, embryo transfer, and intratubal gamete transfer, as well as the necessary personnel and facilities.

> The practice or facility must have a license to perform artificial insemination procedures from a competent authority in accordance with Section 121a of the German Social Code, Book V (SGB V).

22.2 Physicians are obliged to participate in the quality assurance measures introduced by the relevant state medical association in accordance with the respective professional law. The state medical associations are responsible for quality assurance within the scope of the tasks assigned to them by the laws governing the medical professions and medical associations.

Appendix I: Sample treatment plan

Appendix II: Sample follow-up treatment plan

Appendix 10.2 Sample Form for Counseling and Indication Confirmation

Consultation and indication confirmation

Based on the available examination results, the couple

Mrs. ____ and

Mr. ____

according to the guidelines of the Federal Committee of Physicians and Health Insurance Funds, an indication for treatment measures for assisted reproduction.

The following diagnosis(es) led to the indication:

____

____

Planned therapy:

____

____

As there is a sufficient chance of success, I advised the couple on the medical, psychological, and social aspects of assisted reproduction in accordance with sections 7 and 13 to 15 of the directives on "Assisted Reproduction" pursuant to Section 27a, paragraph 4 of the German Social Code, Book V (SGB V).
Possible health risks, physical and emotional stress resulting from the treatment, and the possible chances of success were discussed, and alternatives to having their own child (e.g., adoption) were considered.

________________________   ________________________
Place / Date   Stamp/signature

(c) Bals Pratsch, et al. (2025). Workplace Fertility Center. Springer, Berlin, Heidelberg.
https://doi.org/10.1007/978-3-662-71659-5_6

Appendix 10.3 Sample Treatment Plan

Appendix 1
Sample treatment plan

<table>
<tr>
<td>

Name of health insurance company

Last name, first name of the insured person (female)

W

Date of birth

Insurance number Insured person number   **Status**

Contract physician no.   Date

</td>
<td>

Name of health insurance company

Last name, first name of the insured person (male)

M

Born

Insurance number Insured person number   **Status**

Contract physician no.   Date

</td>
</tr>
</table>

Treatment plan

for artificial insemination measures in accordance with §27a SGB V (German Social Security Code) and the "Directives on Assisted Reproduction" of the Joint Federal Committee for the above-mentioned spouses.

I. Indication(s) in accordance with Nos. 11.1 to 11.5 of the Guidelines on Artificial Insemination:

II. Planned treatment measure:
☐ Insemination in spontaneous cycle (in accordance with No. 10.1)
☐ Insemination after hormonal stimulation (in accordance with No. 10.2)
☐ In vitro fertilization with embryo transfer (according to No. 10.3)
☐ Intratubal gamete transfer (according to No. 10.4)
☐ Intracytoplasmic sperm injection (according to No. 10.5)

Number and type of treatments already performed according to Nos. 10.1 to 10.5

....

III. Cost estimate:
All information is subject to subsequent changes in the diagnostic and therapeutic requirements of individual cases. List of items on a separate sheet if necessary.
Cost estimates must be given as an average cost range in euros.

III a. Costs for services incurred once in the case of reproduction:

Medical treatment (EBM items)

W:	**M:**

Total medical treatment (euros)

W:	**M:**

Material costs and consultation supplies (euros)

W:	**M:**

Total for one-time services incurred in the event of reproduction (euros)

W:	**M:**

III b. Costs per cycle (excluding one-time services incurred in the event of reproduction):

Medical treatment (EBM items)

W:	**M:**

Total medical treatment (euros)

W:	**M:**

Medication costs (euros)

W:	**M:**

Material costs and consultation supplies (euros)

W:	**M:**

Total per cycle case (euros)

W:	**M:**

Place, date, signature, practice/clinic

IV. Approval by health insurance company(ies)

Previous treatments that count toward the maximum number allowed must be taken into account and reduce the number of approved cycles.
If approval is granted for 3 IVF or ICSI cycles, the 3rd IVF or ICSI cycle is subject to the provision that fertilization has taken place in one of the 2 treatment cycles. In the case of insemination in a spontaneous cycle, approval may be granted for up to 8 consecutive cycles.

According to § 27a SGB V, 50% of the costs incurred (including medication costs, see section III b) are the patient's own contribution. A final calculation of the total costs can only be made after the treatment has been completed, depending, among other things, on the contractually agreed point value in cents or euros.

If the treatment method is changed (see Section II) or at the latest one year after approval, a new treatment plan must be submitted.

W: **The treatment/cost plan is** for a maximum of cycles/cycle	**M:** **The treatment/cost plan will be** for a maximum of cycles/cycle

<table>
<tr>
<td>☐ Not approved (separate justification enclosed)

Place, date, signature Health insurance company</td>
<td>☐ Not approved (separate justification enclosed)

Place, date, signature of health insurance company</td>
</tr>
</table>

Appendix 10.4 Sample Form "Record of Processing Activities"

LIST OF PROCESSING ACTIVITIES

EXAMPLE

The sample is filled out as an example; two processing activities are listed.

LIST OF PROCESSING ACTIVITIES

Legal basis: Article 30(1) of the General Data Protection Regulation

Information about the controller

Name: Praxis am Europaplatz
Address: Europaplatz 1a, 23456 Platzstadt
Phone: 0123 456789
Email praxis@europaplatz.de
Website: www.europaplatzpraxis.de

Personal details of the data protection officer

First name and surname: Sabine Müller
Address: Europaplatz 1a, 23456 Platzstadt
Phone: 0123 456788
Email datenschutzbeauftragte@europaplatz.de

Processing activity

Date of creation: March 20, 2018
Date of last change: March 21, 2018

Description of processing activity

Use and application of the practice management system

Purposes of processing

Medical documentation, billing for medical services, quality assurance, appointment management

Description of the categories of data subjects

Patients

Description of data categories

Health data, including genetic data where applicable

Categories of recipients to whom the personal data has been or will be disclosed

Internal: Practice staff
External: other physicians/psychotherapists, associations of statutory health insurance physicians, health insurance companies, the Medical Service of the Health Insurance Funds, medical associations, private medical clearing houses

Deadlines for deletion

10 years after completion of treatment

Processing activity

Date of creation: March 18, 2018
Date of last change: March 22, 2018

Description of processing activity

Maintaining personnel files

Purposes of processing

Implementation of employment relationships

Description of the categories of data subjects

Employees

Description of data categories

Personnel data

Categories of recipients to whom the personal data has been or will be disclosed

Internal: Practice owner Dr. John Doe
External: Health insurance companies, tax offices, pension insurers

Deadlines for deletion

10 years after termination of employment

Appendix 10.5 Statutory Benefit "BKK Fertility Treatment", Patient Information

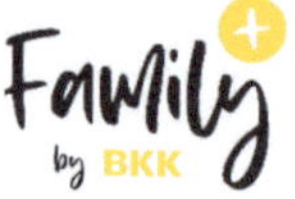

Appendix 5a – Patient information

Dear insured persons,

A quarter of all couples are involuntarily childless. There are many reasons for this. It may be due to organic or hormonal factors or a disease that affects fertility. For the couples affected, the unfulfilled desire to have children usually represents a great psychological and emotional strain within the partnership.

It is good when there is a partner who recognizes these social changes and has a comprehensive, exclusive offer for its insured persons. Together with the Professional Association of Reproductive Medicine in Bavaria (BRB e.V.), the participating company health insurance funds have developed an offer that is designed to support and relieve you on your way to fulfilling your desire to have children.

Take part in the "BKK Kinderwunsch" program—a comprehensive premium offer from the company health insurance funds is available to you!

- Two contributions to a **frozen embryo transfer cycle after transfer** (not in connection with a "freeze-all" within 3 months of the start of the cycle) in the amount of €350.00 each
- Two contributions to a **blastocyst culture after transfer,** each in the amount of €250.00
- **Contribution to the transfer costs** amounting to 50% of the standard statutory health insurance benefit (billed as a benefit in kind directly to the BKK) in the case of a medically necessary **freeze all,** provided that the transfer takes place within 3 months of the start of stimulation
- One-time contribution to a **fourth treatment attempt** beyond the standard benefit **after** transfer*
- If medically necessary, **unbureaucratic and simple** change of procedure from "in vitro fertilization" (IVF) to "intracytoplasmic sperm injection" (ICSI)
- **Increase in the age limit for women from 40 to 42** (first day of cycle before 42nd birthday)*
- **Avoidance of the risk of multiple pregnancies** by transferring a maximum of two embryos (single embryo transfer is recommended if medically possible)
- **Avoidance of additional hormonal stimulation treatment** if cryopreserved fertilized eggs are still available

*For couples wishing to have children where the woman is over 40 years of age or undergoing her fourth treatment attempt, a subsidy is available for the treatment attempt **after transfer** (attempts 1-4 - subsidy amount for the medically indicated procedure: IVF €800 or ICSI €1,000). The remaining costs (e.g., medication and ancillary medical services for artificial fertilization) must be paid **in full privately** for patients over the age of 40 or undergoing their fourth attempt. A so-called termination cycle (planned treatment cycle that is terminated for medical reasons before follicular puncture or after follicular puncture without an identifiable egg cell) is not covered.

You can participate from the age of 25, provided that your husband is under 50. The only requirements for participating in this innovative contract are your signature on the declaration of participation and the approval of your BKK. Participation is voluntary and begins on the day you sign. You are bound to the declaration of participation for one year. Your program-participating physician will provide you with comprehensive information about the content and objectives of the program.

Your right to free choice of doctor within the participating reproductive medicine centers remains unchanged during your participation.

By participating, you agree that embryo transfer will be limited to a maximum of two embryos.

For further information, please refer to the data protection information in accordance with the EU General Data Protection Regulation (GDPR).

The company health insurance funds are happy to support you and wish you every success on your journey. The participating centers will actively support you in this process. Do you have any questions? Please contact your BKK or visit www.bkk-familyplus.de vorbei.

Sincerely, Your company health insurance fund
together with your participating center

As of: January 1, 2025

Appendix 10.6 Brief Information on AG QSReproMed and Data Protection

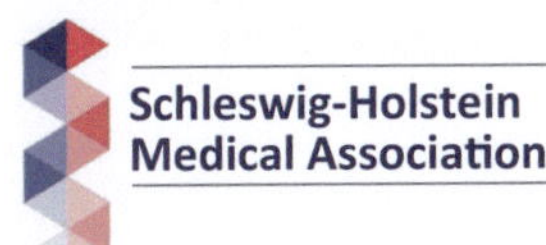

**Schleswig-Holstein
Medical Association**

Brief information on AG QSReproMed and data protection

This brief overview is intended to provide reproductive medicine centers (IVF centers) and their patients with a clear picture of what happens to their data and how data protection requirements are implemented, particularly with regard to the EU-wide General Data Protection Regulation (GDPR).

Version	created on	Processed	Approved by the steering committee of the AG QSReproMed on
1.0.3	Novemb	Pörksen (ÄKSH)	December 21, 2022

1. Who is AG QS ReproMed?

The Working Group on Quality Assurance in Reproductive Medicine (AG QS ReproMed) currently comprises 15 (state) medical associations that have come together to organize joint quality assurance for the more than 110 reproductive medicine treatment centers that fall within their jurisdiction. The data from these centers is evaluated jointly for the working group to ensure a solid statistical basis. The working group determines the rules for how this evaluation is carried out.
The evaluations relating to centers and calendar years in which treatment took place are completely anonymous annual statistics with regard to patients, which are made available to the IVF center concerned, the responsible medical association, and the steering committee of the working group.
Data processing is carried out at the working group's office, which is located at the Schleswig-Holstein Medical Association, address: Bismarckallee 8-12, 23795 Bad Segeberg, tel. 04551-803-615, emailinfo@qsrepromed.de .

2. What data is transferred to the AG QS ReproMed?

Pseudonymized (i.e., assigned a treatment number) medical history and treatment data are transferred from the IVF centers to the working group's office, i.e., no identity data such as last name, first name, addresses, or other contact information, nor insurance numbers of the patients. For data protection reasons, dates of birth are only transmitted on a monthly basis, and the partner's date of birth is not transmitted at all.

A detailed list of the data fields contained in the only interface currently in use is available at www.qsrepromed.de under the link 'transmitted data fields'. An additional, alternative interface definition for the same data with a compatible field list for integration into documentation systems is available to software companies upon request.

These lists comply with the principle of data minimization, i.e., they only contain data fields that are required by the AG office for evaluation.

3. Patient consent

Is patient consent required for the transfer of data? Consent is not required in centers in the following federal states (A):

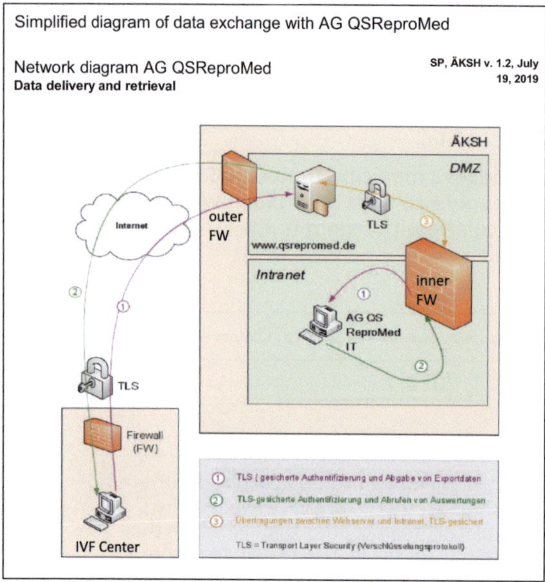

- Brandenburg
- Bremen
- Mecklenburg-Western Pomerania
- Lower Saxony
- North Rhine-Westphalia (Westphalia-Lippe Medical Association)
- Schleswig-Holstein

Here, patients only need to be informed about the data transfer.

Consent is required in centers in the federal states (B):

- Baden-Württemberg
- Bavaria
- Hamburg
- Hesse
- Rhineland-Palatinate
- Saarland
- Saxony
- Saxony-Anhalt
- Thuringia

Here, patients must be asked for their consent to the transfer of pseudonymized data prior to treatment and may revoke this consent at a later date.
Only medical history and treatment data from patients who have given their consent to the transfer will be transferred.

The medical associations of Berlin and North Rhine-Westphalia are not currently participating in the AG QS ReproMed.

4. Can a patient have transferred data deleted retrospectively?

Yes, if consent to the transfer of data was required in advance.
If the treating center is located in a federal state listed in Group B under 3, the patient can also revoke their consent retrospectively. The center then only has to export the information to the AG office again, transmitting the relevant treatment numbers. The AG office will then delete the stored medical history and treatment data based on these treatment numbers.

5. How can a patient view transferred data?

According to the GDPR, affected patients have the right to view this information.
Here, too, a distinction must be made: if a patient was asked for their consent and objected to the transfer of data, no medical history or treatment data relating to them is stored. In all other cases, the following applies:
Since the AG cannot access any patient information, the patient must contact the center treating them. The center must provide the AG office with written information about the patient ID or treatment IDs of any patients who wish to view their stored data.
An email is sufficient for this purpose, but it should be sent by a center employee designated as responsible by the AG office.
The data will be provided in tabular form, either in written form (printout) or as an encrypted email attachment (in Excel, Open Office, or CSV format, as desired). The field contents can be accessed using the documentation of the export field list, which will be provided to you if you do not already have it (source for download: see section 2).

6. How long is the data stored?

Treatment data is stored for at least five and up to a maximum of six years after the start of treatment. There may be exceptions if a medical association leaves the AG. In this case, the data of the centers concerned would be deleted prematurely.

7. Is the data secure?

Data protection and data security are a high priority for the Schleswig-Holstein Medical Association. With the approval of the board, the management of the Medical Association has adopted a data protection and information security guideline and established a data protection and information security management system.
A data protection concept has been created for the QSReproMed working group's office, which documents in detail the technical and organizational measures (TOM) for ensuring data protection and data security. This data protection concept is available to the medical associations of the AG and is part of the order processing agreements (AW) between the participating medical associations as clients and the Schleswig-Holstein Medical Association as contractor; it is made available to the responsible data protection officers upon request. The office provides a state-of-the-art encrypted method for transferring data to its premises.

8. Who handles the data?

Apart from the treatment centers, only the IT staff of the Schleswig-Holstein Medical Association assigned to the AG office, who are of course bound to secrecy, have direct access to the treatment data.
Data security and server operation are ensured by the IT support staff of the Schleswig-Holstein Medical Association.

9. What happens to the data?

The data is used for statistical evaluations, which form the basis of quality assurance. Statistics are compiled for each previous calendar year, which can be used to determine for each center whether the responsible office of the respective Medical Association should or must investigate further.

10. Who is responsible?

The treatment centers are responsible for the proper documentation of the data. The medical associations involved are responsible for data in accordance with the GDPR. They instruct the centers in their area of responsibility to deliver their data exports from the documentation software to the AG office at the Schleswig-Holstein Medical Association. The relevant software company, or its client if applicable, is responsible for the proper functioning of the documentation system.
The participating medical associations contractually ensure (via AW) that the Schleswig-Holstein Medical Association handles the data properly. The Schleswig-Holstein Medical Association is responsible for the proper and secure handling of the data at the office.

11. Contact

Data processing and evaluation

The contact details for the office can be found under 1. Further contact persons can be found a) with regard to the implementation of quality assurance at your state medical association and b) with regard to technical contact persons for the procedure, again at the office.

As data processing is carried out by the IT department of the Schleswig-Holstein Medical Association, the responsible data protection officer on site is the representative of this medical association,

Ms. Marion David, email:datenschutzbeauftragte@aeksh.de , telephone: 04551 803 409.

The competent authority at the state level is the

ULD - Independent State Center for Data Protection Schleswig-Holstein
Holstenstraße 98
24103 Kiel
Postal address: P.O. Box 7116, 24171 Kiel

Appendix 11.1 Psychosocial Counseling for Unfulfilled Desire to Have Children: The BKiD Checklist for Couples

**Psychosocial counseling for infertility:
the BKiD checklist for couples**

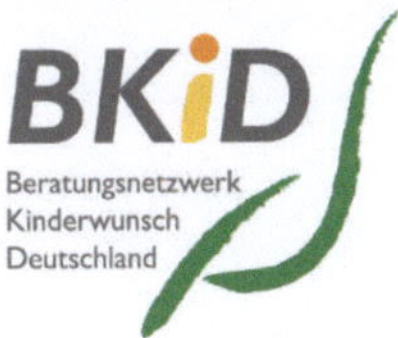

Dear couple, dear person who wants to have children,

Wanting a child and having to wait a long time for one is perceived by many people as a significant psychological burden. Often, the desire to have children is kept secret from others, as the topic is still considered taboo. When this is compounded by complex medical treatment that is not always successful, the situation can push even an otherwise emotionally stable person to the limits of their resilience.

At this point, at the latest, you should consider seeking psychosocial fertility counseling, such as that offered by BKiD counselors. The following BKiD checklist can help you determine whether this counseling can help you.

○ "As a couple, we have no other topic of conversation than our desire to have children and the medical treatment involved."

○ "When I meet pregnant women or women with babies, I want to cross the street; family celebrations often stress me out now."

○ "When my partner gets her period, she is devastated for days. As her partner, I feel helpless and withdraw more and more."

○ "I am enjoying our sex life less and less."

○ "I'm not sure if I'm getting too hung up on wanting children."

○ "Without a child of my own, I feel my life is meaningless."

○ "Since the diagnosis is mine, I am thinking about letting my partner go so that she/he can fulfill her/his desire to have children in a new relationship."

○ "We have distanced ourselves from former friends because they now have children."

○ "My unfulfilled desire to have children and not knowing what the future holds is preventing me from making other important decisions in my life, such as my job."

○ "I find it difficult to draw a line in medical treatment, to allow thoughts of a 'Plan B' or to come to terms with giving up my desire to have children."

○ "I/we are considering treatment with donated sperm or similar."

If you agree with three (or more) of these statements, it would certainly be helpful to seek counseling. But even if you do not identify with these statements, counseling may still be useful if you want to deal with your own situation better or support each other better as a couple. If there is no stamp below: a BKiD counseling specialist can be recommended by your doctor or found online at www.bkid.de.

Glossary

Miscarriage premature termination of pregnancy before viability

Adenomyosis uteri Endometriosis foci in the uterine wall

Adhesion adhesion

Adnexitis Combined inflammation of the fallopian tubes and ovary

Acrosome The acrosome covers the anterior two-thirds of the sperm head like a cap and releases enzymes during fertilization to dissolve the zona pellucida; this enables the sperm to penetrate the egg cell.

Amenorrhea Absence of menstruation for at least 3 months; also absence of menarche

Amniotic cavity Cavity, usually referred to as the amniotic sac from the fetal period onward, develops above the embryonic disc, enlarges by the end of the embryonic period

Androgenization Acne, hirsutism (increased growth of coarse hair, especially on the upper lip, chin, chest, around the navel, and inner thighs), and hair loss due to enhanced effects of male hormones

Antral follicle Follicle with a cavity (antrum) between the granulosa cells, which develops as early as three months before ovulation and can only be detected by vaginal ultrasound once it reaches a size of 3 to 5 mm

ART Term for assisted reproduction or fertilization techniques; these include: intrauterine insemination (IUI), in vitro fertilization (IVF) with advanced methods such as intracytoplasmic sperm injection (ICSI)

Omnibus Act Collection of amendments to existing laws (e.g., Tissue Act)

Asherman syndrome Adhesions between the anterior and posterior walls of the uterus

Frozen embryo transfer (FET) cycle An ART treatment cycle in which embryos are transferred after a thawing procedure; the oocytes were retrieved in a previous IVF cycle and cryopreserved

Trigger shot Injection of hCG, in exceptional cases also a GnRH agonist, to induce ovulation when the follicles are mature (15 to 20 mm in diameter)

Azoospermia No sperm in the ejaculate

Chorionic cavity Cavity that essentially fills the former blastocyst cavity and encloses the amniotic cavity with the embryonic disc up to the implantation site; regresses after the 10th week of gestation

Chromosomes Carriers of genetic information, consisting mainly of DNA

Corpus luteum Corpus luteum, forms after ovulation in the follicular cavity

Dictyotene Resting phase of maturation division (meiosis) lasting for decades, which begins during fetal development between the third and seventh month of pregnancy ("pause" at the onset of meiosis I), continuation of meiosis 12 to 50 years later (from puberty to menopause)

DNA fragmentation index (DFI) Measure of the integrity of DNA (genetic material) in sperm; high DFI indicates breaks in the DNA strands of sperm

Dysmenorrhea Cramp-like lower abdominal pain associated with menstruation

Embryonic period Period from fertilization to the 8th week of development (calculated as the 10th week of gestation)

Embryo Protection Act (ESchG) German criminal law regulating IVF or ICSI treatment, designed in particular to protect against the misuse of techniques for creating human embryos for purposes other than their intended use

Endometrium Uterine lining, which consists of two layers: basalis (lower, constant layer adjacent to the uterine musculature) and functionalis (upper, cyclically variable layer under hormonal influence)

Ectopic pregnancy (EP) Pregnancy outside the uterine cavity

Fertilization A process also referred to as conception; begins with the fusion of the cell membranes of sperm and egg cells and ends with the dissolution of the female and male pronuclei

Fertility preservation Cryopreservation of egg cells and sperm as well as ovarian and testicular tissue prior to germ cell-damaging therapy such as chemotherapy or radiotherapy, or before complete or extensive removal of ovarian or testicular tissue

Fetal period Period from the 10th week of gestation until birth

Follicle Unit consisting of an oocyte surrounded by granulosa cells, which are arranged in layers and begin to form the follicular cavity as early as two to three months before ovulation. These cells produce estrogens.

Fresh cycle An ART treatment cycle in which oocytes are retrieved, fertilized, and after culture, transferred back into the uterus

Galactorrhea Milk discharge

Corpus luteum (yellow body) Former follicular cavity in which the so-called granulosa lutein cells and theca lutein cells develop. These primarily produce progesterone; due to the accumulation of fat in the cells, the corpus luteum appears yellow.

Genome Totality of genetic information stored in the DNA (deoxyribonucleic acid) of an organism

Heterologous (donogenic) treatment Donor treatment

Homologous treatment Partner treatment

Tissue Act (GewebeG) Article law that implements the European Tissue Directive 2004/23/EC into German law, enacting amendments to several laws: Medicinal Products Act (AMG) with the Ordinance on the Manufacture of Medicinal Products and Active Substances (AMWHV), Transplantation Act (TPG) with the associated Tissue Ordinance (TPG-GewV), and Transfusion Act (TFG)

Granulosa cells Layered cells that surround an oocyte, which at the time of ovulation are referred to as cumulus cells. The inner layer of cumulus cells is arranged radially and is called the corona radiata. Granulosa cells produce estrogens.

Hydrosalpinx Scarred fallopian tube with occlusion following infection, filled with fluid

Hyperandrogenemia Elevated androgen levels (DHEAS, free testosterone), provided that blood sampling is performed in the follicular phase (before ovulation)

Hyperprolactinemia Elevated prolactin levels

Hyperthyroidism Overactive thyroid

Hypogonadism Hormone deficiency due to failure of hormone production by the ovaries (estrogen deficiency) or the testes (testosterone deficiency) as a result of dysfunction of the hypothalamus, pituitary gland, or the ovaries or testes themselves

Pituitary gland Hypophysis

Hypothalamus The hypothalamus is a region of the Diencephalon

Hypothyroidism Underactive thyroid

Hysteroscopy Uterine endoscopy

Ideal patient Selection criteria for couples to enable comparison of treatment quality between fertility centers: female age ≤35 years, number of PN cells ≥4–5 (revisions and additions by D·I·R and QSReproMed)

Implantation Embedding of an embryo in the uterine lining around the sixth day after fertilization

Impregnation The mature ovum fuses with the cell membrane with a sperm cell. The sperm nucleus and tail penetrate the ovum

Intracytoplasmic Sperm Injection (ICSI) in contrast to IVF, the penetration of the sperm into the egg is not left to chance, but rather a single sperm is directly injected into an egg cell using an ultra-fine glass needle

In vitro fertilization (IVF) Bringing together a woman's egg cells and a man's sperm in a 'test tube' outside the woman's body: independent penetration of a sperm into the egg cell after the addition of prepared sperm.

Capacitation Proteins are removed from the surface of the sperm, increasing the motility of the sperm cells and enabling them to become capable of fertilization. This process is naturally triggered in the fallopian tube through contact with the epithelium, or in vitro by incubation with culture media.

Cavum Uterine cavity

Klinefelter syndrome most common chromosomal anomaly in men with infertility and other physical and developmental differences; additional X chromosome (47, XXY)

Contamination unwanted contamination of media, surfaces, objects, etc. with microorganisms (such as bacteria, fungi, or viruses) or harmful substances

Cryopreservation Method for preservation at very low temperatures, primarily of cells and tissues; also referred to as freezing

Cryptorchidism Undescended testis

Glossary

Laparoscopy Surgical procedure, also referred to as pelviscopy in gynecology, in which surgical instruments are inserted through small skin incisions to examine and treat the internal reproductive organs.

LH peak sharp increase in luteinizing hormone (LH) that triggers ovulation

MAR test Laboratory method for testing for sperm antibodies in ejaculate (Mixed Antiglobulin Reaction Test)

Meiosis Maturation division in egg and sperm cells: the chromosome set (46,XX or 46,XY) is halved in two steps, so that mature egg and sperm cells have only the single chromosome set (23,X or 23,Y)

Menarche Time of the first menstrual period and onset of fertility

Menopause Time of the last menstrual period and thus the end of fertility

MII oocyte Mature, fertilizable oocyte that has completed only the first step of meiosis (1 polar body extruded) and remains arrested in metaphase II until activation by the entry of a sperm.

Monosomy a specific chromosome is present once instead of twice in the body cells

Myoma Benign muscle nodule of the uterus

Myometrium Muscle layer of the uterine wall

Off-label use Prescription of medications outside the approved indications. Without verification of their safety and efficacy, prescription at the expense of statutory health insurance is not permitted.

Oligomenorrhea Cycle longer than 35 days, but shorter than three months

Oogonia Stem cells of oocyte maturation, which proliferate through mitosis until the fifth month of pregnancy and from which the primary oocytes develop during the fetal period

PN cells Also called pronuclear stages; in the oocyte, the pronuclei become visible 6 to 24 hours after the sperm enters the oocyte and contain the maternal and paternal genetic material

Polyp Benign mucosal growth

Premature Ovarian Insufficiency (POI) Loss of ovarian function before the age of 40

Primordial follicle Unit consisting of follicular epithelial cells (early granulosa cells) and the primary oocyte

Pseudonymization Data records that are assigned a treatment number and stored without identifying information such as name or address

Delayed puberty Delayed puberty: absence of pubertal signs (thelarche and pubarche) or arrest of pubertal development and no menarche by the age of 16 years

Phenotype Appearance of an organism with its visible characteristics and functional properties

Prolactinoma Tumor of the pituitary gland that secretes prolactin

Pubarche Onset of pubic hair as part of puberty

Puberty In girls, starting at around age 10 with breast development (thelarche), pubic hair growth (pubarche), and first menstruation at about 13 to 15 years; puberty in boys from around age 10 to 17 with growth of the testes, penis, pubic hair and body hair, voice deepening, muscle growth, and first ejaculation at about 13 years

Retrograde Ejaculation Semen is ejaculated into the bladder instead of being expelled through the penis.

Sactosalpinx Scarred fallopian tube with irregular wall following infection

Statutory benefits Voluntary benefits in addition to those provided under the Social Code Book (SGB V), which statutory health insurance funds may offer to their insured members

Sertoli-cell-only-syndrome (SCOS) Severe impairment of spermatogenesis characterized by the absence of germinal epithelium in the seminiferous tubules, which contain only Sertoli cells

Spermatogenesis Maturation of sperm cells, which begins at puberty with the two-stage meiotic division via primary and secondary spermatocytes

Spermiogenesis Maturation of sperm morphology after completion of meiosis, from initially round spermatids to spermatozoa, which are composed of a head, midpiece, and tail

Spermatogonia Stem cells of sperm cell maturation, which begin to proliferate mitotically again from puberty onwards and from which, via the spermatocytes, the sperm cells develop

Stimulation treatment Similar terms are ovarian stimulation treatment, hormonal stimulation, gonadotropin stimulation

Synechiae Adhesions

Syncytiotrophoblast Early form of the placenta, develops from the outer *trophoblast cells after implantation,* produces human chorionic gonadotropin (hCG).

Testicular sperm extraction (TESE) Extraction (retrieval) of sperm from testicular tissue that was previously obtained surgically

Theca cells Cells arranged in two layers, located external to the granulosa cells and separated from them by a basement membrane; produce androgens

Thelarche Development of the female breast glands during puberty

Tubuli seminiferi Spermatic tubules in the testis where sperm cells mature

Transfer Transfer, e.g., of embryos into the uterus

Translocation Relocation of chromosome segments to another position within the chromosome set or to another chromosome, with or without gain or loss of genetic material (balanced or unbalanced).

Triploidy Triple set of chromosomes, i.e., each chromosome is present three times in the body cells

Trisomy a specific chromosome is present three times instead of twice in the body cells

Thrombophilia inherited or acquired tendency to form blood clots (thrombi)

Ullrich-Turner syndrome (UTS) most common chromosomal anomaly in women with infertility and other physical and developmental differences; one X chromosome is missing (45, X0)

Uterus bicornis Double malformation of the uterus; defective fusion of the paired Müllerian ducts during embryonic development, from which the uterus arises

Uterus subseptus Uterine cavity partially separated by a septum

Vaginismus Painful vaginal spasm, e.g., during intercourse or a gynecological examination, which the affected woman cannot control voluntarily

Varicocele Enlarged venous plexus along the spermatic cord in the scrotum, usually on the left side

Polluter Pays Principle Principle of causation, medical expenses are only covered by a private health insurance (PHI, "PKV") if the cause of the illness lies with the insured person, e.g., if the cause of involuntary childlessness is attributable to the privately insured partner.

Pronuclear stages Also called pronucleus (PN) cells. In this stage, the maternal and paternal pronuclei are visible in the oocyte; the maternal and paternal chromosomes have not yet "fused."

Zona pellucida Envelope surrounding the oocyte, which has already formed at the beginning of oocyte maturation from the primordial follicle to the primary follicle. It protects the oocyte up to the blastocyst stage.

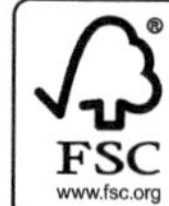